Cardiogenic Shock

Edited by

Steven M. Hollenberg, MD
Sections of Cardiology and Critical Care Medicine
Rush-Presbyterian-St. Luke's Medical Center
Chicago, Illinois

Eric R. Bates, MD
Division of Cardiology, Department of Medicine
University of Michigan
Ann Arbor, Michigan

Futura Publishing Company, Inc.
Armonk, NY

Library of Congress Cataloging-in-Publication Data

Cardiogenic shock / edited by Steven M. Hollenberg, Eric R. Bates.
    p. ; cm.
    Includes bibliographical references and index.
    ISBN 0-87993-702-5 (alk. paper)
    1. Cardiogenic shock. I. Hollenberg, Steven M. II. Bates, Eric R.
    [DNLM: 1. Shock, Cardiogenic—diagnosis. 2. Shock, Cardiogenic—
    therapy. WG 300
    C26747 2002]
    RC685.C18 C367 2002
    616.1′2—dc21
                                                        2001055588

Copyright ©2002
Futura Publishing Company, Inc.

Published by
Futura Publishing Company
135 Bedford Road
Armonk, NY 10504
www.futuraco.com

ISBN #:0-87993-702-5

Every effort has been made to ensure that the information in this book is as up to date and accurate as possible at the time of publication. However, due to the constant developments in medicine, neither the author, nor the editor, nor the publisher can accept any legal or other responsibility for any errors or omissions that may occur.

Printed in the United States of America on acid-free paper.

Preface

The last decade has seen major advances in the management of cardiogenic shock. With aggressive therapy, mortality for this most serious complication of acute myocardial infarction has fallen, as demonstrated in several large databases. This improvement is the result of increasingly active therapy, involving intra-aortic balloon counterpulsation and mechanical revascularization—strategies that have been evaluated in several studies published over the last few years. This book is a timely and comprehensive review of all aspects of cardiogenic shock. The editors and authors are esteemed clinicians and investigators who have furthered our knowledge of the evaluation and management of cardiogenic shock.

All aspects of cardiogenic shock, ranging from pathophysiology to assessment to treatment, are covered in depth. Practical management strategies based on available data are presented. The latest data from randomized trials of treatment strategies- including SHOCK, SMASH, and TACTICS- are discussed. Detailed reviews of related therapies such as ventricular assist devices, as well as special problems such as right ventricular myocardial infarction and rhythm disturbances, are provided. An important vision for the future of potential metabolic support of the myocardium is presented.

Despite the reduction in mortality with early revascularization for cardiogenic shock complicating acute myocardial infarction, a 50% mortality rate at 30 days is unacceptably high. Shock remains the leading cause of death for patients hospitalized with acute myocardial infarction. More basic and clinical investigations are needed to define new effective treatments to reduce further the high mortality rate.

This book provides a detailed overview of the current state of knowledge about cardiogenic shock- an overview that should be invaluable for clinicians treating this entity and for researchers seeking to improve current treatment techniques.

Judith S. Hochman, MD
Professor of Medicine, Columbia University
Director, Cardiac Care Unit and Cardiac Research
St. Luke's/Roosevelt Hospital Center, New York

Dedication

To our families
Susan, Emma, and Rebecca
Nancy, Andrew, Alexis, and Evan

Introduction

Cardiogenic shock has long been a difficult problem for clinicians. The syndrome of cardiogenic shock results from the inability of the heart to deliver enough blood to maintain adequate tissue perfusion. The most common cause is left ventricular pump failure after myocardial infarction, but other important causes include mechanical complications of infarction, right ventricular dysfunction, prolonged cardiopulmonary bypass, valvular disease, and cardiomyopathy. Cardiogenic shock is the leading cause of in-hospital death after myocardial infarction. Despite advances in management of heart failure and acute myocardial infarction, until very recently, clinical outcomes in patients with cardiogenic shock have been frustratingly poor, with reported mortality rates ranging from 50% to 80%.

Recently, however, there has been some cause for optimism. Improved understanding of the pathophysiology of cardiogenic shock has led to renewed emphasis on the notion that not all dysfunctional ischemic myocardium is irretrievably lost; some heart muscle may be stunned or hibernating, and may recover function with hemodynamic support and restoration of flow. This concept, in turn, has underscored the importance of expeditious initiation of supportive measures to maintain blood pressure and cardiac output, including both medications and intra-aortic balloon counterpulsation. Finally, the theory that coronary revascularization would be beneficial by reversing the vicious cycle in which ischemia causes myocardial dysfunction which in turn worsens ischemia, which had been supported by an extensive body of observational and registry studies, has now been strongly buttressed by the results of two randomized controlled trials.

This volume, which outlines current concepts regarding pathogenesis, diagnosis, and management of patients with cardiogenic shock, is organized into three main portions. The first deals with epidemiology and pathophysiology, with consideration of initial diagnostic and therapeutic steps in the evaluation of patients with cardiogenic shock. The second focuses on issues regarding management of patients with cardiogenic shock after myocardial infarction, encompassing use of fibrinolytic therapy, intra-aortic balloon counterpulsation, percutaneous intervention, and surgical revascularization. The last section deals with other considerations, including issues relating to patients with right ventricular infarction, mechanical complications of myocardial infarction, arrhythmias, and mechanical and metabolic support.

A certain fatalism has a tendency to find its way into the treatment of some patients with severe shock, which has the potential to be self-fulfilling. Greater understanding of the rationale for and data supporting the newer modalities of therapy will hopefully lead to increased application of these approaches, and, ultimately, to better outcomes.

Contributors

Francis Q. Almeda, MD, Section of Cardiology, Rush-Presbyterian-St. Luke's Medical Center, Chicago, Illinois

David Antoniucci, MD, Head, Division of Cardiology, Careggi Hospital, Florence, Italy

Carl S. Apstein, MD, Professor of Medicine and Physiology, Director, Cardiac Muscle Research Laboratory, Boston University School of Medicine; Attending Cardiologist, Boston Medical Center, Boston, Massachusetts

Eric R. Bates, MD, Professor of Internal Medicine, Division of Cardiology, Department of Medicine, University of Michigan, Ann Arbor, Michigan

Verdi J. DiSesa, MD, Mary and John Bent Professor and Chairman, Department of Cardiovascular-Thoracic Surgery, Rush-Presbyterian-St. Luke's Medical Center, Chicago, Illinois

Steven M. Hollenberg, MD, Associate Professor of Medicine, Section of Cardiology, Rush-Presbyterian-St. Luke's Medical Center, Chicago, Illinois

Michael P. Hudson, MD, Senior Staff Cardiologist, Director, Coronary Intensive Care Unit, Henry Ford Heart and Vascular Institute, Detroit, Michigan

Russell F. Kelly, MD, Director, Interventional Cardiology, Cook County Hospital, Chicago, Illinois

Lloyd W. Klein, MD, Professor of Medicine, Co-Director, Cardiac Catherization Laboratories and Director, Interventional Cardiology, Rush-Presbyterian-St. Luke's Medical Center, Chicago, Illinois

Sandeep Nathan, MD, Interventional Cardiology Fellow, Rush-Presbyterian-St. Luke's Medical Center, Chicago, Illinois

Zoran S. Nedeljkovic, MD, Fellow in Cardiology, Evans Department of Medicine, Section of Cardiology, Boston University School of Medicine, Boston, Massachusetts

E. Magnus Ohman, MD, Chairman, Division of Cardiology and Professor of Internal Medicine, University of North Carolina, Chapel Hill, North Carolina

Joseph E. Parrillo, MD, Professor of Medicine, Robert Wood Johnson Medical School; Head, Division of Cardiovascular Disease and Critical Care Medicine; Director, Cooper Heart Institute; Director, Cardiovascular Services, Cooper Health System, Camden, New Jersey

Manisha A. Patel, MD, Fellow in Cardiothoracic Surgery, Rush-Presbyterian-St. Luke's Medical Center, Chicago, Illinois

Sergio L. Pinski, MD, Director, Arrhythmia Device Clinic, Rush-Presbyterian-St. Luke's Medical Center; Associate Professor of Medicine, Rush Medical College, Chicago, Illinois

Thomas J. Ryan, MD, Professor of Medicine and Senior Consultant in Cardiology, Evans Department of Medicine, Section of Cardiology, Boston University School of Medicine, Boston, Massachusetts

Joseph G. Salloum, MD, Fellow, Division of Cardiology, University of Texas Houston Health Science Center, Houston, Texas

Kurt W. Saupe, PhD, Assistant Professor, Departments of Medicine and Physiology, University of Wisconsin-Madison, Madison, Wisconsin

Edward B. Savage, MD, Associate Professor of Cardiovascular-Thoracic Surgery, Rush University, Chairman, Division of Cardiothoracic Surgery, Cook County Hospital, Chicago, Illinois

Michael Shapiro, MD, Attending Cardiologist, Cook County Hospital and Rush-Presbyterian-St. Luke's Medical Center; Assistant Professor of Medicine, Rush Medical College, Chicago, Illinois

Richard W. Smalling, MD, PhD, Professor of Medicine, Division of Cardiology, University of Texas Houston Health Science Center, Houston, Texas

Jean-Christophe Stauffer, MD, Division of Cardiology, C.H.U.V., Lausanne, Switzerland

Philip M. Urban, MD, Director of Interventional Cardiology, Cardiovascular Department, Hôpital de la Tour, Geneva, Switzerland

John G. Webb, MD, Director, Cardiac Catheterization and Interventional Cardiology, St. Paul's Hospital, University of British Columbia, Vancouver, British Columbia, Canada

Table of Contents

III. Other Considerations.

Part I.

Diagnosis.

Chapter 1

Epidemiology of Cardiogenic Shock

John G. Webb, MD and Russell F. Kelly, MD

Introduction

Cardiogenic shock may be defined as a state of severe tissue hypoperfusion resulting from cardiac dysfunction. This usually manifests as persistent systemic arterial hypotension with evidence of hypoperfusion, such as cool skin, altered mental status, and diminished urine output. A rigorous definition of shock requires hemodynamic confirmation, as evidenced by sustained systemic hypotension (systolic arterial pressure < 90 mm Hg or mean arterial pressure > 30 mm Hg below basal levels), with adequate left ventricular (LV) filling pressures (pulmonary artery wedge pressure > 15 mm Hg), and a reduced cardiac output (cardiac index < 2.2 L/min/m^2).[1,2] Clinically, the diagnosis of cardiogenic shock is often made without such objective confirmation. Comparison of published reports of cardiogenic shock requires caution, given the wide variability in the criteria used to define shock.[1,3,4]

Cardiogenic shock develops in 5% to 10% of patients hospitalized with acute myocardial infarction (MI), with a reported incidence that has remained constant over the past few decades.[1,5-16] Shock is the major cause of death among patients hospitalized for acute MI, with a reported mortality of 55% to 90%.[5,6,8,9,11,14,17-21] Advances in supportive medical therapy have had, at best, a modest impact on mortality.[20]

While cardiogenic shock may develop in patients with unstable angina without infarction (at least initially), it is uncommon. In the GUSTO-IIb trial, among patients who did not have ST elevation or infarction at the time of randomization, cardiogenic shock developed in only 1.4%.[22] Furthermore, some critically ill patients without a clear-cut cardiac etiology may in fact be in cardiogenic shock. In one study performed in France,

From: Hollenberg SM, Bates ER. *Cardiogenic Shock.* Armonk, NY: Futura Publishing Co., Inc.; ©2002.

patients surviving out-of-hospital arrest underwent emergent coronary angiography.[23] Clinical and electrocardiographic preadmission data indicative of a cardiac cause of the arrest were not required to be included in the study. Of 84 patients studied, coronary artery occlusion was found in 48%, and angioplasty was associated with improved survival.

Clinical Profile

Retrospective studies have described a number of predictors of cardiogenic shock and of mortality. Among patients with MI, shock is more likely to develop in those who are elderly, although shock may occur in any age group.[5-8,11,18,24,25] Women seem to be more likely than men to develop shock,[5,7,11,18,22,24,25] particularly from mechanical causes.[26,27] Most studies have found patients with diabetes mellitus to be at increased risk of shock.[5,7,8,18,22,24] Other risk factors for coronary disease are not more common in shock patients. Patients with cardiogenic shock are also more likely to report a history of peripheral vascular disease and cerebrovascular disease.[7,8,11]

A prior history of MI was more common in patients with shock in the GUSTO-I trial (25%-28% vs. 16%),[17] in the Worcester community study (40%-44% vs. 33%-34%),[5,24] and in many,[8,25] but not all,[11] other reports. A history of angina has been found to be more common in patients who develop shock in some studies,[11,25] but not others.[7,8] Patients who have had prior coronary artery bypass surgery also are at increased risk of developing shock.[17]

Clinical predictors include marked elevation in cardiac enzymes, lactate, or heart rate.[28-30] Although pulmonary congestion is an important finding in many patients with shock,[8] the absence of congestion on physical exam does not exclude the presence of shock;[31] hypoperfusion, evidenced as oliguria and cold extremities, is more important.[32] In the GUSTO-I trial, patients who developed cardiogenic shock after admission (as distinct from those who had shock on arrival) had lower systolic blood pressure than patients who did not develop shock (118 vs. 130 mm Hg) and higher heart rates (81 vs. 75 beats/min). Another study found similar results in patients who developed shock after admission.[8] Diagnostic predictors include persistent occlusion of the infarct-related artery, a marked reduction in cardiac index (< 2.2 L/min/m^2) and ejection fraction ($< 35\%$), and the absence of hyperkinesis of non-acutely infarcted myocardial segments.[33]

The multinational SHOCK Registry enrolled patients with cardiogenic shock complicating acute MI at 36 centers between 1993-1997.[34] This 1190 patient registry represents the largest prospective source of information available, as shown in Tables 1 and 2.

Left ventricular failure was the predominant case of shock in 74.5% of cases. Acute severe mitral regurgitation was diagnosed in 8.3%, ventricular septal rupture in 4.6%, "isolated" right ventricular shock in 3.4%, and tamponade or rupture in 1.7%. ECG infarct location was anterior in 51%, inferior in 38%, posterior in 11%, and lateral in 24%,[1] consistent with other recent series (Table 3).[35,36]

Table 1.

Baseline Characteristics in Shock

SHOCK Registry data in 1190 patients with
post-MI cardiogenic shock.[34]

Age (years)	68.7±11.8
Male sex	59.7%
Transfer to tertiary care center	42.3%
Hypertension	53.1%
Diabetes	32.6%
Smoking history	50.1%
Hyperlipidemia	41.8%
Renal insufficiency	10.9%
Peripheral vascular disease	17.9%
Prior MI	40.2%
Prior congestive heart failure	19.5%
Prior angioplasty	6.2%
Prior coronary bypass surgery	9.6%

MI = myocardial infarction.

Table 2.

Clinical Characteristics in Shock

SHOCK Registry data in 815 patients with
post-MI cardiogenic shock due to LV failure.[34]

Hours from MI to shock (median)	6.2
Chest pain at shock onset	55.9%
Recurrent ischemia pre-shock	19.3%
Re-MI pre-shock	8.3%
Systolic pressure (mm Hg) *	87.8±23.0
Diastolic pressure (mm Hg) *	52.5±17.3
Heart rate	94.9±25.8
Right-heart catheterization	64.2%
Cardiac index (L/min/m^2)	2.1±0.8
Pulmonary wedge pressure (mm Hg)	23.7±8.6
Left ventricular ejection fraction (n=311)	30.4±12.5
Ventilator	74.9%
Inotropic agents	71.7%
Intra-aortic balloon pump	53.1%

*may be on inotropic support

MI = myocardial infarction

Of those with inferior MI, 38.3% had ECG evidence of a prior MI. Only 21.2% of those with predominant LV failure had an inferior MI without prior MI or anterior involvement. Over half of this subgroup (53.4%) had lateral, posterior and/or apical involvement. Although inferior MI occurred often, the association with shock was more likely to be seen in the setting of prior MI or a mechanical complication. When a first

Table 3.

Electrocardiographic Characteristics in Shock

SHOCK Registry data in 815 patients with
post-MI cardiogenic shock due to LV failure.[34]

ST-segment elevation ≥ 2 leads	73.1%
New Q waves in ≥ 2 leads	32.7%
Q waves with ST elevation	14.2%
New left bundle branch block	11.0%
Location of MI	
Anterior	59.9%
Inferior	43.4%
Posterior	17.5%
Lateral	31.5%
Apical	9.8%
Multiple locations	49.1%

MI = myocardial infarction, LV = left ventricular.

inferior MI results in shock, right ventricular MI, mitral insufficiency, septal rupture, or tamponade must be strongly suspected.

The majority of shock patients have ECG findings of transmural MI; ST elevation, Q waves, or new LBBB were present in 79.1% of SHOCK Registry patients. However, 14% to 30% of patients do not, presenting instead with findings of subendocardial MI, ischemia or old left bundle branch block (LBBB).[1,5] In the GUSTO-IIb trial of patients with acute coronary syndromes, for instance, shock occurred in 2.5% of patients without ST elevation versus 4.2% of those with ST elevation.[37]

The risk factors for developing shock in non-ST-elevation infarction seem to be very similar to those discussed above for all patients with shock. Among nearly 8000 non-ST-elevation patients in GUSTO-IIb,[22] those who developed shock were older (73 vs. 65 years) and were more often female (43% vs. 33%) and diabetic (34% vs. 18%) than those who did not develop shock. Prior MI (43% vs. 31%), prior bypass surgery (18% vs. 12%), and prior heart failure (12% vs. 7%) were also more common in shock patients without ST elevation. The GUSTO-IIb study also identified some important differences between shock patients with ST elevation and those without ST elevation.[22] As a group, non-ST-elevation patients were older (73 vs. 70 years) and were more often diabetic (34% vs. 21%), hyperlipidemic (42% vs. 28%), and hypertensive (59% vs. 40%). Other baseline clinical characteristics more common in non-ST-elevation patients included a history of angina (85% vs. 52%), prior MI (44% vs. 24%), prior bypass surgery (18% vs. 4%), and prior heart failure (12% vs. 4%). Striking differences were also apparent on coronary angiography.[22] Multivessel disease was significantly more common in the non-ST-elevation group, and the infarct-related artery location was very different (Table 4). The infarct vessel was more often occluded when ST elevation was present, with 68% of these patients having TIMI grade 0-1 flow, versus 40% of non-ST-elevation patients.

Table 4.

Infarct-Related Artery Location in Patients Undergoing Coronary Angiography for Shock with or without ST Elevation[22]

	ST elevation	no ST elevation
left anterior descending	46%	24%
left circumflex	4%	18%
right coronary	44%	16%
left main	2%	4%
graft	2%	11%
unknown	0	24%
none	1%	2%

The clinical course of subjects with and without ST elevation may differ significantly. In the GUSTO-IIb trial, recurrent ischemia (55% vs. 29%) and reinfarction (32% vs. 12%) were more common in the non-ST-elevation patients, and this was reflected in the finding that the time from the onset of infarction to the appearance of shock was dramatically longer in the non-ST-elevation group (76 vs. 10 hours).[22] Findings in the 14% of patients in the SHOCK trial registry with primary LV failure and non-ST segment elevation infarcts were similar.[1,38] Patients with non-ST segment elevation infarcts tended to have smaller infarcts, earlier time to peak creatine kinase (CK), and more evidence of reperfusion and recurrent ischemia. They tended to be older, with higher rates of female gender, diabetes, hypertension, congestive heart failure (CHF), prior MI and comorbid disease. Although early mortality was lower, mortality at 1 to 2 years was similar.[38]

Mechanical Causes of Cardiogenic Shock

The incidences of the major categories of shock were prospectively assessed in 1422 SHOCK Registry patients.[1,34] Shock was predominantly due to LV failure in 78.5%. Acute severe mitral regurgitation was diagnosed in 6.9%, ventricular septal rupture in 3.9%, "isolated" right ventricular shock in 2.8%, and tamponade or rupture in 1.4%. In all, 12% of shock was largely due to mechanical causes. Other causes of cardiogenic shock, which accounted for approximately 7% of patients in the SHOCK study,[34] include myocarditis, end-stage nonischemic dilated cardiomyopathy, myocardial depression from excessive calcium antagonist or beta-blocker administration, severe myocardial contusion, septic shock with myocardial depression, myocardial stunning after prolonged cardiopulmonary bypass, preexisting valvular heart disease, and hypertrophic cardiomyopathy.[3] It is also important to note that concurrent conditions such as hemorrhage or infection may contribute to shock in 5% to 10% of patients.[1,7,34]

MORTALITY: MAJOR SHOCK CATEGORIES

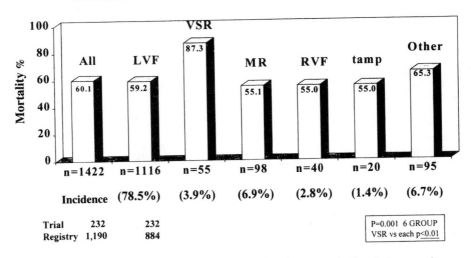

Figure 1. Mortality in cardiogenic shock due to left ventricular failure and mechanical causes. SHOCK Registry data in 1422 patients. LVF = LV failure, MR = severe mitral insufficiency, RVF = isolated RV shock, Tamp = tamponade/rupture, VSR = ventricular septal rupture. (Reproduced with permission.[34])

In-hospital mortality rates for mechanical causes in SHOCK registry patients were significantly different as shown in Figure 1. In the SHOCK Registry analyses, the in-hospital survival rate for mitral insufficiency was 45%[26] and for septal rupture was a disappointing 13%.[34] Surprisingly, the mortality for free wall rupture was 39%,[39] identical to that of shock patients overall.[34]

In contrast to patients with primary LV failure, who most often have anterior infarcts, patients with mitral regurgitation usually have posterior or inferior infarcts that produce mitral incompetence as a result of necrosis of the posteromedial papillary muscle.[26] Nevertheless, anterior MI was present in over one-third of severe mitral insufficiency patients.[26] Shock from mitral regurgitation is more common in women, but other baseline clinical characteristics are generally similar.[26] The SHOCK registry found ST elevation to be less common in patients with mitral regurgitation (41% vs. 63%) and LV ejection fraction to be less severely compromised (36% vs. 30%).[26] Despite this, pulmonary edema on X-ray was more common (81% vs. 58%), and cardiac index and pulmonary capillary wedge pressure were similar in the two groups. Time to shock was significantly longer in the mitral regurgitation patients (13 vs. 6 hours).

In general, patients with ventricular septal or free wall rupture are less likely to have had a prior MI, angina, CHF, diabetes or smoking history. They tend to have less severe coronary disease, and are less likely to have collaterals. The culprit artery is most often occluded. Presumably the larger infarction that may occur in association with sudden occlusion of an artery supplying an area of myocardium not previously ischemic is more predisposed to rupture. Patients with anterior infarcts tend to do better than inferior MI patients, perhaps due to more complex anatomy and surgical repair.[21] Free wall rupture has been reported to complicate as many as 6% of transmural infarcts.[40] Almost one-third of these have been thought to present subacutely and are often unrecognized.[40] This is in keeping with the 2.7% incidence in the SHOCK registry. In contrast to patients without tamponade or rupture, these patients were significantly less likely to have pulmonary edema (17% vs. 53%), diabetes (15% vs. 34%), prior infarction (18% vs. 39%), prior heart failure (4% vs. 21%), peripheral vascular disease (0% vs. 19%), and new Q waves (52% vs. 31%).[39] Three-fourths of the patients had a pericardial effusion, but no hemodynamic characteristics were useful in identifying the presence of free wall rupture or tamponade.[39]

The frequency of unsuspected mechanical complications in shock and the importance of surgical intervention strongly argues for routine and early echocardiography.

Timing Of Shock

Retrospective reports suggest that the majority (80%-90%) of patients who eventually develop shock are not in shock at the time of hospital admission.[5-7,11,14,15,17,18,41] In the Worcester community study, 44% of patients developed shock within the first day, 12% during the second day, 10% on the third day, and the remainder thereafter.[5] Among the 7.1% of patients who developed shock with acute MI in the Multicenter Investigation of the Limitation of Infarct Size (MILIS),[8] shock developed at least 24 hours after hospitalization in half of the cases. In GUSTO-I, 315 patients (11% of the 2972 patients with shock) had shock on arrival to the hospital and 2657 patients (89%) developed shock later.[17] In the prospective SHOCK registry, only one in ten patients (9%) who eventually developed shock due to LV failure was actually in shock at the time of presentation. Approximately one-half (47%) had developed shock within 6 hours of MI and three-quarters (72%) within 24 hours. The remaining one-quarter (28%) developed shock more than 24 hours following MI onset.[42] The median time from hospital admission to shock onset was only 4.6 hours, indicating that the therapeutic window is relatively narrow for most, but not all, patients.[1]

The SHOCK Registry compared the clinical characteristics of the three-quarters of patients presenting with early shock (< 24 hours post-MI) to those presenting with late shock (≥ 24 hours).[43] The demographic, historical, clinical, hemodynamic, and MI management characteristics of the early and late shock groups were similar. Early shock was more often associated with chest pain at shock onset, extensive ST-segment elevation, inferior MI and in-hospital death. Late shock was more often associated with recurrent ischemia, new Q waves and transfer to a tertiary care center. Among relatively nonselected, nontransferred patients, mortality was higher in patients presenting with early shock (in-hospital mortality 70% vs. 59%, p = 0.043). Shock developed earliest when the culprit artery was the left main (median 1.7 hours post-MI), later with the right coronary (3.5 hours) and circumflex (3.9 hours), latest with vein grafts (10.9 hours) and the left anterior descending artery (11.0 hours). Shock also developed earlier in patients with single-vessel disease (5.4 hours) than in patients with triple-vessel disease (7.8 hours).[43]

The left anterior descending artery was the most common culprit vessel, regardless of time of shock onset.[43] However, among late shock (> 24 hours post-MI) patients there was a trend towards an increased frequency of a culprit left anterior descending artery (56.0% vs. 40.6%). In contrast, the right coronary artery was more often the culprit in early shock (< 24 hours) patients (30.3% vs. 20.0%, p = 0.025). That shock might develop promptly following occlusion of the left main coronary artery is intuitive. Excessive vagal tone, mitral insufficiency, and right ventricular involvement may play a role in the setting of inferior MI.[44,45] Following anterior MI, infarct expansion and extension, and ischemia at a distance may play a role in the later development of shock.[4,21]

Although speculative, the goals of reperfusion therapy may vary to some degree in the settings of early and late shock. Early shock more often is due to occlusion of a single major coronary artery and ongoing infarction. In this setting thrombolysis or culprit artery angioplasty may, on occasion, be adequate. However, more complete revascularization[4,33] with multivessel angioplasty or bypass surgery may be particularly desirable in the setting of late shock.

Predictors of Mortality

Reported mortality with medical management of shock ranges from 70%-90%.[21] To put current treatment into perspective it is helpful to look at the SHOCK registry tertiary centers, where 49% of patients underwent coronary angiography and 41% had revascularization; 28% had angioplasty and 16% bypass surgery. The overall in-hospital mortality was 60.3%.[34] This lower mortality may be partly explained by the fact that almost half of these patients were transferred from community hospitals. Patients transferred to a SHOCK Trial center had a lower mortality than direct admissions (54% vs. 67%, p = 0.001). This is attributed to the survival bias associated with transfer; a selection bias frequently seen in other reports as well. Nevertheless, the 67% mortality for direct admissions is lower than that previously reported with shock. To some extent, this may reflect advances in medical management and revascularization. Recent reports suggest a decreasing mortality rate over time with increasing rates of revascularization.[24]

Once pump failure has developed, certain characteristics are associated with a worse outcome. Patients with anterior MI tend to have a higher mortality rate than those with inferior MI (67% vs. 53%, p < 0.05 in the SHOCK Registry).[1] Shock associated with ECG findings of "'non-transmural'" MI tends to be associated with higher mortality.[1,37] Age and comorbidities are predictors of poor outcome.[1,18] Cardiac output and ejection fraction are highly correlated with outcome.[18]

Thrombolysis

Thrombolysis in the setting of acute MI can reduce the likelihood of the subsequent development of shock.[12,13,17,18] The role of thrombolysis in the management of patients who have already developed shock is less clear. Successfully reperfused shock patients have a lower mortality rate than patients with persistent coronary occlusion,[35,46] however, the likelihood of successful reperfusion is low in this setting.[17,47] Although randomized trials have been inconclusive,[41,48] a meta-analysis of several placebo-controlled trials found a trend towards reduced 1-month mortality due to thrombolysis from 61% to 54% in hypotensive, tachycardic patients.[49] This potential of 7 lives saved for every 100 patients treated argues for thrombolysis if early mechanical reperfusion is not an option.

Revascularization

Several uncontrolled, retrospective series have examined the role of balloon angioplasty in cardiogenic shock.[9,17,36,50-63] Pooled data suggest an improved outcome with angioplasty.[4] These reports consistently find that shock patients who undergo angioplasty have a lower mortality rate; (1) than historical controls,[36,50-52,54-64] (2) than nonrandomized shock patients who do not undergo angioplasty,[50,64] (3) if angioplasty is successful than if it is not successful,[36,50,52,61] (4) with a patent infarct artery,[36] and (5) with better cardiac function than patients treated only with medical therapy.[59,62,63] Patency of the infarct artery seems to be the critical factor associated with favorable outcome in shock, regardless of how patency is achieved.[17,18,35] Nonrandomized reports of surgical revascularization in cardiogenic shock have also been encouraging.[4,65-87]

To a large degree, the favorable outcome attributed to revascularization is a consequence of patient selection.[9] Patients undergoing revascularization tend to be younger, less critically ill, have less prior myocardial damage and comorbidity, and are more likely to receive intra-aortic balloon support than patients not undergoing revascularization.[1,9] Angioplasty success rates reported in shock patients (74%) are lower than those reported in nonshock patients, presumably due to the associated hemodynamic instability, arrhythmias, diffuse disease, thrombus, "no reflow" phenomenon, coronary hypoperfusion, intolerance of angiographic contrast, and other factors.[36,50-64]

Two randomized studies have investigated the role of emergency revascularization in a randomized fashion. The first prospective, randomized trial of early percutaneous intervention versus conventional therapy for shock found a nonsignificant trend towards benefit, although the trial was prematurely terminated after enrolling just 55 patients.[88] In the larger, multinational, randomized SHOCK Trial a strategy of emergency early revascularization (with angioplasty or surgery) versus initial medical stabilization in patients with shock due to LV failure resulted in a nonsignificant reduction in 30-day mortality from 56% to 47%. By 1 year, there was a significant 39% improvement in survival.[89,90] This benefit was observed despite the low rates of stent and glycoprotein IIb/IIIa antagonist use in the early revascularization group and the high rates of intra-aortic balloon counterpulsation, thrombolysis, and late revascularization in the initial medical stabilization group.

The method of revascularization may vary. Revascularization in the SHOCK Trial was more often attempted percutaneously in the United States (76% of all emergency revascularization attempts were percutaneous and 24% were surgical). Outside of the United States, treatment modality was roughly equally divided (46% percutaneous and 54% surgical). Nevertheless, 1-year survival rates were identical (Col J and Menon V, personal communication).

The higher 1-year survival with early revascularization was consistent among subgroups; the notable exception was a differential treatment effect by age. There was a marked 18% absolute 1-year survival benefit associated with early revascularization for those < 75 years (52 percent vs. 33 percent) and no difference in survival for those ≥ 75 years old.[90] The apparent lack of benefit for those ≥ 75 years suggest that a routine strategy of early revascularization, as performed in this study, may not be appropriate for the elderly as a group. However, caution is required with such subgroup analyses and other data suggests that early revascularization may be associated with benefit in carefully selected elderly patients.[90]

Angiographic Findings

Cardiogenic shock is most often associated with significant atherosclerotic involvement of all three major coronary arteries. Although predominant involvement of the left anterior descending artery is common, single vessel disease is not.[50-52,65,91-94] In one study of patients with fatal shock, post-mortem examination found significant stenosis of the left anterior descending artery in 80% and triple vessel disease in 68%.[95] Angiographic findings and mortality in patients in the SHOCK registry are shown in Table 5.

Prospective data is available for 147 consecutive patients who survived to protocol driven angiography in the randomized SHOCK Trial[96] as shown in Table 6. Although 49% of patients undergoing protocol angiography had received thrombolysis, TIMI 2 or 3 flow was only identified in 45%.[96] The best 1-year survival was seen when the culprit vessel was the right coronary artery, both in patients treated medically (62.5%) and those treated with early revascularization (71.1%). Survival was poorest when

Table 5.

Angiographic findings and mortality in shock. SHOCK Registry data in 549 patients with post-MI shock due to LV failure[97]

	In-Hospital Mortality
Overall event rate	45.2%
Number of diseased vessels	p=0.002
0 or 1	35.0%
2	39.8%
3	50.8%
Left main disease	p=0.001
Present	62.8%
Absent	49.9%
Culprit vessel	p<0.001
LAD	42.3%
RCA	37.4%
LCX	42.4%
LM	78.6%
SVG	69.7%
Culprit vessel TIMI flow	p=0.035
0 or 1	46.5%
2	49.4%
3	26.0%

MI = myocardial infarction, LV = left ventricular, LAD = left anterior descending, RCA = right coronary artery, LCX = left circumflex coronary artery, LM = left main, SVG = saphenous vein graft.

the culprit was the left main or a vein graft, where no patient survived medical management, and revascularization survival was only 30% and 33%, respectively.

The extent of coronary disease (as assessed by number of diseased vessels or jeopardy score) was strongly predictive of mortality in patients treated with initial medical stabilization in the SHOCK Trial. However, extent of disease did not correlate with mortality in the early revascularization group, where 1-year survival was 55.0%, 54.8%, and 44.4% for one-, two-, and three-vessel disease, respectively (p = 0.274). The impact of this was most dramatic in patients with the worst disease. For example, 1-year survival in patients with three-vessel disease was 44.4% with early revascularization as compared to 32.8% with initial medical management. Similarly, ejection fraction strongly correlated with survival in the medical arm, but this effect appeared markedly blunted in the revascularization arm.[96] Early revascularization appears to blunt the importance of angiographic predictors of survival.

Table 6.

Angiographic Findings in Shock.
Data from 147 consecutive protocol SHOCK Trial
angiograms in patients with post-MI shock due to LV failure.[96]

Culprit vessel	
LAD	46.7%
RCA	29.2%
LCX	13.9%
LM	8.0%
SVG	2.2%
Culprit vessel	
TIMI flow	
0 or 1	55.2%
2	15.7%
3	29.1%
Suitable for CABG	
(# of vessels)	
0	2.2%
1	32.4%
2	37.5%
3	27.9%

MI = myocardial infarction, LV = left ventricular, LAD = left anterior descending, RCA = right coronary artery, LCX = left circumflex coronary artery, LM = left main, SVG = saphenous vein graft, CABG = coronary artery bypass graft.

Late Outcome Following Shock

Improved survival with reperfusion therapy in cardiogenic shock has led to concerns that these additional survivors might have a marginal quality of life with considerable morbidity and limited longevity. Retrospective analyses from the early 1990s reported that shock patients who underwent successful balloon angioplasty and were discharged from hospital had 1-year mortality rates ranging between 4% to 25%.[35,50,52,53,64] Subsequently, the larger, prospective SHOCK trial reported a trend towards reduced 30-day mortality with early revascularization. By 6 months, this apparent benefit was increased, and by 1 year there was a statistically significant (39%) improvement in survival.[89,90]

As shown in Figure 2, it appears that in terms of survival, the benefits of early revascularization may become greater with time.[90] This is in contrast to many other acute phase therapies for MI, such as thrombolysis and primary angioplasty, where survival curves often converge over time.[90] Rehospitalization was required in 19% of patients within the first year, primarily due to CHF. Rehospitalization rates were similar regardless of the approach of early revascularization or initial medical stabilization, and 87% of survivors were in New York Heart Association Class I or II.[90] This would suggest that incremental survivors are not necessarily burdened by excess morbidity.

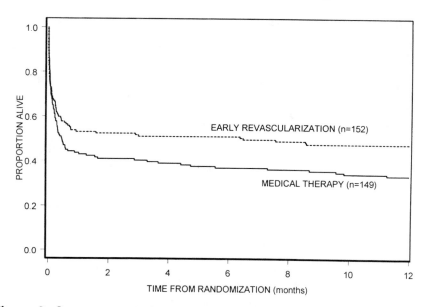

Figure 2. One-year survival in patients with cardiogenic shock in the SHOCK Trial. (Reproduced with permission.[90])

References

1. Hochman JS, Boland J, Sleeper LA, et al. Current spectrum of cardiogenic shock and effect of early revascularization on mortality. Results of an International Registry. SHOCK Registry Investigators. *Circulation* 1995; 91:873-881.
2. Hochman JS, Sleeper LA, Godfrey E, et al. SHould we emergently revascularize Occluded Coronaries for cardiogenic shocK: An international randomized trial of emergency PTCA/CABG-trial design. The SHOCK Trial Study Group. *Am Heart J* 1999; 137:313-321.
3. Hollenberg SM, Kavinsky CJ, Parrillo JE. Cardiogenic shock. *Ann Intern Med* 1999; 131:47-59.
4. Webb JG. Interventional management of cardiogenic shock. *Can J Cardiol* 1998; 14:233-244.
5. Goldberg RJ, Gore JM, Alpert JS, et al. Cardiogenic shock after acute myocardial infarction. Incidence and mortality from a community-wide perspective, 1975 to 1988. *N Engl J Med* 1991; 325:1117-1122.
6. Killip T, 3rd, Kimball JT. Treatment of myocardial infarction in a coronary care unit. A two year experience with 250 patients. *Am J Cardiol* 1967; 20:457-464.
7. Scheidt S, Ascheim R, Killip T, 3rd. Shock after acute myocardial infarction. A clinical and hemodynamic profile. *Am J Cardiol* 1970; 26:556-564.
8. Hands ME, Rutherford JD, Muller JE, et al. The in-hospital development of cardiogenic shock after myocardial infarction: Incidence, predictors of occurrence, outcome and prognostic factors. The MILIS Study Group. *J Am Coll Cardiol* 1989; 14:40-46; discussion 47-48.
9. Himbert D, Juliard JM, Steg PG, et al. Limits of reperfusion therapy for immediate cardiogenic shock complicating acute myocardial infarction. *Am J Cardiol* 1994; 74:492-494.

10. ISIS-2 (Second International Study of Infarct Survival) Collaborative Group. Randomised trial of intravenous streptokinase, oral aspirin, both, or neither among 17,187 cases of suspected acute myocardial infarction: ISIS-2. *Lancet* 1988; 2:349-360.

11. Leor J, Goldbourt U, Reicher-Reiss H, et al. Cardiogenic shock complicating acute myocardial infarction in patients without heart failure on admission: Incidence, risk factors, and outcome. SPRINT Study Group. *Am J Med* 1993; 94:265-273.

12. Meinertz T, Kasper W, Schumacher M, et al. The German multicenter trial of anisoylated plasminogen streptokinase activator complex versus heparin for acute myocardial infarction. *Am J Cardiol* 1988; 62:347-351.

13. Wilcox RG, von der Lippe G, Olsson CG, et al. Trial of tissue plasminogen activator for mortality reduction in acute myocardial infarction. Anglo-Scandinavian Study of Early Thrombolysis (ASSET). *Lancet* 1988; 2:525-530.

14. Holmes DR, Bates ER. Cardiogenic shock during myocardial infarction. The GUSTO experience with thrombolytic therapy (abstract). *Circulation* 1993; 88:I-253.

15. Garrahy PJ, Henzlova MJ, Forman S, et al. Has thrombolysis improved survival from cardiogenic shock? (abstract). *Circulation* 1989; 80 Suppl:II-623.

16. Gruppo Italiano per lo Studio della Sopravvivenza nell'Infarto Miocardico. GISSI-2: A factorial randomised trial of alteplase versus streptokinase and heparin versus no heparin among 12,490 patients with acute myocardial infarction. *Lancet* 1990; 336:65-71.

17. Holmes DR, Jr., Bates ER, Kleiman NS, et al. Contemporary reperfusion therapy for cardiogenic shock: The GUSTO-I trial experience. The GUSTO-I Investigators. *J Am Coll Cardiol* 1995; 26:668-674.

18. Holmes DR, Berger PB, Bates E, et al. Predictors of mortality in cardiogenic shock. The GUSTO experience. *J Am Coll Cardiol* 1995; 25:86A.

19. Califf RM, Bengtson JR. Cardiogenic shock. *N Engl J Med* 1994; 330:1724-1730.

20. International Study Group. In-hospital mortality and clinical course of 20,891 patients with suspected acute myocardial infarction randomised between alteplase and streptokinase with or without heparin. *Lancet* 1990; 336:71-75.

21. Webb J, Hochman J. Pathophysiology and management of cardiogenic shock due to primary pump failure. In: Gersh B, Rahimtoola S, eds. Acute Myocardial Infarction. New York: Chapman & Hall, 1997:308-327.

22. Holmes DR, Jr., Berger PB, Hochman JS, et al. Cardiogenic shock in patients with acute ischemic syndromes with and without ST-segment elevation. *Circulation* 1999; 100:2067-2073.

23. Spaulding CM, Joly LM, Rosenberg A, et al. Immediate coronary angiography in survivors of out-of-hospital cardiac arrest. *N Engl J Med* 1997; 336:1629-1633.

24. Goldberg RJ, Samad NA, Yarzebski J, et al. Temporal trends in cardiogenic shock complicating acute myocardial infarction. *N Engl J Med* 1999; 340:1162-1168.

25. Antoniucci D, Valenti R, Santoro GM, et al. Systematic direct angioplasty and stent-supported direct angioplasty therapy for cardiogenic shock complicating acute myocardial infarction: In-hospital and long-term survival. *J Am Coll Cardiol* 1998; 31:294-300.

26. Thompson CR, Buller CE, Sleeper LA, et al. Cardiogenic shock due to acute severe mitral regurgitation complicating acute myocardial infarction: A report from the SHOCK Trial Registry. *J Am Coll Cardiol* 2000; 36:1104-1109.

27. Menon V, Webb JG, Hillis LD, et al. Outcome and profile of ventricular septal rupture with cardiogenic shock after myocardial infarction: A report from the SHOCK Trial Registry. SHould we emergently revascularize Occluded Coronaries in cardiogenic shocK? *J Am Coll Cardiol* 2000; 36:1110-1116.

28. Sheps DS, Conde C, Cameron B, et al. Resting peripheral blood lactate elevation in survivors of prehospital cardiac arrest: Correlation with hemodynamic, electrophysiologic and oxyhemoglobin dissociation indexes. *Am J Cardiol* 1979; 44:1276-1282.

29. Mavric Z, Zaputovic L, Zagar D, et al. Usefulness of blood lactate as a predictor of shock development in acute myocardial infarction. *Am J Cardiol* 1991; 67:565-568.

30. Kessler KM, Kozlovskis P, Trohman RG, et al. Serum lactate: Prognostic marker for recurrent cardiac arrest? *Am Heart J* 1987; 113:1540-1544.

31. Menon V, White H, LeJemtel T, et al. The clinical profile of patients with suspected cardiogenic shock due to predominant left ventricular failure: A report from the SHOCK Trial Registry. *J Am Coll Cardiol* 2000; 36:1071-1076.

32. Hasdai D, Holmes DR, Jr., Califf RM, et al. Cardiogenic shock complicating acute myocardial infarction: Predictors of death. GUSTO Investigators. Global Utilization of Streptokinase and Tissue-Plasminogen Activator for Occluded Coronary Arteries. *Am Heart J* 1999; 138:21-31.

33. Widimsky P, Gregor P, Cervenka V, et al. Severe diffuse hypokinesis of the remote myocardium--the main cause of cardiogenic shock? An echocardiographic study of 75 patients with extremely large myocardial infarctions. *Cor Vasa* 1988; 30:27-34.

34. Hochman JS, Buller CE, Sleeper LA, et al. Cardiogenic shock complicating acute myocardial infarction--etiologies, management and outcome: A report from the SHOCK Trial Registry. *J Am Coll Cardiol* 2000; 36:1063-1070.

35. Bengtson JR, Kaplan AJ, Pieper KS, et al. Prognosis in cardiogenic shock after acute myocardial infarction in the interventional era. *J Am Coll Cardiol* 1992; 20:1482-1489.

36. O'Neill WW, Erbel R, Laufer N. Coronary angioplasty therapy of cardiogenic shock complicating acute myocardial infarction (abstract). *Circulation* 1985; 72:III-309.

37. Holmes D, Hochman JS. Cardiogenic shock in ST depression versus ST elevation myocardial infarction patients: GUSTO IIB trial (abstract). *Circulation* 1996; 94:I-734.

38. Jacobs AK, French JK, Col J, et al. Cardiogenic shock with non-ST-segment elevation myocardial infarction: A report from the SHOCK Trial Registry. SHould we emergently revascularize Occluded coronaries for Cardiogenic shocK? *J Am Coll Cardiol* 2000; 36:1091-1096.

39. Slater J, Brown RJ, Antonelli TA, et al. Cardiogenic shock due to cardiac free-wall rupture or tamponade after acute myocardial infarction: A report from the SHOCK Trial Registry. *J Am Coll Cardiol* 2000; 36:1117-1122.

40. Lopez-Sendon J, Gonzalez A, Lopez de Sa E, et al. Diagnosis of subacute ventricular wall rupture after acute myocardial infarction: Sensitivity and specificity of clinical, hemodynamic and echocardiographic criteria. *J Am Coll Cardiol* 1992; 19:1145-1153.

41. Gruppo Italiano per lo Studio della Streptochinasi nell'Infarto Miocardico (GISSI). Effectiveness of intravenous thrombolytic treatment in acute myocardial infarction. *Lancet* 1986; 1:397-402.

42. Webb J, Thompson C, Carere R, et al. Early and late development of post-MI shock: Different causes and outcomes (abstract). *Circulation* 1996; 94:I-734.

43. Webb JG, Sleeper LA, Buller CE, et al. Implications of the timing of onset of cardiogenic shock after acute myocardial infarction: A report from the SHOCK Trial Registry. SHould we emergently revascularize Occluded Coronaries for cardiogenic shocK? *J Am Coll Cardiol* 2000; 36:1084-1090.

44. Laster SB, Ohnishi Y, Saffitz JE, et al. Effects of reperfusion on ischemic right ventricular dysfunction. Disparate mechanisms of benefit related to duration of ischemia. *Circulation* 1994; 90:1398-1409.

45. Kinn JW, Ajluni SC, Samyn JG, et al. Rapid hemodynamic improvement after reperfusion during right ventricular infarction. *J Am Coll Cardiol* 1995; 26:1230-1234.

46. Kennedy JW, Gensini GG, Timmis GC, et al. Acute myocardial infarction treated with intracoronary streptokinase: A report of the Society for Cardiac Angiography. *Am J Cardiol* 1985; 55:871-877.

47. Bates ER, Topol EJ. Limitations of thrombolytic therapy for acute myocardial infarction complicated by congestive heart failure and cardiogenic shock. *J Am Coll Cardiol* 1991; 18:1077-1084.

48. Dioguardi N, Lotto A, Levi GF, et al. Controlled trial of streptokinase and heparin in acute myocardial infarction. *Lancet* 1971; 2:891-895.

49. Fibrinolytic Therapy Trialists" (FTT) Collaborative Group. Indications for fibrinolytic therapy in suspected acute myocardial infarction: Collaborative overview of early mortality and major morbidity results from all randomised trials of more than 1000 patients. *Lancet* 1994; 343:311-322.

50. Hibbard MD, Holmes DR, Jr., Bailey KR, et al. Percutaneous transluminal coronary angioplasty in patients with cardiogenic shock. *J Am Coll Cardiol* 1992; 19:639-646.

51. Lee L, Bates ER, Pitt B, et al. Percutaneous transluminal coronary angioplasty improves survival in acute myocardial infarction complicated by cardiogenic shock. *Circulation* 1988; 78:1345-1351.

52. Lee L, Erbel R, Brown TM, et al. Multicenter registry of angioplasty therapy of cardiogenic shock: Initial and long-term survival. *J Am Coll Cardiol* 1991; 17:599-603.

53. Gacioch GM, Ellis SG, Lee L, et al. Cardiogenic shock complicating acute myocardial infarction: The use of coronary angioplasty and the integration of the new support devices into patient management. *J Am Coll Cardiol* 1992; 19:647-653.

54. Shani J, Rivera M, Greengart A, et al. Percutaneous transluminal coronary angioplasty in cardiogenic shock (abstract). *J Am Coll Cardiol* 1986; 7:149A.

55. Heuser RR, Maddoux GL, Ramo BW, et al. Coronary angioplasty in the treatment of cardiogenic shock: The therapy of choice (abstract). *J Am Coll Cardiol* 1986; 7:219A.

56. Brown EJ, Jr., Swinford RD, Gadde P, et al. Acute effects of delayed reperfusion on myocardial infarct shape and left ventricular volume: A potential mechanism of additional benefits from thrombolytic therapy. *J Am Coll Cardiol* 1991; 17:1641-1650.

57. Laramee LA, Rutherford BD, Ligon RW, et al. Coronary angioplasty for cardiogenic shock following myocardial infarction (abstract). *Circulation* 1988; 78 (Suppl II):II-634.

58. Disler L, Haitas B, Benjamin J, et al. Cardiogenic shock in evolving myocardial infarction: Treatment by angioplasty and streptokinase. *Heart Lung* 1993; 16:649-652.

59. Verna E, Repetto S, Boscarini M, et al. Emergency coronary angioplasty in patients with severe left ventricular dysfunction or cardiogenic shock after acute myocardial infarction. *Eur Heart J* 1989; 10:958-966.

60. Meyer P, Blanc P, Baudouy M, et al. [Treatment of primary cardiogenic shock by coronary transluminal angioplasty during the acute phase of myocardial infarction]. *Arch Mal Coeur Vaiss* 1990; 83:329-334.

61. Elchaninoff H, Simpendorfer C, Whitlow PL. Coronary angioplasty improves both early and 1-year survival in acute myocardial infarction complicated by cardiogenic shock (abstract). *J Am Coll Cardiol* 1991; 17:167A.

62. Yamamoto H, Hayashi Y, Oka Y, et al. Efficacy of percutaneous transluminal coronary angioplasty in patients with acute myocardial infarction complicated by cardiogenic shock. *Jpn Circ J* 1992; 56:815-821.

63. Seydoux C, Goy JJ, Beuret P, et al. Effectiveness of percutaneous transluminal coronary angioplasty in cardiogenic shock during acute myocardial infarction. *Am J Cardiol* 1992; 69:968-969.

64. Moosvi AR, Khaja F, Villanueva L, et al. Early revascularization improves survival in cardiogenic shock complicating acute myocardial infarction. *J Am Coll Cardiol* 1992; 19:907-914.

65. DeWood MA, Notske RN, Hensley GR, et al. Intraaortic balloon counterpulsation with and without reperfusion for myocardial infarction shock. *Circulation* 1980; 61:1105-1112.

66. Subramanian VA, Roberts AJ, Zema MJ, et al. Cardiogenic shock following acute myocardial infarction; late functional results after emergency cardiac surgery. *N Y State J Med* 1980; 80:947-952.

67. Berg R, Jr., Selinger SL, Leonard JJ, et al. Immediate coronary artery bypass for acute evolving myocardial infarction. *J Thorac Cardiovasc Surg* 1981; 81:493-497.

68. Rosenkranz ER, Buckberg GD, Laks H, et al. Warm induction of cardioplegia with glutamate-enriched blood in coronary patients with cardiogenic shock who are dependent on inotropic drugs and intra-aortic balloon support. *J Thorac Cardiovasc Surg* 1983; 86:507-518.

69. Kirklin JK, et al. Intermediate-term results of coronary artery bypass grafting for acute myocardial infaraction: Results in 339 patients. *Circulation* 1985; 72 Suppl:II-175-II-178.

70. Phillips SJ, Kongtahworn C, Skinner JR, et al. Emergency coronary artery reperfusion: A choice therapy for evolving myocardial infarction. Results in 339 patients. *J Thorac Cardiovasc Surg* 1983; 86:679-688.

71. Laks H, Rosenkranz E, Buckberg GD. Surgical treatment of cardiogenic shock after myocardial infarction. *Circulation* 1986; 74 (Suppl III):11-16.

72. Guyton RA, et al. Emergency coronary artery bypass for cardiogenic shock. *Circulation* 1987; 76 Suppl:V22-V27.

73. Bolooki H. Emergency cardiac procedures in patients in cardiogenic shock due to complications of coronary artery disease. *Circulation* 1989; 79:I137-I148.

74. Willerson JT, Curry GC, Watson JT, et al. Intraaortic balloon counterpulsation in patients in cardiogenic shock, medically refractory left ventricular failure and/or recurrent ventricular tachycardia. *Am J Med* 1975; 58:183-191.

75. Dunkman WB, Leinbach RC, Buckley MJ, et al. Clinical and hemodynamic results of intraaortic balloon pumping and surgery for cardiogenic shock. *Circulation* 1972; 46:465-477.

76. Mundth ED, Buckley MJ, Leinbach RC, et al. Surgical intervention for the complications of acute myocardial ischemia. *Ann Surg* 1973; 178:379-390.

77. Johnson SA, Scanlon PJ, Loeb HS, et al. Treatment of cardiogenic shock in myocardial infarction by intraaortic balloon counterpulsation surgery. *Am J Med* 1977; 62:687-692.

78. Ehrich DA, Biddle TL, Kronenberg MW, et al. The hemodynamic response to intra-aortic balloon counterpulsation in patients with cardiogenic shock complicating acute myocardial infarction. *Am Heart J* 1977; 93:274-279.

79. Bardet J, Masquet C, Kahn JC, et al. Clinical and hemodynamic results of intraortic balloon counterpulsation and surgery for cardiogenic shock. *Am Heart J* 1977; 93:280-288.

80. O'Rourke MF, Sammel N, Chang VP. Arterial counterpulsation in severe refractory heart failure complicating acute myocardial infarction. *Br Heart J* 1979; 41:308-316.

81. Phillips SJ, Zeff RH, Skinner JR, et al. Reperfusion protocol and results in 738 patients with evolving myocardial infarction. *Ann Thorac Surg* 1986; 41:119-125.

82. Beyersdorf F, Sarai K, Wendt T, et al. Prolonged abnormalities of LV regional wall motion after normal reperfusion in patients with preoperative cardiogenic shock. *Thorac Cardiovasc Surg* 1990; 38:165-174.

83. Allen BS, Buckberg GD, Fontan FM, et al. Superiority of controlled surgical reperfusion versus percutaneous transluminal coronary angioplasty in acute coronary occlusion. *J Thorac Cardiovasc Surg* 1993; 105:864-879; discussion 879-884.

84. Miller MG, Hedley-White J, Weintraub RM, et al. Surgery for cardiogenic shock. *Lancet.* 1974;2(7893):1342-1345.

85. Quigley RL, Milano CA, Smith LR, et al. Prognosis and management of anterolateral myocardial infarction in patients with severe left main disease and cardiogenic shock. The left main shock syndrome. *Circulation* 1993; 88:II65-70.

86. Benetti FJ, Mariani MA, Ballester C. Direct coronary surgery without cardiopulmonary bypass in acute myocardial infarction. *J Cardiovasc Surg (Torino)* 1996; 37:391-395.

87. DeWood M, et al. Acute myocardial infarction: A decade of experience with surgical reperfusion in 701 patients. *Circulation* 1983; 68(Suppl II):8-16.

88. Urban P, Stauffer JC, Bleed D, et al. A randomized evaluation of early revascularization to treat shock complicating acute myocardial infarction. The (Swiss) Multicenter Trial of Angioplasty for Shock-(S)MASH. *Eur Heart J* 1999; 20:1030-1038.

89. Hochman JS, Sleeper LA, Webb JG, et al. Early revascularization in acute myocardial infarction complicated by cardiogenic shock. *N Engl J Med* 1999; 341:625-634.

90. Hochman JS, Sleeper LA, White HD, et al. One-year survival following early revascularization for cardiogenic shock. *JAMA* 2001; 285:190-192.

91. Alonso DR, Scheidt S, Post M, et al. Pathophysiology of cardiogenic shock. Quantification of myocardial necrosis, clinical, pathologic and electrocardiographic correlations. *Circulation* 1973; 48:588-596.

92. Page DL, Caulfield JB, Kaster JA, et al. Myocardial changes associated with cardiogenic shock. *N Engl J Med* 1971; 285:133-137.

93. Swan HJ, Forrester JS, Diamond G, et al. Hemodynamic spectrum of myocardial infarction and cardiogenic shock. A conceptual model. *Circulation* 1972; 45:1097-1110.

94. Blumgart H, Schlesinger M, Davis D. Studies on the relation of the clinical manifestations of angina pectoris, coronary thrombosis and myocardial infarction to the pathologic findings. *Am Heart J* 1940; 19:1097-1110.

95. Wackers FJ, Lie KI, Becker AE, et al. Coronary artery disease in patients dying from cardiogenic shock or congestive heart failure in the setting of acute myocardial infarction. *Br Heart J* 1976; 38:906-910.

96. Sanborn TA, Bergman GW, Webb JG, et al. Core laboratory findings, angioplasty results, and relation to treatment effect: Results from the randomized SHOCK trial. Presented at the Late-Breaking Clinical Trials Session, 48th Annual Scientific Session of the American College of Cardiology, Orlando, FL.

97. Wong SC, Sanborn T, Sleeper LA, et al. Angiographic findings and clinical correlates in patients with cardiogenic shock complicating acute myocardial infarction: A report from the SHOCK Trial Registry. *J Am Coll Cardiol* 2000; 36:1077-1083.

Chapter 2

Pathophysiology of Cardiogenic Shock

Francis Q. Almeda, MD and Joseph E. Parrillo, MD

Introduction

Cardiogenic shock is a condition of insufficient tissue perfusion due to cardiac dysfunction. It is a clinical syndrome that presents with signs and symptoms of diminished cardiac output and tissue hypoxia in the face of adequate intravascular volume. Indeed, it represents one of the most challenging medical emergencies that clinicians face in contemporary medical practice. The most common cause of cardiogenic shock is acute myocardial infarction (MI), and cardiogenic shock accounts for the majority of deaths in patients with acute MI who are able to reach the hospital. The mortality rates for this condition, even in the era of technological medical advances, remain exceedingly high, in the range of 50% to 80%.[1] The diagnosis and management of this complex condition requires a firm understanding of basic and advanced cardiovascular physiology and pathology. This chapter will provide a review of the pathophysiology of cardiogenic shock from its basic underlying principles and mechanisms to its diverse clinical applications.

Definition

The diagnosis of cardiogenic shock can often be suspected at the bedside, but hemodynamic confirmation is necessary to assure the correct diagnosis. The clinical syndrome of cardiogenic shock consists of myocardial dysfunction resulting in diminished cardiac output, and hypotension accompanied by signs of decreased tissue perfusion, such as altered mental status, diminished urine output (< 30 mL/hour), and cool and mottled

From: Hollenberg SM, Bates ER. *Cardiogenic Shock.* Armonk, NY: Futura Publishing Co., Inc.; ©2002.

skin. By definition, it involves a primary insult to the myocardium rather than abnormalities in circulating blood volume or vascular resistance, and exclusion or correction of factors such as acidosis, hypoxia, and hypovolemia. The hemodynamic features of cardiogenic shock include persistent hypotension (systolic blood pressure < 90 mm Hg, or less than 30 mm Hg below baseline levels for more than 30 minutes), a decreased cardiac index (< 2.2 L/min/m^2), and an elevated pulmonary artery occlusion pressure (> 15 mm Hg).[2]

Etiology

Cardiogenic shock may be a result of a primary myopathic process or a mechanical problem (Table 1). The most common cause of cardiogenic shock is acute MI with resultant diminution of left ventricular (LV) function. Autopsy studies show that cardiogenic shock is usually associated with loss of more than 40% of the LV myocardium.[3,4] Thus, cardiogenic shock is more commonly seen with anterior MIs, which generally involve a larger area of myocardium compared with inferior wall infarctions. In the SHOCK Trial Registry,[1] 55% of infarctions were anterior, 46% were inferior, and 50% had multiple sites of involvement by ECG. The cumulative effects of myocardial damage are often significant, and a small MI may result in cardiogenic shock in a patient with a marginal cardiac function at baseline due to previous myocardial injury. Moreover, acute ischemia may result in mechanical complications, such as acute mitral regurgitation due to papillary muscle dysfunction or rupture,[5,6] ventricular septal rupture,[6] or ventricular free wall rupture,[7] which may also lead to cardiogenic shock. Right ventricular infarction, which usually occurs in up to 30% of patients with inferior wall MIs, is a less common but still

Table 1.

Causes of Cardiogenic Shock

Myopathic	Mechanical
• Acute myocardial infarction (Most common)	• Acute mitral regurgitation
• Myocarditis	• Ventricular septal rupture
• Dilated cardiomyopathy	• Ventricular free-wall rupture
• Myocardial depression in septic shock	• Ventricular aneurysm
	• Acute aortic regurgitation (uncommon)
• Right ventricular failure	• Left ventricular outflow tract obstruction (Aortic stenosis, hypertrophic cardiomyopathy)
• Myocardial depression as a sequel of cardiopulmonary arrest or cardiopulmonary bypass	• Left ventricular inflow tract obstruction (Mitral stenosis, left atrial myxoma)

important cause of cardiogenic shock.[8] In the SHOCK Trial Registry,[1] 74.5% of patients had mainly LV dysfunction, 8.3% had acute mitral regurgitation, 4.6% had ventricular septal rupture, 3.4% had isolated right ventricular failure, and 1.7% had pericardial tamponade or cardiac rupture.

Additionally, the late onset of shock may be secondary to infarct extension, reocclusion of a previously patent infarct-related artery, or a severe metabolic imbalance of myocardial oxygen supply and demand compromising the noninfarcted regions.[9]

Other nonischemic causes of cardiogenic shock include acute myocarditis, end-stage dilated cardiomyopathy, acute valvular regurgitation secondary to endocarditis or trauma, severe mitral or aortic stenosis, hypertrophic cardiomyopathy, myocardial contusion, and sequelae of cardiopulmonary arrest or cardiopulmonary bypass.[10] Sepsis may result in myocardial depression, an effect that has been mechanistically linked to cytokines, tumor necrosis factor (TNF) and interleukin-1 (IL-1), and nitric oxide release.[11,12] Sepsis-induced myocardial depression can add to ischemia-induced dysfunction, occasionally resulting in sufficient dysfunction to produce cardiogenic shock.

Basic Cardiovascular Physiology

The underlying mechanism for diminished tissue perfusion in cardiogenic shock is a primary derangement in cardiac function. Maintenance of adequate blood flow to vital organs is dependent mainly on arterial blood pressure, which is determined by cardiac output and peripheral vascular resistance. In cardiogenic shock, the inciting and initiating factor is a decrease in cardiac output, usually due to significant LV impairment.

Cardiac output is a product of stroke volume and heart rate. Stroke volume is dependent on preload, myocardial contractility, and afterload (Figure 1). These factors in turn are influenced by neural and hormonal input from the sympathetic and parasympathetic system, and by circulating vasoactive substances. Cardiac output is significantly affected by ve-

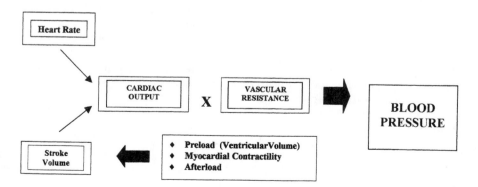

Figure 1. Determinants of systemic blood pressure.

nous return, and this is primarily related to renal mechanisms that control intravascular volume, such as the renin-angiotensin-aldosterone axis, pressure natriuresis, and atrial natriuretic factor.[13]

Resistance to blood flow in any vessel is directly proportional to the length of the vessel and the viscosity of blood, and indirectly proportional to the fourth power of the vessel radius. Thus, small changes in vessel size cause vast changes in the cross-sectional area of the vessel, and result in large changes in resistance to flow. The main site of resistance to flow in the arterial system occurs at the arteriolar level, and this is mainly influenced by arteriolar smooth muscle tone. Arteriolar tone is primarily under a tonic vasoconstrictor stimulus from the sympathetic nervous system, under the influence of both arterial and cardiopulmonary barore-ceptors. This in turn is modulated by catecholamines (epinephrine and norepinephrine) released by the adrenal system. Furthermore, metabolic mediators such as prostaglandins and adenosine result in vasodilation with subsequent increased blood flow in response to increased metabolic demand. Local autoregulation of the vasculature is mediated by the myo-genic response, which is the ability of the blood vessels to constrict and dilate in response to changes in transmural pressure in order to maintain a constant blood flow. Other local autoregulatory systems include the secretion by endothelial cells of nitric oxide (endothelium derived relaxing factor), eicosanoids (molecules derived from arachidonic acid), and endo-thelin-1 and angiotensin II (vasoconstrictor peptides).[14]

Systemic Pathophysiology

Cardiogenic shock is usually the result of MI or myocardial isch-emia.[15] This complex process can be viewed as a progressive downward spiral of events, whereby worsening myocardial function results in wors-ening ischemia, which causes an even greater loss of cardiac function. Adequate perfusion of the myocardium is dependent on the duration of diastole and the pressure gradient between the flow of blood in the coro-nary arteries and the left ventricle. Diastole is usually significantly short-ened during times of ischemia, due to the compensatory tachycardia, and the pressure gradient driving coronary blood flow is often adversely affected due to systemic hypotension on one end and an increased LV end-diastolic pressure at the other end. Furthermore, myocardial oxygen demand is also excessively increased, due to the elevated myocardial wall stress secondary to ischemia. The diminished cardiac output itself may lead to systemic metabolic derangements, such as lactic acidosis, which often contribute further to the cardiac dysfunction. Thus, the sequence of events may be viewed as a vicious cycle of myocardial dysfunction and ischemia which, if uninterrupted, usually results in death. (Figure 2).[16]

Significant impairment of LV function results in a diminution of stroke volume. Several compensatory mechanisms are activated as the body attempts to maintain adequate tissue perfusion. Initial compensa-tory mechanisms include stimulation of the sympathetic nervous system, activation of the renin-angiotensin-aldosterone system, and local vasore-

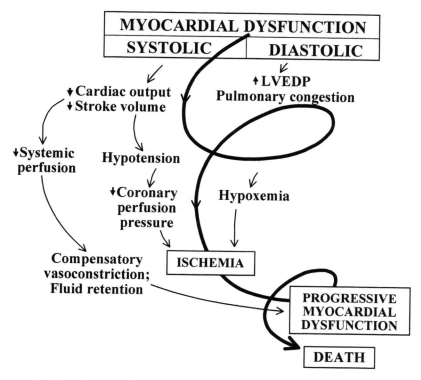

Figure 2. The downward spiral in cardiogenic shock. (Reproduced with permission.[16])

gulation. Sympathetic stimulation results in increased myocardial contractility and heart rate, which increases cardiac output at the expense of increasing myocardial oxygen consumption. The increased catecholamine levels and decreased perfusion of the kidneys results in an increase in renin release and production of angiotensin II, a potent vasoconstrictor, which causes increased aldosterone secretion by the adrenal cortex. Aldosterone raises intravascular volume by increasing sodium and water reabsorption by the kidneys. In addition, secretion of antidiuretic hormone by the posterior pituitary in response to baroreceptor stimulation results in a marked increase in free water reabsorption, further expanding intravascular volume. Activation of the renal mechanisms in an attempt to maintain adequate venous return and preload results in significant fluid retention and may result in pulmonary congestion and hypoxemia. Compensatory increases in peripheral vascular resistance due to sympathetic activation and stimulation by angiotensin II momentarily raise the systemic blood pressure but also result in increased myocardial afterload, which significantly increases myocardial oxygen demand. Local autoregulatory processes result in redistribution of blood from the skeletal muscle, skin, and gastrointestinal tract preferentially to the heart, brain, and kidneys.

Thus, these compensatory mechanisms, while beneficial in the initial stages of cardiogenic shock, all have the net effect of excessively increasing myocardial oxygen consumption, resulting in further deterioration of cardiac function. If uncorrected, the progressive deterioration in cardiac function overwhelms the body's ability to maintain adequate perfusion to the vital organs, resulting in death.[10]

The interruption of this vicious cycle of myocardial dysfunction and ischemia forms the basis for the therapeutic regimens for cardiogenic shock. In the SHOCK Trial Registry,[1] 75% of patients developed cardiogenic shock within 24 hours after presentation, with a median delay of approximately 7 hours from the onset of infarction. The fact that the vast majority of patients with cardiogenic shock present within 24 hours of admission to the hospital highlights the importance of rapid and prompt diagnosis of this condition. Equally important is the immediate initiation of management, which will optimize myocardial perfusion and decrease myocardial ischemia in order to preserve cardiac function and improve clinical outcomes.

Invasive hemodynamic monitoring is essential in monitoring the volume status of the patient, estimating the degree of LV end-diastolic pressure, and excluding right ventricular infarction or mechanical complications. The classic hemodynamic features of cardiogenic shock include the following: persistent hypotension (systolic blood pressure < 90 mm Hg, or less than 30 mm Hg below baseline levels for more than 30 minutes), a decreased cardiac index (< 2.2 L/min/m^2), and an elevated pulmonary occlusion pressure (> 15 mm Hg).[2] Establishing a trend or a sequence of hemodynamic variables for each individual patient is perhaps more important than absolute values *per se*, and creating Frank-Starling ventricular function curves for each patient is often a helpful clinical approach. One must remember that the level of intravascular plasma oncotic pressure is influenced by the levels of both plasma albumin and globulin. Thus, in hypoalbuminemic patients, a lower pulmonary artery occlusion pressure (< 15 mm Hg) may result in significant capillary leakage of fluid leading to pulmonary edema. Pulmonary congestion impairs gas exchange and further exacerbates myocardial ischemia. Conversely, the optimal LV filling pressures may be greater than 15 mm Hg in certain patients, particularly those with significant LV diastolic dysfunction and a history of chronic pulmonary congestion. Thus, the hemodynamic goals for each individual patient must be carefully interpreted in the appropriate clinical context, and must be viewed as an ever-changing dynamic process.

The reduced cardiac output may adversely affect other vital organs of the body, which may result in further deterioration in myocardial performance. Prolonged hypoperfusion of the kidneys may cause acute tubular necrosis with acute renal failure leading to volume overload, acidosis, and electrolyte abnormalities. Severe hepatic congestion due to cardiogenic shock may cause a "shock liver" with marked elevations of liver enzymes and derangement of the coagulation pathway. Ischemia of the gastrointestinal tract may result in significant gastrointestinal bleeding and/or translocation of gastrointestinal organisms into the bloodstream and potential sepsis.

Cardiac Pathophysiology

Both systolic and diastolic dysfunction play a prominent role in the pathophysiology of cardiogenic shock (Figure 2).[17,18] This may be viewed as a complex process, wherein there is an inability of the left ventricle to completely pump blood forward (systolic dysfunction), as well as an impairment in the capability of the left ventricle to relax and fill adequately (diastolic dysfunction). As mentioned earlier, once a critical mass of LV function is lost, (usually approximately 40%)[3,4] then stroke volume begins to diminish significantly. Systolic dysfunction leads to decreased systemic perfusion and hypotension, which results in a reduction in coronary perfusion pressure, and an increase in peripheral vasoconstriction and fluid retention. These compensatory mechanisms result in a vicious cycle, which further worsens the systolic dysfunction. Likewise, myocardial ischemia results in significant diastolic dysfunction, which causes an elevation in LV end-diastolic pressure and myocardial wall stress at a given end-diastolic volume.[19] This abnormal increase in the stiffness of the left ventricle limits adequate LV filling in diastole and may result in pulmonary congestion. This congestion results in progressive hypoxemia and worsens the imbalance of oxygen delivery and oxygen demand in the myocardium, resulting in further ischemia and myocardial dysfunction.[16,17] The compensatory increase in fluid retention to maintain cardiac output may add to the vicious cycle and further increase filling pressures.

Coronary Thrombosis

Acute MI accounts for the majority of patients who present with cardiogenic shock. These patients often have a complete occlusion of a major coronary vessel supplying a significant territory of myocardium. There are about 1.5 million cases of acute MI every year in the United States, resulting in approximately 400,000 to 500,000 deaths annually. The overall mortality rate for patients who present with acute MI is approximately 5% to 30% depending on specific patient characteristics, and about half die before reaching the hospital, usually due to ventricular arrhythmias. The in-hospital mortality is around 10%, and this is most commonly due to cardiogenic shock. Even in the contemporary era of medical advances, cardiogenic shock is associated with an exceedingly high mortality rate, in the range of 50% to 80%.[20]

The pathogenesis of acute coronary syndromes involves a vulnerable plaque that ruptures and fissures and subsequently initiates a cascade of inflammatory and thrombotic mediators in and around the coronary artery wall that result in varying degrees of arterial occlusion and distal microembolization. Significant thrombotic coronary occlusion often develops in arteries that have only a minimal (< 50%) degree of stenosis at baseline.[21] These "mild" lesions may account for up to two-thirds of patients in whom acute coronary syndromes develop.[22] It is this unstable plaque that is "vulnerable," and not necessarily one that is severely stenotic, that is most prone to rupture. Characteristics of a vulnerable plaque include a large lipid core, a predominance of foam and other inflammatory cells, a thin fibrous cap, and a paucity of smooth muscle cells. Thus, plaques that undergo rupture often have a relatively soft core composed of cholesterol esters with a thin protective fibrous covering. Heavy infiltration by macrophages and other inflammatory cells increase the risk of plaque rupture due to secretion of proteolytic enzymes such as plasminogen activators and matrix metalloproteinases that degrade the extracellular matrix and further weaken the fibrous cap.[23] Eccentric plaques are most prone to rupture at the "shoulder" of the lesion at the site of maximal shear stress.[24] Plaque disruption leads to exposure of highly thrombogenic factors to the bloodstream, and further thrombus formation may result in subtotal or complete coronary occlusion. Thus, plaque progression is unpredictable and nonlinear, and severe stenosis may develop rapidly in segments of the coronary vessel that were only mildly stenosed a few months earlier by angiographic examination. Although plaque rupture with subsequent thrombus formation is the predominant pathophysiologic mechanism in acute MI, coronary vasoconstriction mediated by platelet dependent and thrombin dependent factors may also play a contributory role in decreasing coronary blood flow to the myocardium.[25]

Rapid, complete, and sustained relief of coronary obstruction and attainment of normal coronary flow (TIMI III flow) is the ultimate goal in patients who present with an acute MI. From the early studies in fibrinolytic therapy, attainment of optimal reperfusion has been associated with improved outcomes. The angiographic substudy of the GUSTO-I Trial[26] showed that more rapid and complete restoration of coronary flow through the infarct-related artery resulted in improvement in ventricular function and lower mortality among patients with an MI. This was the proposed mechanism by which accelerated tissue plasminogen activator (t-PA) produced the favorable outcome in the GUSTO-I trial compared to streptokinase. Numerous trials have validated this open artery hypothesis. Anderson et al. demonstrated that anterograde flow as defined by TIMI criteria is useful in differentiating different levels of flow with various prognostic consequences, and that normal coronary flow was associated with improved outcomes compared to suboptimal flow.[27]

Intra-aortic balloon counterpulsation or pumping (IABP) has been recognized to be an effective treatment for patients with acute coronary syndromes and cardiogenic shock. (see Chapter 5)[28] The IABP works by correcting the major hemodynamic derangements present in cardiogenic shock, and optimizing the balance between myocardial demand and supply. By deflating in the beginning of systole, the IABP leads to a reduction in left ventricular afterload and myocardial oxygen consumption. By inflating in the beginning of diastole, the balloon improves coronary blood flow and maximizes the coronary perfusion gradient. Thus, the beneficial physiologic effects of IABP placement include a decrease in cardiac afterload, an increase in coronary blood flow, an improvement in cardiac output and renal blood flow, and a reduction in LV end-diastolic pressure, volume, stroke work, and wall tension.[29]

Mechanical Complications (See Chapter 11)

Mechanical complications after acute MI, including acute mitral valve regurgitation, ventricular septal rupture, LV free wall rupture, and LV aneurysm formation, often worsen the pulmonary edema seen in cardiogenic shock (Table 2). These entities usually present within the first week of MI, and should be strongly considered in a patient who presents with an acute ischemic syndrome with sudden and progressive hypotension and pulmonary congestion.

Acute mitral regurgitation results in markedly elevated left atrial pressures due to the inadequate time for the noncompliant left atrium to adjust to the sudden increase in the volume of blood flowing backward from the left ventricle. This increased volume of blood thus results in exceedingly high left atrial pressures, which often lead to significant pulmonary congestion. This is manifested by a large "v" wave seen on the pulmonary capillary occlusion pressure tracing ("wedge") during right heart catheterization. Mitral regurgitation may be secondary to papillary muscle dysfunction or complete or partial rupture of the papillary muscle itself.[30] Severe mitral regurgitation most often involves necrosis of the posteromedial papillary muscle, due to occlusion of its predominantly single vessel blood supply.[31] Relief of myocardial ischemia often improves the degree of papillary muscle dysfunction. Complete or partial rupture of the papillary muscle requires immediate surgical correction. If the blood pressure allows, patients may be temporarily stabilized with afterload reducing agents such as intravenous nitroprusside, which may improve the forward flow of blood and lower left atrial pressure. Some patients may require IABP placement. IABP decreases afterload and enhances LV emptying without producing a decrease in blood pressure. It is a temporary stabilizing measure while preparing a patient for mitral valve surgery. Prompt recognition of severe mitral regurgitation complicating MI due to papillary muscle rupture is essential, since early surgical intervention remains the treatment of choice and may potentially impact on the overall prognosis. The morbidity and mortality of this condition, however, remains frustratingly high.[32]

Ventricular septal rupture is another uncommon, but life-threatening, mechanical complication of acute MI. Ventricular septal rupture usually complicates a first MI, which may be anterior or inferior in location. There is often an absence of collateral blood flow in the face of a totally occluded infarct-related coronary artery, causing severe transmural myocardial necrosis. This catastrophic event usually occurs within 8 days postinfarction, but can occur early; in the SHOCK trial registry,[33] median time from MI to ventricular septal rupture was 16 hours. It may present with new sudden and severe pulmonary edema and systemic hypotension. Clues to the diagnosis include the appropriate clinical scenario and a new harsh holosystolic murmur heard loudest at the left lower sternal border that is often accompanied by a prominent parasternal thrill. Prompt bedside echocardiography with Doppler provides a rapid noninvasive modality for confirming the diagnosis and quantifying the location and severity of the intracardiac shunt. On hemodynamic monitoring, the presence of

Table 2.

Mechanical Complications of Acute Myocardial Infarction.

	Papillary Muscle Rupture	Ventricular Septal Rupture	Ventricular Free Wall Rupture
Clinical Scenario (typical but not invariable)	Inferior myocardial infarction	Usually first infarct; elderly, female patients	Elderly, female, hypertensive patient
Time of Occurrence	2 to 7 days post-infarction	3-8 days post infarction, but may occur earlier (16 hrs)	During first week post-infarction
Clinical Presentation	Pulmonary edema Hypotension	Pulmonary edema; hypotension	Cardiac tamponade; cardiac arrest with pulseless electrical activity
Physical Examination Findings	Holosystolic murmur (may be soft or absent due to low cardiac output)	Holosystolic murmur or parasternal thrill	Cardiac arrest; distant heart sounds; elevated neck veins
Echocardiographic findings	Flail mitral leaflet with severe mitral regurgitation	Visualize shunt and may see defect in septum	Pericardial effusion
Invasive hemodynamic monitoring findings	Large "v" wave on pulmonary capillary wedge tracings	"Step up" in oxygen saturation from right atrium to right ventricle (> 5%); Large "v" wave	Elevation and equalization of diastolic filling pressures
Medical management	Nitroprusside; inotropic support; vasopressors; intraaortic balloon pump placement	Inotropic support; Vasopressors; Intraaortic balloon pump placement	Emergent pericardiocentesis
Definitive treatment	Immediate surgical repair	Immediate surgical repair	Immediate surgical repair

a significant step-up in oxygenation from the right atrium to the right ventricle confirms the diagnosis. Patients may also have a prominent "v" wave on the pulmonary capillary wedge tracings due to the increased blood flow. Patients with a hemodynamically significant ventricular septal rupture may be temporarily stabilized with inotropic support, vasopressors, and IABP placement; prompt surgical repair remains the best therapeutic option in these patients.[33]

Ventricular free wall rupture usually occurs in elderly, female, hypertensive patients. Other risk factors include the late administration of fibrinolytic therapy and large infarctions.[34] Ventricular wall rupture may result in the rapid accumulation of blood in the pericardium often leading to pericardial tamponade. The diagnosis should be suspected in any patient who presents a few days after an acute MI with cardiac arrest and pulseless electrical activity, elevated neck veins, and diminished heart sounds. Due to the rapidity of fluid accumulation in the pericardial space, even a small amount of blood may result in significant hemodynamic compromise. Invasive hemodynamic monitoring would reveal elevation and equalization of diastolic filling pressures in both the right and left side of the heart. Emergent pericardiocentesis may be life-saving. Surgery includes repair of the ventricle using a direct suture method or utilizing a patch to cover the site of rupture.[35]

Left ventricular aneurysms may complicate the clinical course of an acute MI. Depending on the extent of myocardium involved, aneurysms may be associated with refractory congestive heart failure, systemic embolization, or significant episodes of ventricular tachycardia. The diagnosis is suggested by persistent ST segment elevation weeks after infarction, and can be confirmed by two-dimensional echocardiography or left ventriculography. Aneurysms must be distinguished from pseudoaneurysms, which usually have a narrower neck at their base. Surgical repair may be attempted with endoventricular patches or linear repair techniques.[36]

Right Ventricular Infarction (See Chapter 10)

Right ventricular infarction usually occurs in the setting of an acute inferior MI. This is due to the fact that in the majority of cases, the right coronary artery supplies both the lateral wall of the right ventricle through the acute marginal branches, as well the inferior and posterior wall of the left ventricle through the posterior descending artery. Unlike the left ventricle, the right ventricle receives coronary perfusion during both systole and diastole, in the absence of significant right ventricular hypertrophy. Additionally, although the right ventricle has the same cardiac output as the left ventricle, it performs only one-fourth of the stroke work, since the pulmonary vascular resistance is only one-tenth of the systemic resistance, and has only one-sixth of the muscle mass.[37] Thus, the right ventricle has a more favorable oxygen supply ratio than the left ventricle due to perfusion during both systole and diastole, and its lower oxygen requirement due to its smaller muscle mass. The classic clinical presentation of right ventricular infarction includes an elevated jugular venous pressure, clear lung fields, and hypotension.

The degree of hemodynamic compromise that occurs in right ventricular infarction is a function of both the extent of the right ventricular ischemia as well as the constraining influence of the pericardium with the resultant interventricular dependence. Hemodynamic findings associated with severe right ventricular infarction include the following: a right atrial pressure of more than 10 mm Hg and within 5 mm Hg of the of the pulmonary occlusion pressure, a steep and sudden "y" descent in right atrial tracings, and a dip and plateau (square root sign) in the right ventricular pressure tracings. Equalization of right atrial, right ventricular end-diastolic, pulmonary artery diastolic, and pulmonary artery occlusion pressures may occur with right ventricular infarction with excessive dilation of the right ventricular cavity resulting in "engagement" of the pericardium mimicking pericardial tamponade.[38] True pericardial tamponade may be the result of ventricular free wall rupture or hemorrhagic pericarditis with pericardial tamponade. Patients with right ventricular infarction are exquisitely sensitive to changes in intravascular volume. The presence of profound hypotension with the administration of nitrates in a patient with an inferior wall MI is highly suggestive of right ventricular involvement. Loss of atrioventricular synchrony due to atrioventricular block or atrial infarction may also contribute to the hemodynamic compromise. The key components to successful treatment include the maintenance of adequate intravascular volume with normal saline, inotropic support, maintenance of atrioventricular synchrony, and revascularization.

Infarct Extension and Ischemia at a Distance

Progressive myocardial necrosis has been seen in patients with cardiogenic shock. Infarct extension and ischemia at a distance are the two pathophysiologic processes that may contribute significantly to progressive myocardial necrosis. Infarct extension (arbitrarily defined as occurring between 24 hours after infarction and completion of the hospital admission) may result from progression of an intracoronary thrombus, reocclusion of a previously patent infarct related coronary artery, or a severe imbalance of myocardial oxygen demand and supply.[39] Extension of the infarct may also be secondary to occlusion of a side branch from propagation of a coronary thrombus or rupture of another vulnerable plaque. The myocardial cells at the border zone adjacent to the infarcted area are especially susceptible to additional ischemic insults. The findings on pathology include healing MI with surrounding areas of more recent myocardial necrosis, usually within the same vascular distribution. Histologic analysis reveals contraction band necrosis in the areas of recent necrosis.[40]

Patients with large areas of myocardial damage, such as those with extensive anterior infarctions, may undergo mechanical infarct expansion due to remodeling of the infarcted muscle, which may lead to the delayed appearance of cardiogenic shock.[41] The expansion of the infarct leads to LV dilatation, which further compromises coronary blood flow by significantly raising myocardial wall stress and oxygen demand. Infarct expansion usually occurs several hours to days after the index event, and pathologic features include infarct thinning and dilatation. The cellular mechanisms for infarct expansion may include cellular stretch and myocyte slippage. Cellular stretch has been described as an increase in length of the myocytes, while cellular slippage invokes rearrangement of myocyte bundles with myocardial cell size remaining constant. It appears that myocardial cell slippage may be the predominant mechanism involved in this process.

Ischemia that occurs in an area that is remote from the infarcted segment (ischemia at distance) may contribute significantly to LV dysfunction.[42] Patients with cardiogenic shock often have significant multivessel disease. Angiographic data from the SHOCK Trial Registry showed that 15.5% of patients had significant left main lesions and 53.4% had three-vessel coronary artery disease.[43]

Hyperkinesis of the noninfarcted segments is a normal compensatory response that often develops in order to maintain an adequate cardiac output. This compensatory hyperkinesis may be absent or severely limited in patients with a high grade coronary artery stenosis and multivessel disease or previous MI in that territory, and may be an important to contributor to cardiogenic shock and death.[44] Furthermore, cardiogenic shock has been associated with dysfunctional coronary arterial autoregulation and impaired vasodilator reserve, resulting in pressure dependent coronary flow in multiple regions.[45] This renders the patient extremely sensitive to metabolic derangements and systemic hypotension, thus further contributing to impaired ability of the noninfarcted myocardial segments to undergo compensatory hyperkinesis.[46]

Pathophysiology of Myocyte Damage and Death

Cellular death is the final outcome of prolonged tissue hypoperfusion of the vital organs in cardiogenic shock. An excessive reduction in blood flow to the tissues results in cellular dysfunction including membrane disruption, lysosomal enzyme release, and depletion of intracellular energy stores. The major pathophysiologic mechanisms of cellular dysfunction are cellular hypoxia, inflammation, and free radical injury. During significant tissue hypoperfusion, cellular hypoxia is present, and anaerobic rather than aerobic metabolism predominates. Anaerobic glycolysis produces only two molecules of ATP during utilization of one glucose molecule compared to 36 molecules of ATP during aerobic glycolysis. This results in an excessive depletion of intracellular energy reserves. Furthermore, anaerobic metabolism usually results in the overproduction of lactic acid with concomitant intracellular acidosis. Since the main ion transport pumps depend on intracellular energy stores, depletion of intracellular reserves results in a decrease in the transmembrane potential and an excess of intracellular sodium and water. Due to the failure of the major ion transport pumps, the normal gradient of potassium, chloride and calcium is lost. In particular, intracellular accumulation of calcium results in worsening myocardial dysfunction. Early pathologic changes are enlargement of the endoplasmic reticulum and formation of blebs on the surface, which progresses to condensation of the mitochondria. Mitochondrial swelling is an ominous marker of irreversible cellular injury. Cellular death is finally manifested by lysosomal enzyme release, breakdown of the nuclear and plasma membrane, and accumulation of denatured proteins and nuclear material in the cytoplasm.[14]

This cascade of events that ultimately lead to cellular death progresses initially from a reversible phase and eventually enters an irreversible stage. The aggressive management of cardiogenic shock is thus geared towards preventing this downward spiral that leads to irreversible cellular dysfunction.

Although cell necrosis is thought to predominate in myocardial ischemia, there is increasing data to suggest that apoptosis may play a significant part in the pathophysiology of cardiogenic shock. Apoptosis is a physiologic mechanism of "programmed" cell death that functions to remove senescent cells. This mode of cellular death is genetically predetermined and involves several closely linked energy-dependent molecular and biochemical events. This is in contrast to cellular necrosis, which is an "accidental" event that results in cellular death. The biologic hallmark of apoptosis is "fragmentation" in chromosomal DNA. Cells undergoing apoptosis can be differentiated from those undergoing necrosis because apoptotic cells display several distinctive features including a reduction in cell volume, blebbing of the cell membrane, and condensation of nuclear chromatin. Furthermore, unlike myocardial necrosis, apoptosis often occurs in isolated cells without concomitant inflammation.[47] Although myocardial necrosis is the predominant pathophysiologic mechanism in acute MI, there have been accumulating data on the contributing role of apoptosis in this group of patients. Apoptosis has been demonstrated both at the border zone surrounding a core of necrotic infarcted tissue, and at sites distant from the area of infarction.[48,49] The proposed mechanisms for apoptosis include oxidative stress, mechanical stretching of myocardial cells, and inflammatory mediators.

Reversible Myocardial Dysfunction

A core concept in the pathophysiology of cardiogenic shock is the presence of significant areas of nonfunctional but viable myocardium in patients after acute MI. These areas of nonfunctioning myocardium are associated with decreased function and wall motion, but are viable and thus are potentially reversible (Figure 3, Table 3). The two processes are myocardial stunning and hibernating myocardium, which are conceptually distinct but often coexist in the same patient.

Myocardial stunning is a postischemic state of ventricular myocardial hypocontractility that persists even with restoration of normal coronary blood flow.[50, 51] It may persist for hours to days. The pathogenesis of myocardial stunning involves an ischemic event with subsequent coronary reperfusion but a persistence of a wall motion abnormality. Data suggests that this hypocontractile state in the face of normal coronary blood flow may be secondary to an imbalance in calcium regulation and a diminished

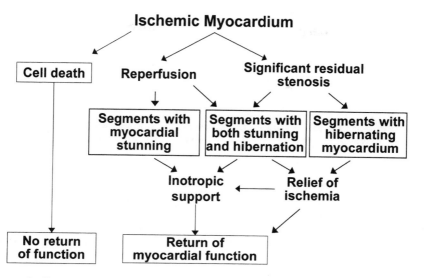

Figure 3. Potential consequences of myocardial ischemia. (Reproduced with permission.[16])

responsiveness of the cardiac myofilaments to calcium,[52] release of oxygen radicals resulting in oxidative stress,[53] microvascular abnormalities, or a combination of these factors. The release of myocardial depressant factors by coronary reperfusion may also play a role in this hypocontractile state.[54] The greater the degree of prior myocardial ischemia, the greater the degree of subsequent myocardial stunning.[51] The stunned ventricle retains its ability to contract in response to inotropic challenge with dobutamine, calcium, isoproterenol, epinephrine, and postextrasytolic potentiation.[55] There is adequate perfusion, which can be documented by techniques such as positron emission tomography using ammonia, and there is sufficient cellular metabolism that can be demonstrated by positron emission tomography showing adequate glucose uptake.[56]

Hibernating myocardium is a state of chronically reduced coronary blood flow associated with a corresponding decrease in myocardial contractility.[57] Rahimtoola initially defined hibernating myocardium as ischemic

Table 3.

A Comparison of Myocardial Stunning and Hibernating Myocardium.

Myocardial Stunning	Hibernating Myocardium
• Myocardial hypocontractility	• Myocardial hypocontractility
• Post-ischemic state	• Ischemic state
• Normal coronary blood flow	• Decreased coronary blood flow
• Reversible in hours to days	• Reversible with revascularization to restore coronary blood flow
• May improve with inotropic support	• May improve with revascularization

myocardium that is supplied by a severely stenosed coronary artery in which contraction is chronically depressed but myocytes remain viable.[58] It is further characterized by an improvement in myocardial function with restoration of myocardial perfusion. Myocardial hibernation, as the name implies, may be viewed as the proverbial "sleeping bear in the wintertime" that slows its metabolic rate in order to match its decreased intake. Likewise, hibernation is a state of equilibrium between function and flow, whereby the myocardium adapts to the chronically reduced blood flow by reducing its contractility, thus achieving a balance between myocardial oxygen supply and demand.[59-61] Recent data suggests that some hibernation may result from repetitive bouts of myocardial stunning.[62] Improvement in function may be seen with revascularization,[63] and this may improve prognosis.[64]

It is important to remember that, although myocardial stunning and hibernation are two pathophysiologically distinct entities, these two conditions may and are often present in the same patient, and that targeting therapy at both conditions may provide the optimal strategy for maximizing cardiac function.[65]

Treatment Implications

The rapid diagnosis and prompt treatment of reversible causes of cardiogenic shock is crucial in management of this complex condition. A better understanding of the underlying pathophysiology of cardiogenic shock will result in the improved diagnosis and treatment of this serious disease entity. Table 4 lists some of the underlying pathophysiologic mechanisms present in cardiogenic shock and the implications for treatment.

In the landmark SHOCK trial, patients with shock due to LV failure complicating MI were randomly assigned to emergency revascularization (152 patients) consisting of angioplasty or coronary artery bypass graft surgery or initial medical stabilization (150 patients) consisting mostly of inotropes or vasopressors, thrombolytic therapy, and IABP. In patients with cardiogenic shock, emergency revascularization did not significantly reduce overall mortality at 30 days between the revascularization and medical therapy groups (46.7% vs. 56% respectively; p = NS). However, at 6 months there was a significant survival benefit for early revascularization compared to medical therapy (50.3% vs. 63.1% respectively; p = 0.027).[66] Moreover, the one year survival was 45.7% for patients treated with early revascularization, compared with 33.6% for patients in the intensive medical stabilization group (95% CI 2.2%, 24.2%; p < 0.03).[67] The authors recommended that early revascularization should be strongly considered for patients with acute MI complicated by cardiogenic shock, particularly those younger than 75 years of age. Therefore, it appears that early revascularization may provide the optimal reperfusion strategy in patients with cardiogenic shock, and thus may interrupt the pathophysiologic vicious cycle (Figure 2) of ischemia causing worsening cardiac function, resulting in worsening ischemia, thereby impacting favorably on long-term mortality.

Table 4.

Pathophysiology and Implications for Treatment of Cardiogenic Shock.

Pathophysiology	Goal	Treatment
Myocardial cell necrosis	Prevent hypoxia; avoid oxygen free radical formation	Restoration of myocardial blood flow
Coronary occlusion	Restore maximal coronary blood flow	Direct angioplasty preferred; thrombolytics.
Systemic hypotension	Improve coronary perfusion pressure	Intraaortic balloon pump (IABP); inotropic agents and vasopressors
Acute mitral regurgitation	Lower left atrial pressure	Afterload reduction with nitroprusside; IABP; surgical correction.
Pulmonary edema	Decrease pulmonary artery occlusion pressure	Intravenous diuretics, afterload reduction
Hibernating myocardium	Restore myocardial perfusion	Myocardial revascularization
Stunned myocardium	Reverse hypocontractility	Inotropic support

Conclusions

Cardiogenic shock is one of the most challenging medical emergencies that face clinicians in contemporary medical practice. It is a complicated condition that has been associated with an exceedingly high mortality rate. The pathophysiology of cardiogenic shock involves a complex interaction of systolic and diastolic dysfunction, resulting in a progressive vicious cycle of myocardial ischemia and worsening myocardial dysfunction. Cardiogenic shock is a clinical syndrome that involves significant pathologic dysfunction at the cellular, myocardial and systemic level. Reversible myocardial dysfunction in the form of stunned or hibernating myocardium often plays a major role in the development and progression of this disease process. A better understanding of the underlying pathophysiology of cardiogenic shock will result in the improved diagnosis and treatment of this serious condition.

References

1. Hochman JS, Boland J, Sleeper LA, et al. Current spectrum of cardiogenic shock and effect of early revascularization on mortality. Results of an International Registry. *Circulation* 1995; 91:873-881.
2. Forrester JS, Diamond G, Chatterjee, K, et al. Medical therapy of acute myocardial infarction by application of hemodynamic subsets (second of two parts). *N Engl J Med* 1976; 295:1404-1413.
3. Harnarayan C, Bennett MA, Penetcost BL, Brewer DB. Quantitative study of infarcted myocardium in cardiogenic shock. *Br Heart J* 1970; 32:728-732.

4. Alonso DR, Scheidt S, Post M, et al. Pathophysiology of cardiogenic shock: Quantification of myocardial necrosis, clinical, pathologic and electrocardiographic correlations. *Circulation* 1973; 48:588-596.

5. Nishimura RA, Schaff HV, Shub C, et al. Papillary muscle rupture complicating acute myocardial infarction: Analysis of 17 patients. *Am J Cardiol* 1983; 51:373-377.

6. Wei JY, Hutchins GM, Bulkley BH. Papillary muscle rupture in fatal acute myocardial infarction: A potentially treatable form of cardiogenic shock. *Ann Intern Med* 1979; 90:149-152.

7. Sutherland FW, Guell FJ, Pathi VL, et al. Postinfarction ventricular free wall rupture: Strategies for diagnosis and treatment. *Ann Thorac Surg* 1996; 61:1281-1285.

8. Zehender M, Kasper W, Kauder E, et al. Right ventricular infarction as an independent predictor of prognosis after acute inferior myocardial infarction. *N Engl J Med* 1993; 328:981-988.

9. Bates ER, Moscucci M. Post-myocardial infarction cardiogenic shock. In: Brown DL, ed. Cardiac Intensive Care. Philadelphia: W.B. Saunders Company, 1998:215-235.

10. Califf RM, Bengtson JR. Cardiogenic shock. *N Engl J Med* 1994; 330:1724-1730.

11. Kumar A, Thota V, Dee L, et al. Tumor necrosis factor alpha and interleukin 1beta are responsible for in vitro myocardial cell depression induced by human septic shock serum. *J Exp Med* 1996; 183:949-958.

12. Lange LG, Schreiner GF. Immune mechanisms of cardiac disease. *N Engl J Med* 1994; 330:1129-1135.

13. West JB. Best and Taylor's Physiologic Basis of Medical Practice: Philadelphia, Williams & Wilkins, 1990:315-317.

14. Hollenberg SM, Parrillo JE. Shock. In: Fauci A, ed. Harrison's Principle's of Internal Medicine: New York, McGraw-Hill, 1998:214-222.

15. Almeda FQ, Parrillo JE. The Contemporary Management of Acute Myocardial Infarction. *Critical Care Clinics* 2001, In Press.

16. Hollenberg SM, Kavinsky CJ, Parrillo JE. Cardiogenic shock. *Ann Intern Med* 1999; 131:47-59.

17. Kones R. Cardiogenic Shock. New York: Futura Publishing Company, 1974.

18. Page DL CJ, Kastor JA, DeSanctis RW, et al. Myocardial changes associated with cardiogenic shock. *N Engl J Med* 1971; 285:133-137.

19. Harizi RC, Bianco JA, Alpert JS. Diastolic function of the heart in clinical cardiology. *Arch Intern Med* 1988; 148:99-109.

20. Ryan TJ, Anderson JL, Antman EM, et al. ACC/AHA guidelines for the management of patients with acute myocardial infarction. A report of the American College of Cardiology/American Heart Association Task Force on Practice Guidelines (Committee on Management of Acute Myocardial Infarction). *J Am Coll Cardiol* 1996; 28:1328-1428.

21. Fishbein MC, Siegel RJ. How big are coronary atherosclerotic plaques that rupture? *Circulation* 1996; 94:2662-2666.

22. Falk E, Shah PK, Fuster V. Coronary plaque disruption. *Circulation* 1995; 92:657-671.

23. Libby P. Molecular bases of the acute coronary syndromes. *Circulation* 1995; 91:2844-2850.

24. Fuster V, Badimon JJ, Chesebro JH. Atherothrombosis: Mechanisms and clinical therapeutic approaches. *Vasc Med* 1998; 3:231-239.

25. Bogaty P, Hackett D, Davies G, et al. Vasoreactivity of the culprit lesion in unstable angina. *Circulation* 1994; 90:5-11.

26. Ross AM, Coyne KS, Moreyra E, et al. Extended mortality benefit of early postinfarction reperfusion. GUSTO-I Angiographic Investigators. *Circulation* 1998; 97:1549-1556.

27. Anderson JL, Karagounis LA, Becker LC, et al. TIMI perfusion grade 3 but not grade 2 results in improved outcome after thrombolysis for myocardial infarction. Ventriculographic, enzymatic, and electrocardiographic evidence from the TEAM-3 Study. *Circulation* 1993; 87:1829-1839.

28. Ohman EM, George BS, White CJ, et al. Use of aortic counterpulsation to improve sustained coronary artery patency during acute myocardial infarction. Results of a randomized trial. *Circulation* 1994; 90:792-799.

29. Weber KT, Janicki JS. Intraaortic balloon counterpulsation. A review of physiological principles, clinical results, and device safety. *Ann Thorac Surg* 1974; 17:602-636.

30. Calvo FE, Figueras J, Cortadellas J, et al. Severe mitral regurgitation complicating acute myocardial infarction. Clinical and angiographic differences between patients with and without papillary muscle rupture. *Eur Heart J* 1997; 18:1606-1610.

31. Sharma SK, Seckler J, Israel DH, et al. Clinical, angiographic and anatomic findings in acute severe ischemic mitral regurgitation. *Am J Cardiol* 1992; 70:277-280.

32. Thompson CR, Buller CE, Sleeper LA, et al. Cardiogenic shock due to acute severe mitral regurgitation complicating acute myocardial infarction: A report from the SHOCK Trial Registry. SHould we use emergently revascularize Occluded Coronaries in cardiogenic shocK? *J Am Coll Cardiol* 2000; 36:1104-1109.

33. Menon V, Webb JG, Hillis LD, et al. Outcome and profile of ventricular septal rupture with cardiogenic shock after myocardial infarction: A report from the SHOCK Trial Registry. *J Am Coll Cardiol* 2000; 36:1110-1116.

34. Honan MB, Harrell FE, Jr., Reimer KA, et al. Cardiac rupture, mortality and the timing of thrombolytic therapy: A meta-analysis. *J Am Coll Cardiol* 1990; 16:359-367.

35. Nunez L, de la Llana R, Lopez Sendon J, et al. Diagnosis and treatment of subacute free wall ventricular rupture after infarction. *Ann Thorac Surg* 1983; 35:525-529.

36. Mills NL, Everson CT, Hockmuth DR. Technical advances in the treatment of left ventricular aneurysm. *Ann Thorac Surg* 1993; 55:792-800.

37. Lee FA. Hemodynamics of the right ventricle in normal and disease states. *Cardiol Clin* 1992; 10:59-67.

38. Kinch JW, Ryan TJ. Right ventricular infarction. *N Engl J Med* 1994; 330:1211-1217.

39. Leor J, Goldbourt U, Reicher-Reiss H, et al. Cardiogenic shock complicating acute myocardial infarction in patients without heart failure on admission: Incidence, risk factors, and outcome. *Am J Med* 1993; 94:265-273.

40. Weisman HF, Healy B. Myocardial infarct expansion, infarct extension, and reinfarction: Pathophysiologic concepts. *Prog Cardiovasc Dis* 1987; 30:73-110.

41. Hands ME, Rutherford JD, Muller JE, et al. The in-hospital development of cardiogenic shock after myocardial infarction: Incidence, predictors of occurrence, outcome and prognostic factors. The MILIS Study Group. *J Am Coll Cardiol* 1989; 14:40-48.

42. Widimsky P, Gregor P, Cervenka V, et al. Severe diffuse hypokinesis of the remote myocardium--the main cause of cardiogenic shock? An echocardiographic study of 75 patients with extremely large myocardial infarctions. *Cor Vasa* 1988; 30:27-34.

43. Wong SC, Sanborn T, Sleeper LA, et al. Angiographic findings and clinical correlates in patients with cardiogenic shock complicating acute myocardial infarction: A report from the SHOCK Trial Registry. *J Am Coll Cardiol* 2000; 36:1077-1083.

44. Grines CL, Topol EJ, Califf RM, et al. Prognostic implications and predictors of enhanced regional wall motion of the noninfarct zone after thrombolysis and angioplasty therapy of acute myocardial infarction. The TAMI Study Groups. *Circulation* 1989; 80:245-253.

45. McGhie AI, Golstein RA. Pathogenesis and management of acute heart failure and cardiogenic shock: Role of inotropic therapy. *Chest* 1992; 102:626S-632S.

46. Webb JG. Interventional management of cardiogenic shock. *Can J Cardiol* 1998; 14:233-244.

47. Colucci WS. Apoptosis in the heart. *N Engl J Med* 1996; 335:1224-1226.

48. Olivetti G, Quaini F, Sala R, et al. Acute myocardial infarction in humans is associated with activation of programmed myocyte cell death in the surviving portion of the heart. *J Mol Cell Cardiol* 1996; 28:2005-2016.

49. Bartling B, Holtz J, Darmer D. Contribution of myocyte apoptosis to myocardial infarction? *Basic Res Cardiol* 1998; 93:71-84.

50. Bolli R. Myocardial 'stunning" in man. *Circulation* 1992; 86:1671-1691.

51. Bolli R. Basic and clinical aspects of myocardial stunning. *Prog Cardiovasc Dis* 1998; 40:477-516.

52. Atar D, Gao WD, Marban E. Alterations of excitation-contraction coupling in stunned myocardium and in failing myocardium. *J Mol Cell Cardiol* 1995; 27:783-791.

53. Jeroudi MO, Hartley CJ, Bolli R. Myocardial reperfusion injury: Role of oxygen radicals and potential therapy with antioxidants. *Am J Cardiol* 1994; 73:2B-7B.

54. Brar R, Schaer GL, Hollenberg SM, et al. Release of soluble myocardial depressant activity by reperfused myocardium (abstract). *J Am Coll Cardiol* 1996; 27:386A.

55. Becker LC, Levine JH, DiPaula AF, et al. Reversal of dysfunction in postischemic stunned myocardium by epinephrine and postextrasystolic potentiation. *J Am Coll Cardiol* 1986; 7:580-589.

56. Conti CR. The stunned and hibernating myocardium: A brief review. *Clinic Cardiol* 1991; 14:708-712.

57. Wijns W, Vatner SF, Camici PG. Hibernating myocardium. *N Engl J Med* 1998; 339:173-181.

58. Rahimtoola SH. A perspective on the three large multicenter randomized clinical trials of coronary bypass surgery for chronic stable angina. *Circulation* 1985; 72:V123-V135.

59. Kloner RA, Przyklenk K, Patel B. Altered myocardial states. The stunned and hibernating myocardium. *Am J Med* 1989; 86:14-22.

60. Kloner RA, Przyklenk K. Stunned and hibernating myocardium. *Annu Rev Med* 1991; 42:1-8.

61. Marban E. Myocardial stunning and hibernation. The physiology behind the colloquialisms. *Circulation* 1991; 83:681-688.

62. Shen YT, Vatner SF. Mechanism of impaired myocardial function during progressive coronary stenosis in conscious pigs. Hibernation versus stunning? *Circ Res* 1995; 76:479-488.

63. Topol EJ, Weiss JL, Guzman PA, et al. Immediate improvement of dysfunctional myocardial segments after coronary revascularization: Detection by intraoperative transesophageal echocardiography. *J Am Coll Cardiol* 1984; 4:1123-1134.

64. Bonow RO. The hibernating myocardium: Implications for management of congestive heart failure. *Am J Cardiol* 1995; 75:17A-25A.

65. Heyndrickx G, Vatner SF, Wijns W. Stunning, Hibernation, and Preconditioning: Clinical Pathophysiology of Myocardial Ischemia. Philadelphia: Lippincott-Raven Publishers, 1997.

66. Hochman JS, Sleeper LA, Webb JG, et al. Early revascularization in acute myocardial infarction complicated by cardiogenic shock. SHOCK Investigators. *N Engl J Med* 1999; 341:625-634.

67. Hochman JS, Sleeper LA, White HD, et al. One-year survival following early revascularization for cardiogenic shock. *JAMA* 2001; 285:190-192.

Chapter 3

Clinical Assessment and Initial Management of Cardiogenic Shock

Steven M. Hollenberg, MD

Introduction

Shock is a syndrome comprising an array of symptoms, signs, and laboratory abnormalities that result from systemic hypoperfusion and consequent cellular and organ dysfunction. After recognizing the presence of shock, the clinician must perform the clinical assessment required to understand its cause while initiating supportive therapy before shock causes irreversible damage to vital organs. The challenge is that since speed is important to achieve a good outcome, evaluation and therapy must begin simultaneously. While the evaluation must be thorough, neither overzealous pursuit of a diagnosis before stabilization has been achieved nor overzealous empiric treatment without establishing the underlying pathophysiology is desirable.

A practical approach is to make a rapid initial evaluation on the basis of a limited history, the physical examination, and specific diagnostic procedures. Cardiogenic shock is diagnosed after documentation of myocardial dysfunction and exclusion of alternative causes of hypotension. Supportive therapy to maintain blood pressure, oxygenation, and tissue perfusion should be initiated concomitantly with the diagnostic evaluation. Such support is crucial to stabilize the patient with cardiogenic shock to allow time for the institution of definitive interventions aimed at reversing the underlying pathology.

From: Hollenberg SM, Bates ER. *Cardiogenic Shock.* Armonk, NY: Futura Publishing Co., Inc.; ©2002.

Initial Evaluation

History and Physical Examination

Obtaining a full history in patients in extremis is neither practical nor entirely necessary. Nonetheless, a directed history is invaluable in the expeditious evaluation of a patient with shock. Predictors of the predilection to develop cardiogenic shock after myocardial infarction (MI) include age, history of previous infarction, diabetes, peripheral vascular disease, and cerebrovascular disease,[1-3] all obtainable in the initial history. In addition, historical information can often furnish important clues in the differential diagnosis of shock; specifics are provided below.

Bedside clinical assessment can provide a reasonably good indication of global perfusion. Hemodynamic criteria for cardiogenic shock include sustained hypotension, with systolic pressure below 90 mm Hg for at least 30 minutes, along with decreased cardiac output and increased filling pressures.[4] Any given level of arterial pressure, however, must be interpreted in light of the chronic blood pressure; thus, in patients with severe chronic hypertension, a decrease in mean arterial pressure of 40 mm Hg may produce tissue hypoperfusion even if mean pressure still exceeds 60 mm Hg.[5] Conversely, patients with chronically low blood pressures may not develop shock until the mean arterial pressure drops below 50 mm Hg. Tachycardia is almost invariably present in patients with shock in the absence of chronotropic incompetence or medications which decrease heart rate.

Patients with shock are usually ashen or cyanotic, and can have cool skin and mottled extremities. Cerebral hypoperfusion may be manifested by a clouded sensorium, restlessness, or agitation. Pulses are rapid and faint, and may be irregular in the presence of arrhythmias. Patients are tachypneic and pulmonary rales are usually present, although their absence does not exclude the diagnosis.[6] The jugular veins are usually distended, and a precordial heave resulting from left ventricular (LV) dyskinesis may be palpable. The heart sounds may be distant, and third and/or fourth heart sounds are usually present. Murmurs indicative of valvular disease, mitral regurgitation, or ventricular septal defect may be heard, but these murmurs may be soft or inaudible due to low cardiac output, and are difficult to hear in the presence of pulmonary congestion, and so their absence does not exclude mechanical complications. Oliguria is present in most patients with shock.

The most common etiologies of cardiogenic shock are listed in Table 1. Consideration of pertinent historical and physical findings in these conditions follows.

Cardiogenic Shock Due to Left Ventricular Dysfunction In Acute Myocardial Infarction

Left ventricular (LV) dysfunction resulting from acute MI is the most common cause of cardiogenic shock.[4,7] Historical clues include a history

Table 1.

Causes of Cardiogenic Shock

ACUTE MYOCARDIAL INFARCTION
Pump Failure
Large infarction
Smaller infarction with pre-existing left ventricular dysfunction
Infarct extension
Reinfarction
Infarct expansion
Mechanical complications
Acute mitral regurgitation due to papillary muscle rupture
Ventricular septal defect
Free-wall rupture
Pericardial tamponade
Right ventricular infarction

OTHER CONDITIONS
End-stage cardiomyopathy
Myocarditis
Myocardial contusion
Prolonged cardiopulmonary bypass
Septic shock with severe myocardial depression
Left ventricular outflow tract obstruction
Aortic stenosis
Hypertrophic obstructive cardiomyopathy
Obstruction to left ventricular filling
Mitral stenosis
Left atrial myxoma

of recent and/or past episodes of chest discomfort. A history of pre-existing LV dysfunction, in addition to being a predisposing factor for the development of cardiogenic shock, is also important in guiding management. Although shock may occur upon occlusion of a major coronary artery, it most often evolves more gradually, due to infarct extension, reocclusion of a previously patent infarct artery, or decompensation of myocardial function in the noninfarct zone.[4]

The classic presentation of cardiogenic shock resulting from LV dysfunction includes hypotension, tachycardia, dyspnea, jugular venous distension, pulmonary congestion, ventricular gallops, and signs of peripheral hypoperfusion. In 1967, Killip reported a mortality of 81% in 47 patients with acute MI presenting with shock and pulmonary edema (Killip Class IV).[8] The importance of physical examination findings in determining prognosis in MI was confirmed in a recent analysis of the GUSTO-I trial, in which altered sensorium, cold, clammy skin, and oliguria, along with hemodynamic data, were independent predictors of mortality in the shock population.[9]

Recent analysis of patients from the SHOCK trial registry has revealed that approximately one-quarter of patients with severe acute LV dysfunction manifest hypotension and hypoperfusion in the absence of clinical pulmonary congestion.[6] Patients with predominant LV dysfunction were classified into groups depending on the presence or absence of peripheral hypoperfusion (defined by oliguria, cold peripheries, or both) and pulmonary congestion (rales on physical examination or pulmonary congestion on chest roentgenogram). Of the 571 patients for whom data were available, 367 (64%) had both congestion and hypoperfusion, 14 (3%) had neither, 32 (6%) had isolated pulmonary congestion, and 158 (28%) had isolated hypoperfusion.[6] These patients had only slightly lower pulmonary capillary wedge pressure than patients with both hypoperfusion and congestion (22 ± 7 vs. 24 ± 9 mm Hg, p = 0.012), and equally low cardiac indices (2.1 ± 0.8 vs. 1.9 ± 0.6 L/min/m^2, p = 0.22). In-hospital mortality was high in both groups of patients (70% for patients with hypoperfusion only, 60% for patients with hypoperfusion and congestion).[6] These data are in accordance with findings from patients with cardiogenic shock in the GUSTO trial, in whom low cardiac output and high pulmonary capillary wedge pressure predicted mortality.[9] Thus, it is clear that the absence of pulmonary congestion in the presence of hypoperfusion neither rules out cardiogenic shock, nor confers a lower risk of mortality.

Mechanical Complications of Acute Myocardial Infarction

Ischemic mitral regurgitation is usually associated with inferior MI and ischemia or infarction of the posterior papillary muscle.[10] Papillary muscle rupture typically occurs 1 to 7 days after acute MI (SHOCK trial registry median, 12.8 hours) and presents dramatically with pulmonary edema, hypotension, and signs of peripheral hypoperfusion. When a papillary muscle ruptures, the murmur of acute mitral regurgitation may be limited to early systole because of rapid equalization of pressures in the left atrium and left ventricle. More importantly, the murmur may be soft or inaudible, especially when cardiac output is low.[11]

Ventricular septal rupture may occur with either anterior or inferoposterior infarction. Patients tend to be older (mean age 72 in SHOCK trial registry)[12] and female. Patients who have ventricular septal rupture present acutely with shock and pulmonary edema, and can be difficult to distinguish from those with ruptured papillary muscles on clinical grounds alone, but a pansystolic murmur and a parasternal thrill are present.

Ventricular free wall rupture usually occurs during the first week after MI (median in SHOCK trial, 16-18 hours); the classic patient is elderly, female, and hypertensive.[13] Free wall rupture presents as a catastrophic event with a pulseless rhythm due to pericardial tamponade.

Right Ventricular Infarction

Right ventricular infarction occurs in up to 30% of patients with inferior infarction and is clinically significant in 10%.[14] The classic clinical presentation includes hypotension, elevated jugular venous pressure, and clear lung fields. The complete triad, however, is not always evident,[15] and a high index of suspicion is warranted in the appropriate clinical situation. Kussmaul's sign, an inspiratory rise in jugular venous pressure, is sensitive and specific in this context.[15] Hypotension in response to the administration of nitroglycerin in a patient with evidence of inferior ischemia is highly suggestive. ST elevation in right-sided ECG lead V_{4R} is diagnostic.

Dilated Cardiomyopathy/Myocarditis

Patients with cardiogenic shock on the basis of dilated cardiomyopathy usually have a history of symptomatic heart failure. Patients with myocarditis may have a more sudden onset of symptoms, and may have a history suggestive of an antecedent viral syndrome.[16] Physical examination demonstrates tachycardia and hypotension, usually with a narrow pulse pressure indicative of low stroke volume. Jugular venous distension, S_3 and S_4 gallops, and peripheral edema are usually noted. The holosystolic murmurs of mitral and tricuspid regurgitation are often present.

Valvular Heart Disease

Cardiogenic shock as a presentation of end-stage valvular heart disease is uncommon, but the diagnosis merits consideration, and clinical findings can be subtle when cardiac output is low. Severe aortic stenosis usually presents with antecedent symptoms of angina or syncope, but decompensation can occur, often in the setting of atrial fibrillation.[17] The carotid upstrokes are usually delayed and diminished; a late-peaking systolic ejection murmur is present but may not be loud. Chronic aortic regurgitation causes cardiomegaly, but when left ventricular decompensation ensues, the diastolic murmur may decrease in intensity. Similarly, cardiomegaly is a prominent feature of chronic mitral regurgitation, but the murmur may be subtle in the latter stages. End-stage mitral stenosis follows a history of symptomatic heart failure.[18] Physical findings are those of pulmonary hypertension and right-sided failure: jugular venous distension, right ventricular heave, a loud P_2, right ventricular S_3 and S_4, tricuspid regurgitation, hepatomegaly with or without ascites, and peripheral edema.

Acute valvular regurgitation, on the other hand, presents more dramatically. Acute aortic regurgitation may result from acute infective endocarditis, acute aortic dissection, tears of myxomatous valve leaflets, and valve disruption from blunt or perforating chest trauma. When acute aortic regurgitation causes hemodynamic decompensation, many of the classic signs, such as wide pulse pressure and low diastolic pressure, may be greatly attenuated or absent.[11] Aortic diastolic pressure may be relatively well maintained as the LV diastolic pressure rises, and pulse pressure may be narrow due to reduced forward stroke volume. Diastolic pressure equilibration may shorten the diastolic murmur. A third heart sound is almost always present. Acute mitral regurgitation may result from chordal rupture in patients with myxomatous valves, acute infective endocarditis, and blunt or perforating chest trauma resulting in leaflet tear or chordal rupture, as well as papillary muscle rupture or dysfunction in the setting of inferior infarction. Acute mitral regurgitation is manifested by pulmonary edema. Left ventricular ejection into the "low pressure" left atrium can lead to an acute reduction in cardiac output with subsequent hypotension, tachycardia, narrow pulse pressure, and cardiogenic shock.[11]

Other Diagnostic Tests

A 12-lead electrocardiogram should be performed immediately upon presentation. This may reveal evidence of infarction or arrhythmias. Conversely, an entirely normal electrocardiogram makes it unlikely that myocardial ischemia is the cause of cardiogenic shock. Other initial diagnostic tests should include a chest radiograph and measurement of arterial blood gases, electrolytes, complete blood count, and cardiac enzymes.

An imbalance between oxygen supply and oxygen demand results in anaerobic glycolysis, with conversion of pyruvate to lactate. In shock resulting from decreased oxygen delivery, blood lactate levels can thus be used as an index of global perfusion.[19] The trend of lactate concentrations may be a better indicator than a single value.[20] In patients with decompensated congestive heart failure, in whom the assessment of disease severity on clinical grounds may be challenging, the presence of lactic acidosis can provide an indication of previously unsuspected hypoperfusion.[21]

To the physician confronted with a critically ill patient, echocardiography can be a key element in successful differential diagnosis.[22] This is particularly true in the evaluation of patients with suspected cardiogenic shock, and early echocardiography should be performed routinely.[5] Expeditious evaluation of global and regional left ventricular performance is crucial for management of congestive heart failure, with or without suspected myocardial ischemia. Echocardiography is simple, safe, and permits systemic interrogation of cardiac chamber size, left and right ventricular function, valvular structure and motion, atrial size, and the anatomy of the pericardial space. Doppler interrogation can be used to noninvasively assess right and left ventricular filling pressures, pulmonary artery pressures, stroke volume, and cardiac output.

Echocardiography provides information on LV chamber size, presence of thinned and akinetic segments characteristic of previous infarction, overall systolic performance, and regional wall motion abnormalities. Echocardiography is extremely useful for the rapid diagnosis of mechanical causes of shock after MI such as papillary muscle rupture and acute mitral regurgitation, acute ventricular septal defect, and free wall rupture and tamponade.[23] Unsuspected severe mitral regurgitation is not uncommon. In some cases, echocardiography may reveal findings compatible with right ventricular infarction.

Echocardiography can also reveal alternative diagnoses, such as valvular abnormalities, pericardial tamponade, or hypertrophic cardiomyopathy. Acute right heart failure, manifested by a dilated and hypokinetic right ventricle without hypertrophy suggestive of chronic pulmonary hypertension, can suggest pulmonary embolism.[24,25]

Transthoracic echocardiographic images may be suboptimal due to a poor acoustic window in critically ill patients, particularly those who are obese, have chronic lung disease, or are on positive pressure ventilation. Contrast echocardiography may be used to improve image quality.[26] Transesophageal echocardiography can also provide better visualization, and can be performed safely at the bedside.[27]

Hemodynamic Monitoring

Pulmonary artery catheterization provides simultaneous assessment of filling pressures and cardiac output, and can be quite useful for initiating and monitoring therapy. The hemodynamic profile of cardiogenic shock includes a pulmonary capillary occlusion pressure greater than 15 mm Hg and a cardiac index less than 2.2 $L/min/m^2$.[28] Invasive hemodynamic monitoring can reveal unrecognized volume depletion in patients with suspected cardiogenic shock.[5,29] Hemodynamic monitoring can also be useful in the diagnosis of mechanical complications of infarction. Right heart catheterization may reveal an oxygen step-up diagnostic of ventricular septal rupture or a large "v" wave that suggests severe mitral regurgitation, although v waves may be present in acute ventricular septal defect. Equalization of diastolic filling pressures may suggest pericardial tamponade. The hemodynamic profile of right ventricular infarction includes high right-sided filling pressures in the presence of normal or low occlusion pressures.[30]

Pulmonary artery catheterization can also be used to assess the adequacy of global perfusion. Mixed venous oxygen saturation is an indicator of the balance between oxygen delivery and consumption. In a patient with a stable oxygen demand, in the absence of hypoxemia and anemia, desaturation of hemoglobin in mixed venous blood can reflect decreased cardiac output.[31] Mixed venous oxygen saturation can be measured by withdrawing a blood sample from the pulmonary artery, or continuous measurement of mixed venous oxygen saturation can be achieved using an oximetric pulmonary artery catheter.

The pulmonary artery catheter provides hemodynamic data not easily inferred from physical examination or laboratory evaluation. Even though it is clear the pulmonary artery catheter is a diagnostic tool, whether its use translates into definable benefits for patients has recently come into question,[32] prompting a critical look at the available data concerning its risks and benefits. Catheterization prompts changes in therapy in many patients, but most of the data regarding outcomes are retrospective; prospective randomized trials are lacking. In this context, it should be noted that retrospective analyses have not demonstrated an increase in mortality in the subgroup of patients with cardiogenic shock after infarction[33] or in critically ill patients with congestive heart failure.[32] Although prospective trials may never be able to demonstrate conclusively that acquisition of hemodynamic data leads to decreases in mortality, the benefits of more rapid diagnosis seem clear, and optimization of supportive therapy is often best guided by hemodynamic assessment.[34]

Initial Management

General Considerations

Patients with shock should be treated in an intensive care unit (Table 2). Continuous electrocardiographic monitoring should be performed for detection of rhythm disturbances, and pulse oximetry should be used to detect fluctuations in arterial oxygenation. Laboratory measurements such as arterial blood gases, serum electrolytes, complete blood counts, coagulation parameters, and lactate concentrations should be done early and repeated as indicated.[5] Bladder catheterization is routine, and central venous access usual, although the diagnostic workup should not be delayed to insert a central line.

In shock states, measurement of blood pressure using an arterial cannula provides the most appropriate and reproducible measurement of arterial pressure. Noninvasive monitoring by auscultation or oscillometric methods is commonly inaccurate in hypotensive patients, and these methods measure arterial pressure only intermittently. Arterial cannulation allows for beat-to-beat analysis so that decisions regarding therapy can be based on immediate and reproducible blood pressure information.[5]

Maintenance of adequate oxygenation and ventilation are critical. Many patients require intubation and mechanical ventilation early in their course, if only to reduce the work of breathing and facilitate sedation

---

Table 2.

Stabilization of the Patient with Cardiogenic Shock

Monitoring in intensive care unit
    Continuous ECG monitoring
    Pulse oximetry
Establish venous access
Reverse hypoxia and acidosis
    Mechanical ventilation
    Non-invasive ventilation in selected situations
Treat pain and anxiety
Correct electrolyte abnormalities
Correct arrhythmias
Optimize ventricular filling
Vasopressor support to restore adequate perfusion pressure
    Dopamine
    Norepinephrine
    Phenylephrine

and stabilization before cardiac catheterization. Some recent studies have suggested that use of continuous positive airway pressure in patients with cardiogenic pulmonary edema can decrease the need for intubation.[35] Nonetheless, the studies are small and need to be evaluated with some caution; failure of noninvasive ventilation occurred at least half of the time. If patients do not manifest rapid clinical improvement with noninvasive ventilation, the strategy should be reconsidered.

Electrolyte abnormalities should be corrected, because hypokalemia and hypomagnesemia predispose to ventricular arrhythmias. Relief of pain and anxiety with morphine sulfate (or fentanyl if systolic pressure is compromised) can reduce excessive sympathetic activity and decrease oxygen demand, preload, and afterload. Arrhythmias and heart block may have major effects on cardiac output, and should be corrected promptly with antiarrhythmic drugs, cardioversion, or pacing. Measures that are routinely used and have been proven to improve outcome after MI, such as nitrates, beta-blockers, and angiotensin-converting enzyme inhibitors,[36] have the potential to exacerbate hypotension in cardiogenic shock, and should be withheld until the patient stabilizes.

Following initial stabilization and restoration of adequate blood pressure, tissue perfusion should be assessed. If tissue perfusion remains inadequate, inotropic support or intra-aortic balloon pumping should be initiated. If tissue perfusion is adequate but significant pulmonary congestion remains, diuretics may be employed. Vasodilators can be considered as well, depending on the blood pressure. If tissue perfusion is adequate and no pulmonary congestion is present, then no further resuscitative measures are needed (See Figure 1). In each of these situations, however, expeditious cardiac catheterization should be performed and the patient assessed for revascularization; prompt reperfusion is the key to achieving a good outcome in patients with cardiogenic shock.

Fluids

The initial approach to the hypotensive patient should include fluid resuscitation unless frank pulmonary edema is present. Patients are commonly diaphoretic and relative hypovolemia may be present in as many as 20% of patients with cardiogenic shock.[37] In the original description of hemodynamic subsets in MI by Forrester et al., approximately 20% of patients had low cardiac index and low pulmonary capillary wedge pressure; most had reduced stroke volume and compensatory tachycardia.[28] Some of these patients would be expected to respond to fluid infusion with an increase in stroke volume, although the magnitude of such a response depends on the degree of ischemia and cardiac reserve.

Fluid infusion is best initiated with predetermined boluses titrated to clinical endpoints of heart rate, urine output, and blood pressure. Ischemia produces diastolic as well as systolic dysfunction, and thus elevated filling pressures may be necessary to maintain stroke volume in patients with cardiogenic shock. Patients who do not respond rapidly to initial fluid boluses or those with poor physiologic reserve should be considered for invasive hemodynamic monitoring.

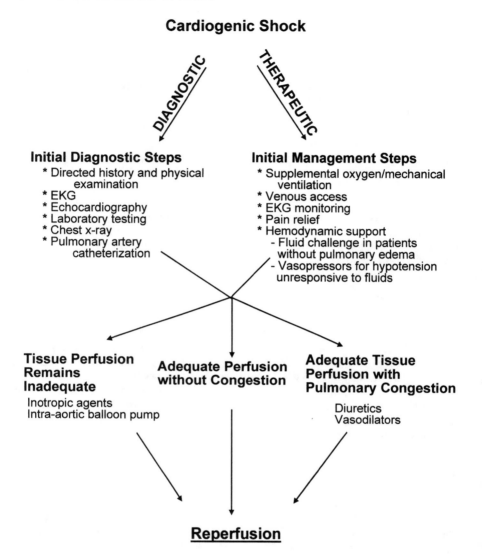

Figure 1. Diagnostic and therapeutic steps in cardiogenic shock. (Reproduced with permission.[4])

Optimal filling pressures vary from patient to patient; hemodynamic monitoring can be used to construct a Starling curve at the bedside, identifying the filling pressure at which cardiac output is maximized. Maintenance of adequate preload is particularly important in patients with right ventricular infarction.

Vasopressor Agents

When arterial pressure remains inadequate, therapy with vasopressor agents may be required to maintain coronary perfusion pressure.

Maintenance of adequate blood pressure is essential to break the vicious cycle of progressive hypotension with further myocardial ischemia.

Dopamine, which acts directly on myocardial β_1-adrenergic receptors and acts indirectly by releasing norepinephrine, has both inotropic and vasopressor effects. Dopamine also acts on specific dopamine receptors in the renal and splanchnic circulation to produce vasodilation.[38] The net effect of dopamine administration is dependent on the dosage, with effects on contractility predominating at doses less than 10 μg/kg/min, and alpha-adrenergic effects predominating above 20 μg/kg/min. Because dopamine increases both blood pressure and cardiac output, it is usually preferable as the initial choice in patients with systolic pressures less than 80 mm Hg.[4,39]

When hypotension remains refractory, norepinephrine, a natural catecholamine with potent alpha-adrenergic and less pronounced β_1-adrenergic effects, may be necessary to maintain organ perfusion pressure.[31] Its predominant effect is vasoconstriction, with little change in cardiac output. Norepinephrine is more potent than dopamine and may be more effective at reversing hypotension in patients with shock. Norepinephrine is usually started at 1-2 μg/min and titrated to effect.

Both dopamine and norepinephrine can cause tachycardia and increased peripheral resistance, which may exacerbate myocardial ischemia. Catecholamines are also arrhythmogenic. Phenylephrine, a selective α-1 adrenergic agonist, may be a good choice when tachyarrhythmias limit therapy with other vasopressors; doses start at 50 μg/min and range to 200 μg/min.

Vasopressor infusions need to be titrated carefully in patients with cardiogenic shock to maximize coronary perfusion pressure with the least possible increase in myocardial oxygen demand. It is also mandatory to ensure that filling pressures are optimal. Hemodynamic monitoring is useful in this regard.

Inotropic Agents

In patients with inadequate tissue perfusion and adequate intravascular volume, cardiovascular support with inotropic agents should be initiated. Dobutamine, a selective β_1-adrenergic receptor agonist, can improve myocardial contractility and increase cardiac output, and is the initial agent of choice in patients with systolic pressures greater than 80 mm Hg.[4] Dobutamine may exacerbate hypotension in some patients, and can precipitate tachyarrhythmias. Use of dopamine may be preferable if systolic pressure is less than 80 mm Hg, although tachycardia and increased peripheral resistance may worsen myocardial ischemia.[4,39] In some situations, a combination of dopamine and dobutamine can be more effective than either agent alone.[40]

Milrinone is a phosphodiesterase inhibitor that increases intracellular cyclic AMP by mechanisms not involving adrenergic receptors, producing both positive inotropic and vasodilatory actions.[41] This effect may be important in patients with chronic heart failure, in whom chronic elevation of circulating catecholamine levels can produce down-regulation of beta-adrenergic receptors.[42] Milrinone has minimal chronotropic and arrhythmogenic effects compared to catecholamines.[43] In addition, because milrinone does not stimulate adrenergic receptors directly, its effects may be additive to those of the catecholamines. Milrinone, however, has the potential to cause hypotension and has a long half-life; in patients with tenuous clinical status, its use is often reserved for situations in which other agents have proven ineffective.[29] Standard administration of milrinone calls for a bolus loading dose of 50 μg/kg followed by an infusion of 0.5 μg/kg/min, but many clinicians eschew the loading dose (or halve it) in patients with marginal blood pressure.

Infusion of inotropic agents can increase myocardial oxygen demand and produce tachyarrhythmias in patients with cardiogenic shock. Invasive hemodynamic monitoring can be extremely useful in allowing optimization of therapy in these unstable patients, because clinical estimates of filling pressure can be unreliable;[44] in addition, changes in myocardial performance and compliance and therapeutic interventions can change cardiac output and filling pressures precipitously. Optimization of filling pressures and serial measurements of cardiac output (and other parameters, such as mixed venous oxygen saturation) allow for titration of the dosage of vasoactive agents to the minimum dosage required to achieve the chosen therapeutic goals.[34]

Intra-aortic balloon counterpulsation (IABP) reduces systolic afterload and augments diastolic perfusion pressure, increasing cardiac output and improving coronary blood flow.[45] These beneficial effects, in contrast to those of inotropic or vasopressor agents, occur without an increase in oxygen demand, and decreased afterload is accomplished without lowering blood pressure. In patients with cardiogenic shock and compromised tissue perfusion, IABP can be an essential support mechanism to stabilize patients and allow time for definitive therapeutic measures to be undertaken.[46,47] Full consideration of IABP therapy can be found in Chapter 5.

Patients with Adequate Tissue Perfusion and Pulmonary Congestion

In patients whose primary abnormality after initial resuscitation from cardiogenic shock is pulmonary congestion but who appear to have adequate tissue perfusion, diuretics may be used. Bolus doses of loop diuretics are usually used, but continuous infusion may be more effective in patients with tenuous hemodynamics.[48] Vasodilators should be used with extreme caution in the acute setting due to the risk of precipitating further hypotension and decreasing coronary blood flow.

After blood pressure has been stabilized, however, vasodilator therapy can decrease both preload and afterload. Sodium nitroprusside is a balanced arterial and venous vasodilator that decreases filling pressures and can increase stroke volume in patients with heart failure by reducing afterload.[49] Nitroglycerin is an effective venodilator that reduces the pulmonary capillary occlusion pressure and can decrease ischemia by reducing LV filling pressure and redistributing coronary blood flow to the ischemic zone.[50] Both agents may cause acute and rapid decreases in blood pressure and dosages must be titrated carefully; invasive hemodynamic monitoring can be useful in optimizing filling pressures when these agents are used.

Conclusions

Expeditious initiation of a focused diagnostic assessment and institution of supportive therapy is the key to achieving a good outcome in the initial management of patients with cardiogenic shock. Measures to maintain blood pressure, oxygenation, and tissue perfusion should be initiated concomitantly with the diagnostic evaluation. Such measures are temporizing, but are vital to reverse the vicious cycle in which myocardial ischemia causes hypotension, which in turn worsens ischemia. Such support is crucial to stabilize the patient and permit the institution of definitive measures aimed at the underlying pathology.

References

1. Hands ME, Rutherford JD, Muller JE, et al. The in-hospital development of cardiogenic shock after myocardial infarction: Incidence, predictors of occurrence, outcome and prognostic factors. The MILIS Study Group. *J Am Coll Cardiol* 1989; 14:40-46.

2. Leor J, Goldbourt U, Reicher-Reiss H, et al. Cardiogenic shock complicating acute myocardial infarction in patients without heart failure on admission: Incidence, risk factors, and outcome. SPRINT Study Group. *Am J Med* 1993; 94:265-273.

3. Hochman JS, Buller CE, Sleeper LA, et al. Cardiogenic shock complicating acute myocardial infarction--etiologies, management and outcome: A report from the SHOCK Trial Registry. SHould we emergently revascularize Occluded Coronaries for cardiogenic shocK? *J Am Coll Cardiol* 2000; 36:1063-1070.

4. Hollenberg SM, Kavinsky CJ, Parrillo JE. Cardiogenic shock. *Ann Intern Med* 1999; 131:47-59.

5. Hollenberg SM, Parrillo JE. Shock. In: Fauci AS, Braunwald E, Isselbacher KJ, et al., eds. Harrison's Principles of Internal Medicine. New York: McGraw-Hill, 1997:214-222.

6. Menon V, White H, LeJemtel T, et al. The clinical profile of patients with suspected cardiogenic shock due to predominant left ventricular failure: A report from the SHOCK Trial Registry. SHould we emergently revascularize Occluded Coronaries in cardiogenic shocK? *J Am Coll Cardiol* 2000; 36:1071-1076.

7. Hochman JS, Boland J, Sleeper LA, et al. Current spectrum of cardiogenic shock and effect of early revascularization on mortality. Results of an International Registry. *Circulation* 1995; 91:873-881.

8. Killip T, Kimball JT. Treatment of myocardial infarction in a coronary care unit. A two year experience with 250 patients. *Am J Cardiol* 1967; 20:457-464.

9. Hasdai D, Holmes DR, Califf RM, et al. Cardiogenic shock complicating acute myocardial infarction: Predictors of death. GUSTO Investigators. Global Utilization of Streptokinase and Tissue-Plasminogen Activator for Occluded Coronary Arteries. *Am Heart J* 1999; 138:21-31.

10. Voci P, Bilotta F, Caretta Q, et al. Papillary muscle perfusion pattern. A hypothesis for ischemic papillary muscle dysfunction. *Circulation* 1995; 91:1714-1718.

11. Khan SS, Gray RJ. Valvular emergencies. *Cardiol Clin* 1991; 9:689-709.

12. Menon V, Webb JG, Hillis LD, et al. Outcome and profile of ventricular septal rupture with cardiogenic shock after myocardial infarction: A report from the SHOCK Trial Registry. SHould we emergently revascularize Occluded Coronaries in cardiogenic shocK? *J Am Coll Cardiol* 2000; 36:1110-1116.

13. Slater J, Brown RJ, Antonelli TA, et al. Cardiogenic shock due to cardiac free-wall rupture or tamponade after acute myocardial infarction: A report from the SHOCK Trial Registry. Should we emergently revascularize occluded coronaries for cardiogenic shock? *J Am Coll Cardiol* 2000; 36:1117-1122.

14. Zehender M, Kasper W, Kauder E, et al. Right ventricular infarction as an independent predictor of prognosis after acute inferior myocardial infarction. *N Engl J Med* 1993; 328:981-988.

15. Dell'Italia LJ, Starling MR, O'Rourke RA. Physical examination for exclusion of hemodynamically important right ventricular infarction. *Ann Intern Med* 1983; 99:608-611.

16. Felker GM, Thompson RE, Hare JM, et al. Underlying causes and long-term survival in patients with initially unexplained cardiomyopathy. *N Engl J Med* 2000; 342:1077-1084.

17. Selzer A. Changing aspects of the natural history of valvular aortic stenosis. *N Engl J Med* 1987; 317:91-98.

18. Bonow RO, Carabello B, de Leon AC, Jr., et al. Guidelines for the management of patients with valvular heart disease: Executive summary. A report of the American College of Cardiology/American Heart Association Task Force on Practice Guidelines (Committee on Management of Patients with Valvular Heart Disease). *Circulation* 1998; 98:1949-1984.

19. Weil MH, Afifi AA. Experimental and clinical studies on lactate and pyruvate as indicators of the severity of acute circulatory failure. *Circulation* 1970; 41:989-1001.

20. Vincent JL, Dufaye P, Berre J. Serial lactate determinations during circulatory shock. *Crit Care Med* 1983; 11:449-451.

21. Ander DS, Jaggi M, Rivers E, et al. Undetected cardiogenic shock in patients with congestive heart failure presenting to the emergency department. *Am J Cardiol* 1998; 82:888-891.

22. Kaul S, Stratienko AA, Pollock SG, et al. Value of two-dimensional echocardiography for determining the basis of hemodynamic compromise in critically ill patients: A prospective study. *J Am Soc Echocardiogr* 1994; 7:598-606.

23. Nishimura RA, Tajik AJ, Shub C, et al. Role of two-dimensional echocardiography in the prediction of in- hospital complications after acute myocardial infarction. *J Am Coll Cardiol* 1984; 4:1080-1087.

24. Ribeiro A, Lindmarker P, Juhlin-Dannfelt A, et al. Echocardiography Doppler in pulmonary embolism: Right ventricular dysfunction as a predictor of mortality rate. *Am Heart J* 1997; 134:479-487.

25. Kasper W, Konstantinides S, Geibel A, et al. Prognostic significance of right ventricular afterload stress detected by echocardiography in patients with clinically suspected pulmonary embolism. *Heart* 1997; 77:346-349.

26. Reilly JP, Tunick PA, Timmermans RJ, et al. Contrast echocardiography clarifies uninterpretable wall motion in intensive care unit patients. *J Am Coll Cardiol* 2000; 35:485-490.

27. Pearson AC, Castello R, Labovitz AJ. Safety and utility of transesophageal echocardiography in the critically ill patient. *Am Heart J* 1990; 119:1083-1089.

28. Forrester JS, Diamond G, Chatterjee K, et al. Medical therapy of acute myocardial infarction by application of hemodynamic subsets. *N Engl J Med* 1976; 295:1356-1362,1404-1413.

29. Califf RM, Bengtson JR. Cardiogenic shock. *N Engl J Med* 1994; 330:1724-1730.

30. Kinch JW, Ryan TJ. Right ventricular infarction. *N Engl J Med* 1994; 330:1211-1217.

31. Task Force of the American College of Critical Care Medicine, Hollenberg SM, Ahrens TS, et al. Practice parameters for hemodynamic support of sepsis in adult patients. *Crit Care Med* 1999; 27:639-660.

32. Connors AF, Jr., McCaffree DR, Gray BA. Evaluation of right-heart catheterization in the critically ill patient without acute myocardial infarction. *N Engl J Med* 1982; 308:263-267.

33. Zion MM, Balkin J, Rosenmann D, et al. Use of pulmonary artery catheters in patients with acute myocardial infarction. Analysis of experience in 5,841 patients in the SPRINT registry. *Chest* 1990; 98:1331-1335.

34. Hollenberg SM, Hoyt JW. Pulmonary artery catheters in cardiovascular disease. *New Horiz* 1997; 5:207-213.

35. Pang D, Keenan SP, Cook DJ, et al. The effect of positive pressure airway support on mortality and the need for intubation in cardiogenic pulmonary edema: A systematic review. *Chest* 1998; 114:1185-1192.

36. Ryan TJ, Anderson JL, Antman EM, et al. ACC/AHA guidelines for the management of patients with acute myocardial infarction. A report of the American College of Cardiology/American Heart Association Task Force on Practice Guidelines. *J Am Coll Cardiol* 1996; 28:1328-1428.

37. Alpert JS, Becker RC. Mechanisms and management of cardiogenic shock. *Crit Care Clin* 1993; 9:205-218.

38. Goldberg LI, Hsieh YY, Resnekov L. Newer catecholamines for treatment of heart failure and shock: An update on dopamine and a first look at dobutamine. *Prog Cardiovasc Dis* 1977; 17:327-340.

39. McGhie AI, Golstein RA. Pathogenesis and management of acute heart failure and cardiogenic shock: Role of inotropic therapy. *Chest* 1992; 102:626S-632S.

40. Richard C, Ricome JL, Rimailho A, et al. Combined hemodynamic effects of dopamine and dobutamine in cardiogenic shock. *Circulation* 1983; 67:620-626.

41. Jaski BE, Fifer MA, Wright RF, et al. Positive inotropic and vasodilator actions of milrinone in patients with severe congestive heart failure. Dose-response relationships and comparison to nitroprusside. *J Clin Invest* 1985; 75:643-649.

42. Bristow MR, Ginsburg R, Minobe W, et al. Decreased catecholamine sensitivity and β-adrenergic-receptor density in failing human hearts. *N Engl J Med* 1982; 307:205-211.

43. Benotti JR, Grossman W, Braunwald E, et al. Effects of amrinone on myocardial energy metabolism and hemodynamics in patients with severe congestive heart failure due to coronary artery disease. *Circulation* 1980; 62:28-34.

44. Hansen RM, Viquerat CE, Matthay MA, et al. Poor correlation between pulmonary arterial wedge pressure and left ventricular end-diastolic volume after coronary aftery bypass graft surgery. *Anesthesiology* 1986; 64:764-770.

45. Willerson JT, Curry GC, Watson JT, et al. Intraaortic balloon counterpulsation in patients in cardiogenic shock, medically refractory left ventricular failure and/or recurrent ventricular tachycardia. *Am J Med* 1975; 58:183-191.

46. Bates ER, Stomel RJ, Hochman JS, et al. The use of intraaortic balloon counterpulsation as an adjunct to reperfusion therapy in cardiogenic shock. *Int J Cardiol* 1998; 65 Suppl 1:S37-42.

47. Sanborn TA, Sleeper LA, Bates ER, et al. Impact of thrombolysis, intra-aortic balloon pump counterpulsation, and their combination in cardiogenic shock complicating acute myocardial infarction: A report from the SHOCK Trial Registry. SHould we emergently revascularize Occluded Coronaries for cardiogenic shocK? *J Am Coll Cardiol* 2000; 36:1123-1129.

48. Dormans TP, van Meyel JJ, Gerlag PG, et al. Diuretic efficacy of high dose furosemide in severe heart failure: Bolus injection versus continuous infusion. *J Am Coll Cardiol* 1996; 28:376-382.

49. Cohn JN, Burke LP. Nitroprusside. *Ann Intern Med* 1979; 91:752-757.

50. Flaherty JT, Becker LC, Bulkley BH, et al. A randomized trial of intravenous nitroglycerin in patients with acute myocardial infarction. *Circulation* 1983; 68:576-588.

Part II.

Management.

Chapter 4

Fibrinolytic Therapy for Cardiogenic Shock Complicating Acute Myocardial Infarction

Eric R. Bates, MD

Fibrinolytic Therapy

Fibrinolytic therapy has been shown to restore infarct artery patency, reduce infarct size, preserve left ventricular (LV) function, and decrease mortality in patients with acute myocardial infarction (MI).[1-4] It represents the first major advance in the field of acute MI since electrical defibrillators were developed and coronary care units were organized in the 1960s. The greatest survival benefit in normotensive patients has been demonstrated in those with the most jeopardized myocardium (e.g., anterior infarction, new left bundle branch block [LBBB]). It would be reasonable to hope that patients with cardiogenic shock, the highest risk subset of patients with acute MI, would have the most to gain from fibrinolytic therapy.

Coronary Thrombosis

Although James Herrick was not the first to describe coronary thrombosis, he is given credit for describing the clinical features of acute MI secondary to sudden obstruction of the coronary artery.[5] Nevertheless, the pathophysiology of acute MI remained controversial until 1980, when DeWood and colleagues[6] demonstrated angiographic occlusion of the infarct artery in 87% of patients with ST segment elevation within 4 hours of symptom onset. Thrombosis was seen in only 65% of patients studied between 12-24 hours because of spontaneous fibrinolysis, explaining the inability of previous autopsy studies to detect thrombus consistently. Moreover, patients were sent directly to coronary artery bypass graft surgery, where intraluminal thrombus was found. Subsequently Chazov et al.[7] and Rentrop et al.[8] demonstrated immediate arteriographic recanalization following intracoronary infusion of streptokinase. Other trials quickly established clinical efficacy, leading first to approval by the United States Food and Drug Administration of intracoronary streptokinase and urokinase and then, in November 1987, to approval of both intravenous streptokinase and alteplase for the acute treatment of acute MI. More recently, pathologic and angioscopic observations have confirmed that fissuring or rupture of a vulnerable atherosclerotic plaque initiates coronary thrombosis and acute MI.[9]

Myocardial Reperfusion

Reimer et al.[10] demonstrated in a dog model that myocardial necrosis following acute coronary artery occlusion occurs over several hours. Myocytes in the sub-endocardium are irreversibly injured first, with a wavefront of cell death moving progressively toward the epicardium. The amount of ischemic muscle at risk for necrosis that becomes irreversibly injured is therefore dependent on the duration of arterial occlusion; conversely, myocardial salvage is dependent on time to reperfusion. Clinical trials have confirmed the concept that "time is muscle." Enzymatically determined infarct size, LV function, and mortality rates are all related to time to reperfusion.[1,2]

The success of any reperfusion strategy depends upon early, complete, sustained infarct artery patency, and restoration of normal coronary artery blood flow and microvascular perfusion. Early patency can salvage ischemic myocardium, preserving LV function. Late patency may not reduce infarct size, but a number of other potential benefits may be realized including limitation of infarct expansion, reduced arrhythmogenicity, improved collateral circulation, better myocardial diastolic function, enhanced efflux of toxic metabolites, faster healing, and decrease in mural thrombus formation.[11] Presumably, these factors explain the mortality reduction seen with fibrinolytic therapy when it is administered in a time frame beyond which myocardial salvage can be expected.

More recently, it has been shown that epicardial coronary artery patency alone is not sufficient to achieve successful reperfusion. Normal microvascular reperfusion has to be restored. This can be documented clinically by rapid resolution of ST segment elevation[12] or angiographically by the TIMI frame count.[13] Failure to achieve microvascular reperfusion is associated with infarct sizes and clinical complications equivalent to those seen with persistently occluded infarct arteries.[14]

Indications and Contraindications for Fibrinolytic Therapy

Patients with ischemic chest pain from 20 minutes to 12 hours in duration not quickly relieved by nitroglycerin are candidates for fibrinolytic therapy if they have ST segment elevation ≥ 1 mm in two contiguous leads or new LBBB and are at low risk for bleeding.[3] An accurate history and ECG interpretation are critically important in excluding patients without acute MI from the bleeding risks of fibrinolytic therapy. In particular, patients with aortic dissection, pericarditis, gastroesophageal reflux disease, and early repolarization changes must be diagnosed correctly. Patients with minor hemorrhage, menstruation, nontraumatic cardiopulmonary resuscitation, or diabetic retinopathy can be treated.

Treating certain subgroups has been somewhat controversial. Although age is the most important predictor of mortality, and almost half of all deaths occur in those over 75 years of age, fewer candidates in this subgroup are treated.[15] Presumably this is due to concern about increasing hemorrhagic risk. Nevertheless, data from the Fibrinolytic Therapy Trialists (FTT) Collaborative Group overview support a mortality reduction in appropriate candidates.[1,15] In general, patients with inferior acute MI have a lower risk for death than patients with anterior acute MI. However, those with reciprocal precordial ST segment depression, right ventricular involvement, or third degree atrioventricular block are high risk and should be aggressively treated.[16] Patients without these findings may have myocardial salvage even if they do not have a survival advantage with treatment. Finally, patients who present late may benefit from treatment if they have ongoing chest pain and a persistent ECG injury current.[17] Resolution of chest pain and ECG changes suggest either spontaneous reperfusion or completion of the infarction.

Contraindications for fibrinolytic therapy are listed in Table 1.[3] They relate mostly to situations where bleeding risk is increased. Fibrinolytic therapy is contraindicated in patients with only ST segment depression, except those with acute posterior MI.

Complications

The major complication of fibrinolytic therapy is bleeding. Noncerebral bleeding has been defined as severe if it results in hemodynamic compromise requiring intervention, or moderate if transfusion is required without hemodynamic compromise. The most common cause of bleeding is cardiac catheterization. In the GUSTO-I trial,[18] 1% of patients had severe bleeding and 12% had moderate bleeding. Advanced age, lighter body weight, and female gender were associated with increased bleeding. Bleeding and transfusion rates are at least halved in studies where arterial puncture is not performed.

Intracerebral hemorrhage occurs in 0.5% to 1.0% of patients.[19] Excessive heparin anticoagulation probably contributes to some of these events. Others may be secondary to dose administration errors, which may be reduced with bolus fibrinolytic therapy. Over half of these patients die and are included in the mortality statistics. Some of this risk is balanced by a decreased incidence of embolic stroke from LV mural thrombus in these patients.

Infarct artery reocclusion is highest in the first 24 hours, occurs in 10% of patients during the hospitalization, and may occur in 30% by 3

Table 1.

Contraindications and Cautions for Thrombolytic Use in Myocardial Infarction[3]

Contraindications
- Previous hemorrhagic stroke at any time; other strokes or cerebrovascular events within 1 year
- Known intracranial neoplasm
- Active internal bleeding (does not include menses)
- Suspected aortic dissection

Cautions/relative contraindications
- Severe uncontrolled hypertension on presentation (blood pressure > 180/110 mm Hg)
- History of prior cerebrovascular accident or known intracerebral pathology not covered in contraindications
- Current use of anticoagulants in therapeutic doses (INR ≥ 2-3); known bleeding diathesis
- Recent trauma (within 2-4 weeks), including head trauma or traumatic or prolonged (> 10 min) CPR or major surgery (< 3 weeks)
- Noncompressible vascular punctures
- Recent (within 2-4 weeks) internal bleeding
- For streptokinase/anistreplase: prior exposure (especially within 5 d-2 y) or prior allergic reaction
- Pregnancy
- Active peptic ulcer
- History of chronic severe hypertension

months.[20,21] This event is unpredictable by any clinical criteria and negates any possible benefit from fibrinolytic therapy on LV salvage or clinical endpoints.

Fibrinolytic Agents

Five fibrinolytic agents have been approved for intravenous use in the United States to treat acute MI. Fibrin specific agents (alteplase, reteplase, tenecteplase) result in higher reperfusion rates, but also in increased risk for hemorrhagic stroke. Bolus injection agents (reteplase, tenecteplase) are easier to administer and are associated with lower dose error rates.

Streptokinase. Tillet and Garner[22] discovered in 1933 that a filtrate of beta-hemolytic strains of streptococcus could dissolve human thrombus. Streptokinase is a single-chain nonenzyme protein which forms a 1:1 stoichiometric complex with plasminogen. The streptokinase-plasminogen activator complex then converts plasminogen to plasmin, which initiates fibrinolysis. Intravenous streptokinase was initially used in the late 1950s for acute MI[23] and was tested in several multicenter trials in the 1960s and 1970s.[24] Unfortunately, improvement in LV function and mor-

Table 2.

Dosages of Fibrinolytic Agents		
Streptokinase (SK)	1.5 million units over 60 minutes	
Anistreplase (APSAC)	30 units over 5 minutes	
Alteplase (rt-PA)	15 mg bolus, 0.75 mg/kg over 30 minutes up to 50 mg, 0.5 mg/kg over 60 minutes up to 35 mg.	
Reteplase (r-PA)	10 MU bolus x 2, 30 minutes apart	
Tenecteplase (TNK-t-PA)	Weight adjusted	
	< 60 kg	30 mg bolus
	≥ 60-70 kg	35 mg bolus
	≥ 70-80 kg	40 mg bolus
	≥ 80-90 kg	45 mg bolus
	> 90 kg	50 mg bolus

tality were inconsistently found because of inadequate doses and late implementation of therapy. The conventional dose (Table 2) was derived empirically by Schroeder and colleagues.[25] Sixty- and 90-minute patency rates are approximately 60% and 2- to 3-hour patency rates are 70%.[26] When compared with placebo, streptokinase reduced mortality in both the GISSI-1 trial[27] (13% vs. 10.7%) and the ISIS-II trial[28] (12% vs. 9.2%).

Anistreplase (APSAC). Anistreplase (anisoylated plasminogen strepto-kinase activator complex) is a stoichiometric combination of streptokinase and human lys-plasminogen. The anisoyl group reversibly bound to the catalytic center of the plasminogen moiety slowly undergoes deacylation prior to direct plasminogen activation. The delayed onset of action permits the agent to be administered over a few minutes. Patency rates are equivalent to those seen with a 3-hour alteplase dose, with a 90-minute patency rate of 70%.[26] The APSAC Intervention Mortality Study[29] (AIMS) was stopped prematurely after 1258 patients were randomized to anistreplase or placebo because of a 47% mortality reduction (6.4% vs. 12.1%).

Alteplase (rt-PA). Tissue plasminogen activator (t-PA) is a naturally occurring single chain serine protease normally secreted by vascular endo-thelium. It was first obtained from the Bowes melanoma cell line and is now produced by recombinant DNA techniques. Native t-PA and alteplase (rt-PA) have a binding site for fibrin, which causes a great affinity for attaching to thrombus and preferentially lysing it, although systemic plasminogen activation occurs at clinical doses.

Neuhaus and colleagues[30] developed the weight-adjusted front-loaded dosing strategy (Table 2) which has proven superior to the 3-hour infusion or the double bolus regimen. Sixty-minute patency rates are approximately 74%, with 90-minutes and 2- to 3-hour patency rates at about 85%.[26] The ASSET trial[31] and the LATE trial[17] demonstrated significant mortality reduction with alteplase versus placebo when symptom duration was less than 6 hours (7.2% vs. 9.8%) or 6-12 hours (8.9% vs. 12%), respectively. Superior infarct artery patency and flow rates were shown for alteplase compared with streptokinase in the GUSTO-I trial,[32,33] which resulted in a lower mortality rate with alteplase.

Reteplase (r-PA). Recombinant plasminogen activator is a non-glycosylated deletion mutant of wild-type t-PA, expressed in *Escherichia coli*. It is created by deleting the finger, epidermal growth factor, and kringle-1 domains from the alteplase molecule. These modifications decrease fibrin specificity and prolong the half-life of the agent. In the RAPID-I and RAPID-II trials,[34,35] patency and flow rates were higher for reteplase than alteplase, but in the GUSTO-III trial,[36] the mortality and stroke outcomes were equivalent. The major advantage of this agent is the double bolus administration, which obviates the need for the infusion pump and dose adjustment needed with alteplase.

Tenecteplase (TNK-t-PA). Tenecteplase is a triple-combination mutant of the wild-type t-PA molecule with amino acid substitutions at three sites. Threonine (T) is replaced by an asparagine at position 103, creating a new glycosylation site. An asparagine (N) at position 117 is replaced by glutamine, removing a glycosylation site. Finally, four amino acids [lysine, histadine, and two arginines (K)] at positions 296-299 are replaced by four alanine residues. The substitutions lead to a prolonged half-life, increased fibrin specificity, and increased resistance to inhibition by plasminogen activator inhibitor-1 (PAI-1). Unlike reteplase, which is given in two fixed dose boluses, tenecteplase is administered as a weight adjusted single bolus. In the ASSENT-2 trial,[37] mortality and stroke rates were equivalent between alteplase and tenecteplase.

Facilitated Fibrinolysis

Preliminary studies have suggested that more potent antithrombin therapy with low molecular weight heparin[38] or direct thrombin inhibitors,[39] or more potent antiplatelet therapy with a glycoprotein IIb/IIIa[40,41] receptor antagonist might improve outcomes with fibrinolytic therapy. Equivalent safety and superior reductions in morbidity and mortality will have to be demonstrated before new strategies can replace traditional fibrinolytic therapy.

Adjunctive Therapy

Adjunctive drug therapy is required (Table 3).[3] First, aspirin should be given immediately and continued indefinitely on a daily basis. The reduction in mortality by 20% in the ISIS-II trial[28] was equivalent to that seen with streptokinase, and the effect was additive to streptokinase. Second, unfractionated heparin adjusted to maintain an activated partial thrombin time of 1.5-2.0 times control should be given for 48 hours in patients undergoing fibrinolytic therapy with alteplase, reteplase, or ten-

Table 3.

Adjunctive Drug Therapy	
• ASA 160-325 mg po qd	
• Beta adrenergic blockers	
1. Atenolol	5 mg IV x 2 over 10 min; 50 mg po 10 minutes later; then 50-100 mg po daily.
2. Metoprolol	5 mg IV x 3 over 15 min; 50 mg po 10 minutes later; then 50-100 mg po twice daily.
• Heparin	
1. Alteplase, reteplase, tenecteplase	60 U/kg bolus (maximum 4000 U) 12 U/kg infusion (maximum 1000 U/hr). aPTT 50-70 sec for 48 hours.
2. Streptokinase	Withhold for at least 6 hrs until aPTT < 70 sec. Treat only those at high risk for systemic emboli (large or anterior MI, atrial fibrillation, previous embolus, or LV thrombus).
• ACE Inhibitor	Captopril 12.5-50 mg po thrice daily. Enalapril 2.5-10 mg po twice daily.
• Nitroglycerin	10-200 mcg/min infusion.

ecteplase. Patients treated with the nonselective agents streptokinase or APSAC should not be treated for at least 6 hours because the early massive production of fibrin split products produces systemic anticoagulation. Heparin can be started after the activated partial thrombin time has fallen below 70 seconds in high risk patients. Third, beta-blocker therapy should be started in patients without bradycardia, heart block, hypotension, congestive heart failure, or bronchospasm. Finally, ACE inhibitor therapy should be given within 24 hours to patients with anterior acute MI or congestive heart failure in the absence of hypotension. Additionally, nitroglycerin can be infused to reduce ischemic chest pain and control blood pressure. Calcium channel blockers, magnesium, and routine lidocaine are not recommended.

Cardiogenic Shock

Development of Cardiogenic Shock After Fibrinolytic Therapy

Cardiogenic shock, not arrhythmia, is the most common cause of death in patients hospitalized with acute MI. Unfortunately, neither the incidence nor the mortality rate associated with cardiogenic shock has been reduced by modern cardiac intensive care interventions, including vasopressor and inotropic drug infusions, hemodynamic monitoring, and intra-aortic balloon counterpulsation or pumping (IABP).[42]

Cardiogenic shock usually develops insidiously over several hours; only a minority of patients present to the emergency department in hemodynamic collapse. Therefore, successful reperfusion potentially could reduce the incidence of cardiogenic shock in high risk patients by restoring blood flow to ischemic but still viable myocardium. Predictors for subsequent development of cardiogenic shock include age > 65 years, LV ejection fraction < 35%, large infarct size estimated by ECG or enzyme criteria, diabetes mellitus, and history of prior acute MI.[43]

Three controlled trials have demonstrated a reduction in the incidence of cardiogenic shock in patients treated with fibrinolytic therapy. In the APSAC Multicenter trial,[44] 313 patients with symptom duration < 4 hours were randomized to either heparin or APSAC. In those who survived for at least 24 hours, APSAC reduced the incidence of cardiogenic shock from 9.5% to 3.2% (p = 0.03). The AIMS was a double-blind, placebo-controlled trial which enrolled 1258 patients. In-hospital cardiogenic shock rates were 4.6% in the placebo group and 2.6% in the APSAC group (p = 0.07).[45] Finally, the Anglo-Scandinavian Study of Early Thrombolysis (ASSET) trial[31] randomized 5011 patients with symptom duration < 5 hours to a 3-hour infusion of alteplase or placebo. Alteplase reduced the incidence of shock from 5.1% to 3.8% (p < 0.05).

Several comparative fibrinolytic trials have shown no mortality difference between treatment groups and, interestingly, no difference in the incidence of cardiogenic shock. The GISSI-2/International trial[46] was a more than 8000 patient extension of the GISSI-2[47] trial to provide adequate statistical power for detecting differences in mortality. A total of 20,891 patients were randomized to streptokinase or a 3-hour infusion of alteplase within 6 hours of symptom onset. Cardiogenic shock developed in 5.9% and 5.6% of the patients, respectively. The ISIS-3 study[48] randomized 41,299 patients to streptokinase, APSAC, or a 4-hour duteplase infusion within 24 hours of symptom onset. The respective incidences of cardiogenic shock were 7.1%, 7.1%, and 6.7%. The GUSTO-III trial[36] randomized 15,059 patients within 6 hours of the onset of symptoms to reteplase or front-loaded alteplase. Cardiogenic shock occurred in 4.6% of patients treated with reteplase and 4.4% of patients treated with alteplase. Finally, the ASSENT-2 trial[37] compared tenecteplase versus front loaded alteplase in 16,949 patients within less than 6 hours of onset of symptoms. Cardiogenic shock occurred, respectively, in 3.9% and 4.0% of patients.

Conversely, several comparative fibrinolytic trials have shown a superior mortality benefit for one agent and a corresponding reduction in the incidence of cardiogenic shock. In the rt-PA-APSAC Patency Study (TAPS),[49] cardiogenic shock developed less frequently with front-loaded alteplase (1.9%) than with APSAC (8.1%). The GUSTO-I trial[32] enrolled 41,021 patients within 6 hours of symptom onset. Cardiogenic shock occurred less often (p < 0.001) with front-loaded alteplase (5.1%), than with streptokinase and intravenous heparin (6.3%), streptokinase and subcutaneous heparin (6.9%), or a combination of alteplase and streptokinase (6.1%). The INJECT trial[50] randomized 6010 patients to double bolus reteplase or streptokinase. Patients treated with reteplase had significantly lower rates of cardiogenic shock (4.7% vs. 6.0%; p < 0.05).

In summary, fibrinolytic therapy appears to decrease the risk of developing cardiogenic shock after acute MI, and the treatment strategies with the highest patency rates are associated with the lowest rates of both cardiogenic shock and mortality.

Treatment Results with Fibrinolytic Therapy for Patients with Hypotension

Several studies that did not document the presence of cardiogenic shock did classify patients by baseline blood pressure. There were 631 patients in the ISIS-2 study[28] with systolic blood pressure < 100 mm Hg who were treated with either streptokinase or placebo. Those treated with streptokinase had a lower 5-week vascular mortality rate (27.3% vs. 35.0%).

AIMS[45] treated half of the patients with APSAC and enrolled 125 patients with systolic blood pressure < 100 mm Hg. Again, a survival advantage for those treated with fibrinolysis was seen at 30 days (15% vs. 23%) and at 1 year (15% vs. 32%).

The FTT Collaborative Group[1] pooled results from nine controlled fibrinolytic trials enrolling more than 1000 patients with suspected MI. In 2,466 patients with systolic blood pressure < 100 mm Hg, fibrinolytic therapy reduced 35-day mortality from 35.1% to 28.9% (2p < 0.01). This represented a savings of 62 lives per 1000 patients treated, compared with the 19 lives saved per 1000 patients treated in those with systolic blood pressure 100-149 mm Hg. Thus, it is evident that hypotension conveys an increased mortality risk, but not as high as the mortality risk associated with cardiogenic shock. Additionally, mortality reduction with fibrinolytic therapy is much more impressive in hypotensive patients than in those with cardiogenic shock.

Use of Fibrinolytic Therapy for Cardiogenic Shock

The Worcester Heart Attack Study[51] is an observational longitudinal study of 9076 patients hospitalized with acute MI in metropolitan Worcester, MA during eleven 1-year periods between 1975 and 1997. In the five periods since 1990, while fibrinolytic therapy was administered to 20%-25% of patients without cardiogenic shock, it was given to 20%-33% of patients with cardiogenic shock.

The second National Registry of Myocardial Infarction (NRMI-2) documented outcomes in 426,253 patients in 1662 United States hospitals between 1994 and 1997.[52] Patients with cardiogenic shock (n = 26,280) were equally likely to be treated with fibrinolytic therapy (19%) as those without cardiogenic shock.

The SHOCK Registry[53] enrolled 856 patients between 1993 and 1998 from 36 centers participating in a randomized trial of cardiogenic shock. Fibrinolytic therapy was given to 34%. In the randomized SHOCK trial[54] (n = 302), 94% of patients were eligible for fibrinolytic therapy and 56% received it.

Unfortunately, the multicenter registries do not distinguish between patients with cardiogenic shock on presentation and those who develop cardiogenic shock after hospital admission. Additionally, the treatment frequencies from the SHOCK investigators are higher than routine community use because of the treatment bias of these physicians interested in aggressively treating patients with this diagnosis. Therefore, precisely how many patients with cardiogenic shock, either on presentation or after admission, are currently being treated with fibrinolytic therapy is unknown.

Treatment Results With Fibrinolytic Therapy

Intracoronary streptokinase. Mathey et al.[55] were the first investigators to report successful fibrinolysis in patients with cardiogenic shock. They infused streptokinase at a rate of 2,000 U/min for a mean duration of 29 ± 15 minutes in six patients. Reperfusion was successful in three patients and all three survived.

The Society for Cardiac Angiography subsequently enrolled 1029 patients from 35 laboratories in an intracoronary streptokinase registry between July, 1981 and August, 1984.[56] The overall reperfusion rate was 71% and the hospitality mortality rate was 8.2%. An average of 235,000 ± 102,000 U of streptokinase was infused over 57 ± 23 minutes. Successful reperfusion was associated with an in-hospital mortality rate of 5.5% versus 14.7% when reperfusion was unsuccessful. In 44 patients with cardiogenic shock, the mortality rate was 66%, but patency was achieved in only 44%. In the 19 patients with successful reperfusion, the mortality rate was 42%; in 25 patients in whom reperfusion was unsuccessful, the mortality rate was 84% (p < 0.0001).

Randomized trial results. Most trials of fibrinolytic therapy excluded patients with cardiogenic shock. In an analysis of 94 trials involving 81,005 patients, only three reported subset data on cardiogenic shock.[57]

The first placebo-controlled, randomized trial of intravenous fibrinolytic therapy that demonstrated clear therapeutic efficacy was the GISSI-1 trial.[27] A total of 11,806 patients received either intravenous streptokinase or placebo, with 280 patients classified as Killip Class 4 on admission. Overall, 21-day mortality was reduced by 18% in patients receiving streptokinase (10.7% vs. 13%, p = 0.002). However, there was no reduction in mortality in Killip Class IV patients (69.9% vs. 70.1%). Other subset analyses in the study showing no treatment benefit in patients with nonanterior acute MI, age > 65 years, and treatment > 6 hours after onset of symptoms were subsequently refuted by larger studies.

The GISSI-2/International Study Group[46] compared streptokinase with a 3-hour infusion of alteplase. A total of 173 patients were Killip Class IV on admission. Mortality rates were high for both groups (65% vs. 78%), but they were worse with alteplase.

In the GUSTO-1 study,[58] streptokinase was compared with a 90-minute infusion of alteplase. Mortality rates for patients with cardiogenic shock were lower than in previous studies (56% vs. 59%), but the interpretation of the data is limited by the fact that 19% of patients underwent balloon angioplasty and 24% had intra-aortic balloon pump counterpulsation.

It is interesting to note that in both the GISSI-2/International trial[46] and the GUSTO-1 trial,[58] patients with cardiogenic shock treated with streptokinase fared better than patients treated with alteplase, despite the fact that alteplase has been shown to be the superior fibrinolytic agent. Possible explanations for this observation include a prolonged lytic state with streptokinase in a setting of low coronary blood flow, which might reduce the risk of reocclusion, and greater thrombus penetration by a less fibrin-specific agent because of less binding on the surface of the thrombus.

Other results. The FTT overview[1] did not detail patients by Killip class, but did describe patients with both a systolic blood pressure < 100 mm Hg and a heart rate > 100 beats/min. Fibrinolytic therapy reduced mortality from 61.1% to 53.8%.

The SHOCK Registry[59] evaluated 856 patients with cardiogenic shock regarding fibrinolytic therapy utilization. Patients treated with fibrinolytic therapy had a lower in-hospital mortality rate than those who did not receive fibrinolytic therapy (54% vs. 64%, p = 0.005), even after adjustment for age and revascularization status (odds ratio 0.70, p = 0.027). This result is in conflict with the randomized clinical trial data where no clear benefit was seen. Although the much larger sample size may explain the results, it is also possible that baseline differences resulted in treatment differences.

The results of these trials do not support an obvious treatment benefit for fibrinolytic therapy in patients with cardiogenic shock. The explanation for this lack of efficacy appears to be the low reperfusion rate achieved in this subset of patients.

Reperfusion Failure with Fibrinolytic Therapy

As mentioned above, Kennedy et al.[56] initially reported on the low patency rate and high mortality rate seen with intracoronary streptokinase therapy in patients with cardiogenic shock. Similarly, Bengston and colleagues[60] noted a patency rate of only 48% after intravenous thrombolytic therapy in 69 patients with cardiogenic shock.

The primary defect in cardiogenic shock is impaired myocardial contractility and low cardiac output. This results in systemic hypotension and elevation of LV filling pressures. The resultant decrease in coronary perfusion pressure and myocardial perfusion further decreases myocardial contractility and perpetuates the vicious cycle of mechanical and neurohormonal events that lead to progressive cardiogenic shock and death.

Becker[61] summarized possible hemodynamic, mechanical, and metabolic explanations for the limitations of fibrinolytic therapy in cardiogenic shock. Coronary blood flow decreases when mean arterial pressure falls below 65 mm Hg and ceases when mean arterial pressure falls below 30 mm Hg. The combination of both low coronary blood flow and reduced coronary perfusion pressure decreases both the delivery of the fibrinolytic agent to the thrombus and the penetration of the agent into the thrombus. Vasoconstriction and passive collapse of the arterial wall are mechanical factors that may further reduce coronary blood flow and fibrinolytic drug delivery in a low perfusion state. Finally, acidosis may decrease the conversion of plasminogen to plasmin or even dissociate the plasminogen–streptokinase complex, impairing fibrinolytic efficacy.

Prewitt and coworkers[62] tested the influence of aortic blood pressure on the rate and extent of coronary fibrinolysis in a canine model. Coronary thrombosis was induced by injection of a radioactive thrombus through a catheter placed in the left anterior descending artery. Phlebotomy was performed to adjust the systolic blood pressure to either 130 mm Hg or 75 mm Hg. Intracoronary alteplase was infused for 30 minutes and a gamma camera was used to measure the rate and extent of thrombus dissolution. Both were decreased in the hypotensive dogs. Infusing norepinephrine to restore the systemic pressure to 130 mm Hg in the hypotensive dogs normalized the rate and extent of fibrinolysis. In a similar experiment,[63] increasing diastolic blood pressure and peak diastolic blood flow with IABP enhanced clot lysis in hypotensive dogs. Postulated mechanisms included enhanced delivery of alteplase to the thrombus and mechanical fragmentation of the thrombus providing a greater surface area for alteplase binding and fibrinolysis. Since cardiac output did not change significantly in these experiments, blood pressure appeared to be the important variable.[64]

Other factors besides failure to reperfuse the infarct artery or microvasculature contribute to the high mortality rate in cardiogenic shock. These include extensive myocardial necrosis, infarct expansion or aneurysm formation, ventricular dilation, persistent metabolic acidosis, increased preload and afterload, infarct extension, infarct artery reocclusion, and metabolic fatigue of noninfarct zones.[64]

Adjunctive Intra-aortic Balloon Pump Counterpulsation

Intra-aortic balloon pump counterpulsation in cardiogenic shock can stabilize patients hemodynamically, but in the absence of myocardial reperfusion, it does not reduce mortality. Since poor reperfusion rates with fibrinolytic therapy appear to be due to reduced coronary blood flow and perfusion pressure, the addition of IABP counterpulsation should be beneficial, as suggested by the Prewitt experiments.[62,63] On average, IABP counterpulsation results in a 10% to 40% increase in cardiac output, a 70% increase in diastolic blood pressure, and a significant increase in coronary blood flow velocity in critically ill patients.[64]

Stomel et al.[65] retrospectively analyzed 64 patients with cardiogenic shock treated at a community hospital with either fibrinolysis alone, IABP counterpulsation alone, or both. There were 36 patients who did not undergo subsequent revascularization. Only 2 of 26 (8%) of these patients treated with either fibrinolysis or balloon counterpulsation alone survived, compared with 4 of 10 (40%) patients treated with both interventions.

The GUSTO-I trial[66] enrolled 315 patients with cardiogenic shock and treated them with fibrinolytic therapy. Intraaortic balloon pump counterpulsation was used early in 62 patients. These patients had a strong trend toward improved 30-day and 1-year mortality.

The second National Registry of Myocardial Infarction (NRMI-2)[67] identified 21,718 patients with acute MI who presented with or developed in-hospital cardiogenic shock. Thirty-two percent (6992) received IABP counterpulsation. When patients treated with fibrinolytic therapy were analyzed, those also treated with IABP counterpulsation had a significantly lower mortality rate than those who were not treated (49% vs. 69%, p < 0.001).

The SHOCK Trial Registry[59] also examined the potential benefit of combining IABP counterpulsation with fibrinolytic therapy. Compared with fibrinolytic therapy alone (n = 132), such patients (n = 160) had a lower mortality rate (47% vs. 63%, p = 0.007).

The Thrombolysis and Counterpulsation to Improve Cardiogenic Shock Survival (TACTICS) trial[68] was stopped prematurely because of poor patient recruitment after only 57 patients had been enrolled. It was the first attempt at a prospective randomized trial on this subject. There was a statistically insignificant trend toward a survival advantage consistent with the magnitude of benefit shown in the previous retrospective studies.

Hudson and colleagues[69] analyzed 3500 patients with cardiogenic shock enrolled in the GUSTO-1 and GUSTO-3 studies. IABP counterpulsation use was associated with improved 30-day survival (45% vs. 58%; p = 0.001).

Unfortunately, most of these studies are confounded by selection bias for IABP counterpulsation and some are confounded by the use of PTCA. For instance, in the SHOCK Registry,[59] 68% of patients treated with IABP and fibrinolytic therapy underwent revascularization with PTCA or CABG versus only 20% in the fibrinolysis only group. Thus, it remains to be proven that this strategy has clinical efficacy, although it makes theoretical sense.

Adjunctive Revascularization

Most trials evaluating revascularization in cardiogenic shock have retrospectively compared PTCA to no PTCA therapy in patients who usually did not get fibrinolytic therapy. Only the GUSTO-I trial evaluated this question in patients who had previously received fibrinolytic therapy.[58,70,71] In the initial report,[58] shock occurred in 2972 patients (7.2%): 315 (11%) had shock on arrival and 2657 (89%) developed shock after hospital admission. Angioplasty was performed in only 22% of patients, and reduced the 30-day mortality in patients with shock on admission

(43% vs. 61%; p = 0.028) and in patients who developed shock after hospital admission (32% vs. 61%; p < 0.001).

To avoid the bias associated with including patients who die before PTCA could be performed, an additional analysis focused on 2200 patients who survived for 1 hour after the onset of shock.[70] Mortality at 30 days was lower in the 406 patients who underwent early cardiac catheterization compared with the 1794 patients who did not get the diagnostic test (38% vs. 62%). Early PTCA was performed in 197 patients and was successful in 148. Thirty-day mortality was lower in those with successful PTCA (35% vs. 55% when PTCA was unsuccessful). A subsequent report from this trial evaluated 1321 30-day survivors of cardiogenic shock, 88% of whom survived to 1 year.[71] Data were available on 578 patients who had undergone revascularization (PTCA or CABG) within 30 days and 728 patients who had not. After adjustment of baseline differences, revascularization was associated with reduced 1-year mortality (odds ratio 0.6; p = 0.007).

Conclusion

Mortality from cardiogenic shock remains frustratingly high. Although fibrinolytic therapy decreases mortality and morbidity in most subgroups of patients with MI, it does not appear to have a significant benefit in patients who have already developed cardiogenic shock, probably because of hypotension and low reperfusion rates. Attempts to increase reperfusion rates by increasing blood pressure with aggressive inotropic and pressor therapy and intra-aortic balloon counterpulsation are logical, but have not been adequately tested. To date, emergency revascularization is the only intervention that has been shown to consistently reduce mortality rates in patients with cardiogenic shock.

References

1. Fibrinolyic Therapy Trialists' (FTT) Collaborative Group. Indications for fibrinolytic therapy in suspected acute myocardial infarction: Collaborative overview of early mortality and major morbidity results from all randomized trials of more than 1000 patients. *Lancet* 1994; 343:311-322.
2. White HD, Van de Werf FJJ. Thrombolysis for acute myocardial infarction. *Circulation* 1998; 97:1632-1646.
3. Ryan TJ, Anderson JL, Antman EM, et al. ACC/AHA guidelines for the management of patient with acute myocardial infarction. *J Am Coll Cardiol* 1996; 28:1328-1428.
4. Ryan TJ, Antman EM, Brooks NH, et al. 1999 update: ACC/AHA guidelines for the management of patients with acute myocardial infarction. *Circulation* 1999; 100:1016-1030.
5. Herrick JB. Clinical features of sudden obstruction of the coronary arteries. *JAMA* 1912; 59:2015-2020.
6. DeWood MA, Spores J, Notske R, et al. Prevalence of total coronary occlusion during the early hours of transmural infarction. *N Engl J Med* 1980; 303:897-902.

7. Chazov EI, Mateeva LS, Mazaev AV, et al. Intracoronary administration of fibrinolysis in acute myocardial infarction. *Ter Arkh* 1976; 48:8-19.

8. Rentrop KT, Blanke H, Karsch KR, et al. Acute myocardial infarction: Intracoronary application of nitroglycerine and streptokinase. *Clin Cardiol* 1979; 2:354-363.

9. Falk E, Shah PK, Fuster V. Coronary plaque disruption. *Circulation* 1995; 92:1565-1569.

10. Reimer KA, Lowe JE, Rasmussen MM, Jennings RB. The wave-front phenomenon of ischemic death. I. Myocardial infarct size vs duration of coronary occlusion in dogs. *Circulation* 1977; 56:786-794.

11. Kim CB, Braunwald E. Potential benefits of late reperfusion of infarcted myocardium. The open artery hypothesis. *Circulation* 1993; 88:2426-2436.

12. Schröder R, Dissmann R, Bruggemann T, et al. Extent of early ST segment elevation resolution: A simple but strong predictor of outcome in patients with acute myocardial infarction. *J Am Coll Cardiol* 1994; 24:384-391.

13. Gibson CM, Murphy SA, Rizo MJ, et al. Relationship between TIMI frame count and clinical outcomes after thrombolytic administration. *Circulation* 1999; 99:1945-1950.

14. Roe MT, Ohman EM, Maas AC, et al. Shifting the open-artery hypothesis downstream: The quest for optimal reperfusion. *J Am Coll Cardiol* 2001; 37:9-18.

15. White HD. Thrombolytic therapy in the elderly. *Lancet* 2000; 356:2028-2030.

16. Bates ER. Revisiting reperfusion therapy in inferior myocardial infarction. *J Am Coll Cardiol* 1997; 30:334-342

17. LATE Study Group. Late Assessment of Thrombolytic Efficacy (LATE) study with alteplase 6-12 hours after onset of acute myocardial infarction. *Lancet* 1993; 342:759-766.

18. Berkowitz SD, Granger CB, Pieper KS, et al. Incidence and predictors of bleeding after contemporary thrombolytic therapy for myocardial infarction. *Circulation* 1997; 95:2508-2516.

19. Gore JM, Granger CB, Simoons ML, et al. Stroke after thrombolysis. Mortality and functional outcomes in the GUSTO-I trial. *Circulation* 1995; 92:2811-2818.

20. Ohman EM, Califf RM, Topol EJ, et al. Consequences of reocclusion after successful reperfusion therapy in acute myocardial infarction. TAMI Study Group. *Circulation* 1990; 82:781-791.

21. Meijer A, Verheugt FW, Werter CJ, et al. Aspirin versus coumadin in the prevention of reocclusion and recurrent ischemia after successful thrombolysis: A prospective placebo-controlled angiographic study. APRICOT Study. *Circulation* 1993; 87:1524-1530.

22. Tillet WS, Garner RI. The fibrinolytic activity of hemolytic streptococci. *J Exp Med* 1933; 58:485-502.

23. Fletcher AP, Alkjaersig N, Smyrniotis FE, et al. The treatment of patients suffering from early myocardial infarction with massive and prolonged streptokinase therapy. *Trans Assoc Am Physicians* 1958; 71:287-296.

24. Yusuf S, Collins R, Peto R, et al. Intravenous and intracoronary fibrinolytic therapy in acute myocardial infarction: Overview of results on mortality, reinfarction and side-effects from 33 randomized controlled trials. *Eur Heart J* 1985; 6:556-585.

25. Schröder R, Biamino G, von Leitner ER, et al. Intravenous short-term infusion of streptokinase in acute myocardial infarction. *Circulation* 1983; 67:536-548.

26. Granger CB, White H, Bates ER, et al. Patency profiles and left ventricular function after intravenous thrombolysis: A pooled analysis. *Am J Cardiol* 1994; 74:1220-1228.

27. Gruppo Italiano per lo Studio della Streptokinasi nell'Infarto Miocardico. Effectiveness of intravenous thrombolytic treatment in acute myocardial infarction. *Lancet* 1986; 1:397-401.

28. Second International Study of Infarct Survival Collaborative Group. Randomized trial of intravenous streptokinase, oral aspirin, both, or neither among 17,187 cases of suspected acute myocardial infarction. ISIS-2. *Lancet* 1988; 2:349-360.

29. AIMS Trial Study Group. Effect of intravenous APSAC on mortality after acute myocardial infarction: Preliminary report of a placebo-controlled clinical trial. *Lancet* 1988; 1:545-549.

30. Neuhaus K-L, Feuerer W, Jeep-Tebbe S, et al. Improved thrombolysis with a modified dose regimen of recombinant tissue-type plasminogen activator. *J Am Coll Cardiol* 1989; 14:1556-1559.

31. Wilcox RG, von der Lippe G, Olsson CG, et al. Trial of tissue plasminogen activator for mortality reduction in acute myocardial infarction: Anglo-Scandinavian Study of Early Thrombolysis (ASSET). *Lancet* 1988; 1:525-530.

32. The GUSTO Investigators. An international randomized trial comparing four thrombolytic strategies for acute myocardial infarction. *N Engl J Med* 1993; 329:673-682.

33. The GUSTO Angiographic Investigators. The effects of tissue plasminogen activator, streptokinase, or both on coronary artery patency, ventricular function, and survival after acute myocardial infarction. *N Engl J Med* 1993; 329:1615-1622.

34. Smalling RW, Bode C, Kalbfleisch J, et al. More rapid, complete, and stable coronary thrombolysis with bolus administration of reteplase compared with alteplase infusion in acute myocardial infarction. *Circulation* 1995; 91:2725-2732.

35. Bode C, Smalling RW, Berg G, et al. Randomized comparison of coronary thrombolysis achieved with double-bolus reteplase (recombinant plasminogen activator) and front-loaded, accelerated alteplase (recombinant tissue plasminogen activator) in patients with acute myocardial infarction. *Circulation* 1996; 94:891-898.

36. The GUSTO-III Investigators. A comparison of reteplase with alteplase for acute myocardial infarction. *N Engl J Med* 1997; 337:1118-1123.

37. ASSENT-2 Investigators. Single-bolus tenecteplase compared with frontloaded alteplase in acute myocardial infarction: The ASSENT-2 double-blind randomised trial. *Lancet* 1999; 354:716-722.

38. Ross AM, Molhoek P, Lundergan C, et al. Randomised comparison of enoxaparin, a low-molecular-weight heparin, with unfractionated heparin adjunctive to recombinant tissue plasminogen activator thrombolysis and aspirin: Second trial of Heparin and Aspirin Reperfusion Therapy (HART-II). *Circulation* 2001; 104:648-652.

39. White HD, Aylward PE, Frey MJ, et al. Randomized, double-blind comparison of hirulog versus heparin in patients receiving streptokinase and aspirin for acute myocardial infarction (HERO). *Circulation* 1997; 96:2155-2161.

40. Antman EM, Gibson CM, de Lemos JA, et al. Combination reperfusion therapy with abciximab and reduced dose reteplase: Results from TIMI 14. The Thrombolysis in Myocardial Infarction (TIMI) 14 Investigators. *Eur Heart J* 2000; 21:1944-1953.

41. SPEED Group. Trial of abciximab with and without low-dose reteplase for acute myocardial infarction. *Circulation* 2000; 101:2788-2794.

42. Bates E, Topol E. Limitations of thrombolytic therapy for acute myocardial infarction complicated by congestive heart failure and cardiogenic shock. *J Am Coll Cardiol* 1991; 18:1077-1084.

43. Hands ME, Rutherford JD, Muller JE, et al. The in-hospital development of cardiogenic shock after myocardial infarction: Incidence, predictors of occurrence, outcome and prognostic factors. *J Am Coll Cardiol* 1989; 14:40-46.

44. Meinertz T, Kasper W, Schumacher M, et al. The German multicenter trial of anisoylated plasminogen streptokinase activator complex versus heparin for acute myocardial infarction. *Am J Cardiol* 1988; 62:347-351.

45. AIMS Trial Study Group. Long-term efects of intravenous anistreplase in acute myocardial infarction: Final report of the AIMS study. *Lancet* 1990; 335:427-431.

46. The International Study Group. In-hospital mortality and clinical course of 20,891 patients with suspected acute myocardial infarction randomised between alteplase and streptokinase with or without heparin. *Lancet* 1990; 336:71-75.

47. Gruppo Italiano per lo Studio Della Sopravvivenza nell'infarto Miocardico. GISSI-2: A factorial randomised trial of alteplase versus streptokinase and heparin versus no heparin among 12,490 patients with acute myocardial infarction. *Lancet* 1990; 336:65-71.

48. Third International Study of Infarct Survival Collaborative Group. ISIS-3: A randomized comparison of streptokinase vs tissue plasminogen activator vs anistreplase and of aspirin plus heparin vs aspirin alone among 41,299 cases of suspected acute myocardial infarction. *Lancet* 1192: 339:753-770.

49. Neuhaus K-L, Von Essen R, Tebbe U, et al. Improved thrombolysis in acute myocardial infarction with front-loaded administration of alteplase: Results of the rt-PA-APSAC Patency Study (TAPS). *J Am Coll Cardiol* 1992; 19:885-891.

50. International Joint Efficacy Comparison of Thrombolytics. Randomised, double-blind comparison of reteplase double-bolus administration with streptokinase in acute myocardial infarction (INJECT): Trial to investigate equivalence. *Lancet* 1995; 346:329-336.

51. Goldberg RJ, Samad NA, Yarzebski J, et al. Temporal trends in cardiogenic shock complicating acute myocardial infarction. *N Engl J Med* 1999; 340:1162-1168.

52. Goldberg RJ, Gore JM, Thompson CA, et al. Recent magnitude of and temporal trends (1994-1997) in the incidence and hospital death rates of cardiogenic shock complicating acute myocardial infarction: The second National Registry of Myocardial Infarction. *Am Heart J* 2001; 141:65-72.

53. Hochman JS, Buller CE, Sleeper LA, et al. Cardiogenic shock complicating acute myocardial infarction—etiologies, management and outcome: A report from the SHOCK Trial Registry. *J Am Coll Cardiol* 2000; 36:1063-1070.

54. Hochman JS, Sleeper LA, Webb JG, et al. Early revascularization in acute myocardial infarction complicated by cardiogenic shock. *N Engl J Med* 1999; 341:625-634.

55. Mathey DG, Kuck KH, Tilsner V, et al. Nonsurgical coronary artery recanalization in acute transmural myocardial infarction. *Circulation* 1981; 63:489-497.

56. Kennedy JW, Gensini GG, Timmis GC, et al. Acute myocardial infarction treated with intracoronary streptokinase: A report of the Society for Cardiac Angiography. *Am J Cardiol* 1985; 55:871-877.

57. Col NF, Gurwitz JH, Alpert JS, et al. Frequency of inclusion of patients with cardiogenic shock in trials of thrombolytic therapy. *Am J Cardiol* 1994; 73:149-157.

58. Holmes DR, Jr, Bates ER, Kleiman NS, et al. Contemporary reperfusion therapy for cardiogenic shock. *J Am Coll Cardiol* 1995; 26:668-674.

59. Sanborn TA, Sleeper LA, Bates ER, et al., for the SHOCK Investigators. Impact of thrombolysis, aortic counterpulsation, and their combination in cardiogenic shock: A report from the SHOCK Trial Registry. *J Am Coll Cardiol* 2000; 36:1123-1129.

60. Bengston JR, Kaplan AJ, Pieper KS, et al. Prognosis in cardiogenic shock after acute myocardial infarction in the interventional era. *J Am Coll Cardiol* 1992; 20:1482-1489.

61. Becker RC. Hemodynamic, mechanical, and metabolic determinants of thrombolytic efficacy: A theoretic framework for assessing the limitations of thrombolysis in patients with cardiogenic shock. *Am Heart J* 1993; 125:919-925.

62. Prewitt RM, Gu S, Garger PJ, et al. Marked systematic hypotension depresses coronary thrombolysis induced by intracoronary administration of recombinant tissue-type plasminogen activator. *J Am Coll Cardiol* 1992; 20:1626-1633.

63. Prewitt RM, Gu S, Schick U, et al. Intraaortic balloon counterpulsation enhances coronary thrombolysis induced by intravenous administration of a thrombolytic agent. *J Am Coll Cardiol* 1994; 23:794-798.

64. Levine GN, Hochman JS. Thrombolysis in acute myocardial infarction complicated by cardiogenic shock. *J Throm Thrombo* 1995; 2:11-20.

65. Stomel RJ, Rasak M, Bates ER. Treatment strategies for acute myocardial infarction complicated by cardiogenic shock in a community hospital. *Chest* 1994; 105:997-1002.

66. Anderson RD, Ohman EM, Holmes DR, Jr, et al. Use of intraaortic balloon counterpulsation in patients presenting with cardiogenic shock: Observations from the GUSTO-I study. *J Am Coll Cardiol* 1997; 30:708-715.

67. Barron HV, Every NR, Parsons LS, et al. The use of intra-aortic balloon counterpulsation in patients with cardiogenic shock complicating acute myocardial infarction: data from the National Registry of Myocardial Infarction 2. *Am Heart J* 2001; 141:933-939.

68. Ohman EM, Nannas J, Stomel RJ, et al. Thrombolysis and counterpulsation to improve cardiogenic shock survival (TACTICS): Results of a prospective randomized trial. *Circulation* 2000; 102:II-600 (abst).

69. Hudson MP, Granger CB, Stebbins AL, et al. Cardiogenic shock survival and use of intra-aortic balloon counterpulsation: Results from the GUSTO-I and III trials. *Circulation* 1999; 100:370 (abst).

70. Berger PB, Holmes DR, Jr., Stebbins AL, et al. Impact of an aggressive invasive catheterization and revascularization strategy on mortality in patients with cardiogenic shock in the Global Utilization of Streptokinase and Tissue Plasminogen Activator for Occluded Coronary Arteries (GUSTO –I) Trial: An observational study. *Circulation* 1997; 96:122-127.

71. Berger PB, Tuttle RH, Holmes DR, Jr., et al. One-year survival among patients with acute myocardial infarction complicated by cardiogenic shock, and its relation to early revascularization: Results from the GUSTO-I trial. *Circulation* 1999; 99:873-878.

Chapter 5

Intra-aortic Balloon Counterpulsation for Cardiogenic Shock Complicating Acute Myocardial Infarction

Michael P. Hudson, MD and E. Magnus Ohman, MD

Introduction

Cardiogenic shock results from inadequate cardiac pumping function and insufficient tissue perfusion. Pathophysiologic causes of this impaired cardiac pumping function include acute myocardial infarction (MI) with or without mechanical complications, cardiomyopathy, prolonged cardiopulmonary bypass, myocarditis, and sepsis-associated myocardial depression.[1] Regardless of etiology, cardiogenic shock will usually progress as an inexorable downward spiral towards worsening organ perfusion, impaired homeostatic function, irreversible organ damage, and death unless effective therapeutic interventions are initiated. Intra-aortic balloon pump (IABP) counterpulsation has been applied in a variety of clinical conditions associated with the development and presence of cardiogenic shock (Table 1). This chapter will explore the therapeutic use of IABP counterpulsation in patients with cardiogenic shock complicating acute MI.

Historical Development

The development of IABP counterpulsation is a direct response to the failures and shortcomings of cardiogenic shock pharmacological therapies.

From: Hollenberg SM, Bates ER. *Cardiogenic Shock*. Armonk, NY: Futura Publishing Co., Inc.; ©2002.

Table 1.

Clinical Conditions Treated with IABP Counterpulsation

Cardiogenic shock ± acute myocardial infarction
Unstable angina refractory to medical therapy
Severe congestive heart failure/Cardiomyopathy
Right ventricular failure or infarction
Bridge to heart transplantation
Supporting or following high-risk percutaneous coronary intervention
Following coronary bypass surgery
Valvular heart disease (aortic stenosis, mitral regurgitation)

IABP = intra-aortic balloon pump.

Sympathomimetic vasopressor agents (dopamine, norepinephrine, epinephrine, and dobutamine) and vasodilators (nitroprusside, phosphodiesterase inhibitors) produce favorable hemodynamic effects by stimulation of specific myocardial and endothelial receptors. These potent vasoactive agents are recommended for initial hemodynamic stabilization of cardiogenic shock patients.[2] Unfortunately, these agents rarely normalize circulatory function and often lead to increased myocardial oxygen demand, worsening ischemia, or reduced systemic arterial pressure despite other intended hemodynamic effects.[3] Not surprisingly, pharmacological therapies have failed to improve cardiogenic shock survival in observational and randomized controlled studies.

IABP counterpulsation emerged in the late 1960s after two decades of experimental and technical innovation.[4] Kantrowitz and Kantrowitz first attempted to augment diastolic aortic pressure and increase coronary blood flow in 1953 by returning blood from the femoral artery to the aorta via an external tubing circuit.[5] In 1958, Harkin described the concept of arterial counterpulsation and developed a system in which blood was removed from one femoral artery during systole and returned during diastole into the opposite femoral artery.[6] In the same year, Kantrowitz and McKinnon incorporated the diaphragm as a pumping source to augment aortic diastolic pressure.[7] In 1962, Moulopoulos pioneered the use of an expandable carbon-dioxide balloon positioned in the descending aorta to improve hemodynamics.[8] After several technical improvements, Kantrowitz et al. reported the first successful clinical application of IABP counterpulsation for cardiogenic shock in 1967.[9] In 1984, Nanas et al. reported the use of a high-volume counterpulsation device similar to current models.[10] Early prototypes required surgical cutdown, direct arterial visualization, and surgical insertion and removal of the catheter. During the early-mid 1980s, catheter and insertion refinements led to smaller-diameter sheaths and catheters plus "over-wire" systems that could be inserted and removed percutaneously over conventional guidewires.

Hemodynamic Principles

IABP counterpulsation provides mechanical circulatory assistance jointly by lowering aortic pressure in systole and increasing aortic pres-

Table 2.

Hemodynamic Effects of IABP Counterpulsation

Diastolic aortic pressure	↑↑
Cardiac output	↑
Mean arterial pressure	↑
Left ventricular stroke work index	↑↑
Left ventricular ejection fraction	↑
Coronary blood flow	↑ or ↓
Peripheral vascular resistance	↓↓
Left ventricular wall tension	↓↓
Pulmonary capillary wedge pressure	↓↓
Myocardial oxygen demand	↓
Left ventricular volume	↓
Central venous pressure	↓
Systolic aortic pressure	↓
Heart rate	↓

Slight (↑ increase, ↓ decrease)
Moderate (↑↑ increase, ↓↓ decrease)
IABP = intra-aortic balloon pump; LV = left ventricular.

sure in diastole. In synchrony with the patient's electrocardiogram, a predetermined and self-contained volume of gas (helium or CO_2) is pumped into the aortic balloon during cardiac diastole and withdrawn during systole. Diastolic balloon inflation displaces blood from the aorta, causing increased aortic diastolic pressure and mean arterial pressure. The balloon then deflates just prior to the onset of systole, creating an empty or potential space in the aorta and a reduction in systemic vascular resistance and afterload. This afterload reduction allows greater emptying of the left ventricle and leads to beneficial decreases in end-systolic volume, end-diastolic volume, and left ventricular (LV) wall tension. Reduced LV volumes and wall tension combined with augmented diastolic arterial pressure produce favorable increases in myocardial oxygen supply and decreases in myocardial oxygen demand. The cumulative hemodynamic and metabolic effects of IABP counterpulsation are depicted in Table 2. Individual responses depend on balloon volume, heart rate, cardiac rhythm, blood pressure, balloon inflation/deflation rates, and myocardial loading conditions, but certain effects are well-substantiated in animal and human studies. In the setting of cardiogenic shock, IABP counterpulsation decreases systolic pressure approximately 10%, augments diastolic pressure from 30% to 80%, and increases cardiac output by 10% to 40%.[3,][11-15] There is controversy over whether IABP counterpulsation increases coronary blood flow. IABP counterpulsation increases diastolic and mean aortic pressure. Since coronary blood flow occurs mostly during diastole, it is not surprising that several studies have shown increased coronary blood flow and perfusion during IABP counterpulsation.[11] Animal studies show conflicting results, with some studies showing increased coronary flow rates only in the setting of hypotension.[16, 17] Human clinical studies, meanwhile, have showed inconsistent but generally favorable results. Several investigators have failed to demonstrate increased coronary blood flow after IABP counterpulsation, particularly in patients with severe coronary stenoses or in the distal coronary vasculature.[18-20] In 1972, Mueller and colleagues published results in 10 patients with cardiogenic shock demonstrating a mean increase of 23 mL/100 g/min in coronary blood flow (68 vs. 91 mL/100 g/min, p < 0.001) after IABP therapy, accompanied by favorable changes in myocardial lactate metabolism.[15] More recently, Kern et al. studied 19 patients with cardiogenic shock secondary to acute MI, unstable angina, mitral regurgitation, and high-risk angioplasty.[11] Peak phasic, mean coronary flow velocity, and diastolic coronary flow velocity integral were increased significantly during IABP counterpulsation, (115% ± 115%, 67% ± 61%, and 103% ± 81%, respectively, all p < 0.001). The most dramatic increases were noted in patients with basal systolic blood pressures less than 90 mm Hg, suggesting a potent therapeutic means of ischemia relief in the hypotensive patient.

Clinical Management of the Intra-Aortic Balloon Pump

Insertion of IABP

The IABP was originally inserted surgically through the common femoral artery. Following surgical cutdown, a prosthetic graft was anastomosed to the artery and the cylindrical balloon was advanced via the graft and positioned in the descending aorta. Surgical implantation was associated with high rates of infection, bleeding, and vascular complications, and necessitated surgical repair of the artery after IABP removal.[21] Equally important, surgical insertion was not amenable to high-risk, urgent clinical situations.

Percutaneous IABPs became available in the late 1970s and allowed prompt bedside insertion and nonoperative removal. These IABP devices are typically inserted via the femoral artery after identification of the inguinal landmarks and palpation of the femoral and distal arterial pulses. The inguinal region should be cleansed with an antibacterial solution and draped in a sterile fashion. A 0.5-cm skin incision located 2 cm below the inguinal ligament is then made. Using a modified Seldinger technique, a needle is advanced at a 45° angle to cannulate the common femoral artery. Once pulsatile blood return is obtained, a J-tipped guidewire is advanced through the needle lumen and advanced to the descending aorta under fluoroscopic guidance. Progressively larger dilators are passed over the wire into the vessel to create a tract allowing advancement of the 8-10 Fr arterial sheath. The deflated intra-aortic balloon is prepared and passed over the guidewire to a position just inferior to the origin of the left subclavian artery and cephalad to the renal arteries. Sheathless insertion may also be done by omitting sheath placement and passing the balloon directly over the guidewire. After correct positioning is confirmed by fluoroscopy, the guidewire is removed, air is purged from the system, the balloon is connected to console tubing, and the sheath/balloon

Table 3.

Contraindications to IABP Counterpulsation

Absolute Contraindications
      Suspected aortic dissection
      Distal aortic occlusion or severe stenosis
      Moderate-severe aortic valve insufficiency
      Abdominal or thoracic aortic aneurysm
Relative Contraindications
      Severe peripheral vascular disease
      Aortic, iliofemoral arterial grafts
      Contraindication to heparin or anticoagulation
      Tachyarrythmias (heart rate > 150 beats/min)
      Mild aortic valve insufficiency
      Irregular ventricular rhythms due to frequent ectopy or atrial fibrillation

IABP = intra-aortic balloon pump.

catheter is sutured to the anterior thigh. Balloon counterpulsation can then be initiated, with careful inspection of the hemodynamic tracing and adjustment of the proper timing and assist ratio. During the course of insertion, the guidewire and balloon should never be advanced forcibly through resistance. If tortuosity is encountered, the contralateral femoral site should be attempted, or surgical cutdown and insertion via the left axillary artery may be attempted.

Contraindications to IABP

Relative risks and benefits of IABP counterpulsation vary by patient and clinical scenario. Absolute and relative contraindications to IABP counterpulsation are listed in Table 3. Presence of these contraindications significantly increases the risks and diminishes the potential therapeutic benefit of IABP counterpulsation. Aortic valve insufficiency is a contraindication because diastolic balloon inflation will not augment diastolic pressure and coronary flow, but instead will propel blood volume into the decompensated left ventricle. Aortic dissection or aneurysm is a contraindication because of the increased risk of vascular damage, rupture, or embolism. Tachyarrhythmias reduce clinical efficacy by reducing the ability of the console to track and coordinate balloon inflation/deflation with the cardiac cycle.

Timing

Once the IABP has been inserted, adjustment of balloon timing then becomes critical to optimize hemodynamic benefit. Timing refers to the positioning of the inflation and deflation points on the arterial waveform. The balloon is inflated at the beginning of diastole (time of aortic valve closure), which may be identified on the arterial pressure tracing by the

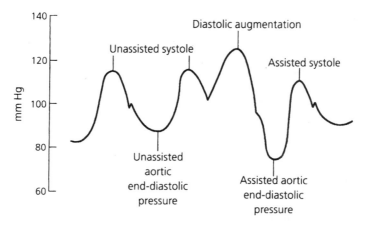

Figure 1. Arterial waveform variations during IABP therapy (1:2 Assist Ratio). Figure depicts two complete cardiac cycles, including an initial unassisted systolic arterial tracing followed by an assisted cardiac cycle. Note the diastolic augmentation after balloon inflation in the assisted beat, followed by decreased end diastolic and end systolic pressures in the subsequent unassisted cycle.

dicrotic notch. Deflation is timed, then, to occur immediately before aortic valve opening just prior to the next systole. IABP timing is ordinarily synchronized with the cardiac cycle by means of the electrocardiogram. In such cases, a native or pacemaker R wave is the trigger event for IABP timing. Alternatively, the systolic upstroke of the arterial waveform or an internal mechanical trigger may determine IABP timing. Current IABP models provide automatic and manual timing modes with digital display of an inflation marker or inflation interval, which may be adjusted according to the waveform appearance. Precise timing is adjusted with the balloon control console while observing the displayed arterial pressure tracings so as to maximally augment diastolic pressure and reduce aortic end-diastolic pressure (see Figure 1).

Assist Ratio

An assist ratio describing the proportion of cardiac cycles that are augmented must be chosen. A 1:1 assist ratio indicates that each cardiac cycle is assisted while a 1:2 ratio indicates every other cardiac cycle is assisted. Ratios between 1:1 and 1:3 are generally used and maximal hemodynamic assistance usually occurs at a 1:1 assist ratio. In certain circumstances, particularly arrhythmias and tachycardias, a lower assist ratio may improve hemodynamic response. It is always advisable to individualize parameters to the patient and to test several timing and assist ratio settings.

Anticoagulation

Anticoagulation therapy is generally recommended throughout the course of IABP counterpulsation therapy in order to reduce the risk of thrombotic and embolic complications. No comparative trials of anticoagulation regimens or counterpulsation settings exist for patients receiving IABP therapy. Thrombotic complications can likely be reduced by shortening the duration of IABP support and avoiding prolonged periods of balloon inactivity. Unless specific contraindications exist, we recommend administration of intravenous heparin adjusted to an activated partial thromboplastin time (aPTT) of 50-70 seconds or therapeutic doses of low molecular weight heparins (i.e., enoxaparin 1 mg/ kg q 12 hr) throughout IABP counterpulsation. Bleeding complications, either related or unrelated to IABP therapy, occur frequently during IABP counterpulsation. Lower doses of intravenous heparin (50-100 U/ hour) or no anticoagulation may be adequate in patients with ongoing bleeding complications or diathesis; however, clinicians should begin preparation for IABP removal in such patients.

Nursing Care

IABP counterpulsation requires that a patient be kept in bed and supine. Minimal movement of the pelvis and lower extremities is required to avoid catheter dislodgment and vascular injury. Agitation and even delirium may occur during IABP counterpulsation.[22] Extensive patient counseling and explanation of what to expect may alleviate anxiety and improve compliance. The patient's lower leg should be secured with a cloth or leather restraint. Sedation with benzodiazepines and haloperidol are frequently required.

IABP Discontinuation

Discontinuation of IABP counterpulsation may be accomplished by several methods, ideally after stabilization or correction of the circulatory abnormalities. Anticoagulation should be withheld for 2 to 4 hours before sheath/ balloon removal. Some intensive care units or catheterization labs may wish to check activated clotting times and defer sheath/ balloon removal until the activated clotting time is less than 150-200 seconds. Most simply, the balloon pump can be turned off and removed. Others advocate gradual weaning of the assist ratio or balloon volume over several hours with repeated monitoring of hemodynamic status. In most cases, if the patient can hemodynamically tolerate 1:2 or 1:3 assist ratio, then the device can be removed. We generally recommend a short period of 1:2 or 1:3 support followed by IABP removal 30 to 60 minutes later as long as arterial pressure is maintained. At time of IABP removal, the console is turned off, the balloon deflated and tubing aspirated. Sheath and balloon are removed as one unit with bleeding allowed momentarily to expel possible clots. Proximal and direct manual pressure are then applied for minimum of 15 minutes to achieve hemostasis. If the IABP needs to be removed urgently in an anticoagulated patient, replacement of a 9-11 Fr sheath over a guidewire is recommended.

Complications

Patients should be monitored closely for complications after balloon insertion with specific attention directed towards vital signs, catheter entry site, lower extremity vascular exam, and lower extremity skin exam. Percutaneous insertion of IABPs can be achieved in more than 90% of patients; however, vascular and hemorrhagic complications remain a significant problem. Possible complications, as shown in Table 4, are due to hemorrhage, perforation of the aorta, dissection of the femoral/iliac artery or aorta, ischemic injury to the lower extremities, embolism, thrombocytopenia, and hemolysis.[23]

Estimated rates of overall complications, thromboembolic events, and hemorrhagic events are difficult to extrapolate from published studies due to variability in IABP insertion, duration, catheter/balloon diameter, underlying condition, adjunctive therapies, and study definitions. The largest study of surgically placed IABPs reported an overall complication rate of 44% (death < 1%, vascular injury 22%, hemorrhage 13%, limb ischemia 14%) in 733 IABP patients.[24] Other surgical studies using 10-12 Fr size catheter systems reported overall complication rates of 30% to 45% and detectable limb ischemia in 40% of patients, necessitating balloon removal in 30% of patients.[25]

Nonrandomized trials have compared complication rates between surgical and percutaneous insertion. The largest trial by Collier et al. included 400 patients and reported an overall complication rate of 29%, with similar rates of major ischemic complications in both groups and more frequent

---

Table 4.

Complications Associated with Intra-aortic Balloon Counterpulsation

Major Complications
  Death
  Hemorrhage leading to hypotension or blood transfusion
  Sepsis
  Limb ischemic requiring amputation or surgical vascular repair
  Spinal cord ischemia/ infarct
  Mesenteric or renal ischemia or infarction
  Aortic dissection
  Gas or thrombotic embolism
  Balloon entrapment requiring surgical removal
Minor Complications
  Groin hematoma
  Minor hemorrhage
  Delirium
  Arterial thrombosis
  Fever/ Bacteremia
  Cellulitis/ Access site infection
  Ischemic foot or leg ulcer
  Ischemic or traumatic neuropathy
  Pseudoaneurysm
  Claudication

minor ischemic complications with the percutaneous technique.[26] Despite these findings, percutaneous placement of the IABP has become the standard technique due to ease of insertion.

Several observational studies have reported complication rates for IABP counterpulsation in the current reperfusion era. In a Global Utilization of Streptokinase and Tissue-Plasminogen Activator for Occluded Coronary Arteries I (GUSTO-1) substudy of patients with cardiogenic shock treated initially with thrombolysis, moderate and severe/ life-threatening hemorrhage were increased in patients treated with early IABP therapy versus no IABP therapy, (for moderate hemorrhage, 47% vs. 12%, p = 0.0001, for severe, 10% vs. 5%, p = 0.16, respectively).[27] In the PAMI-II (Primary Angioplasty in Myocardial Infarction II) trial, prophylactic insertion of IABP in high-risk AMI patients treated with primary angioplasty also resulted in higher rates of hemorrhagic complications (36% vs. 27%, p = 0.05) largely due to increased access site bleeding.[28] No differences were reported in this study in the rate of red blood cell transfusion, fall in hematocrit, or major vascular complications.

Innovations and miniaturization of catheter design and greater use of sheathless percutaneous insertion technique may reduce future IABP complication rates.[29] Nevertheless, most observational and randomized trials show increased rates of hemorrhagic and thromboembolic complications associated with IABP therapy. Pooled analysis suggests overall complication rates of 15% to 57%, vascular complication rates of 5% to 33%, and bleeding rates of 2% to 26%.[4] Multivariate regression analysis has identified peripheral vascular disease, femoral bruit, absent distal pulses, diabetes, female gender, prolonged support, smoking, percutaneous insertion, and hypertension as clinical factors associated with increased complications.[30, 31]

Clinical Studies

IABP Studies in the Pre-Reperfusion Era

Cardiogenic shock complicates 5% to 8% of all thrombolytic-treated myocardial infarctions and represents the leading cause of death after AMI hospitalization. Before the advent of reperfusion therapy, studies of IABP counterpulsation in AMI patients primarily focused on hemodynamic outcomes. In 1973, Scheidt and colleagues prospectively treated 87 cardiogenic shock patients with IABP counterpulsation at a median of 13 hours following infarct onset.[12] Heart rate fell from 110 ± 24 to 103 ± 21 beats per minute; cardiac output increased 500 mL per minute from 2.4 to 2.9 L/min. Systolic arterial pressure fell from 76 to 57 mm Hg. Diastolic arterial pressure rose significantly, from 53 to 83 mm Hg, with no change in mean arterial pressure. Unfortunately, no control group was included in this series to assess treatment efficacy or safety. Sixty percent of the patients expired during IABP support, and the in-hospital mortality rate was 83%.

Two randomized, controlled trials of IABP counterpulsation in high-risk AMI patients were conducted in the prethrombolytic era. Neither trial enrolled patients with clearly defined cardiogenic shock. O'Rourke and colleagues randomized thirty patients with AMI and acute heart failure to IABP support (n = 14) versus conventional therapy (n = 16) between 1976 and 1979.[32] IABP counterpulsation was begun 7.1 hours (range 4.8 to 13.7 hours) after AMI symptom onset and continued for a mean of 4.5 days. Infarct size, as measured by either peak or cumulative creatine kinase, was not reduced in the IABP versus control groups, (1794 ± 846 IU/ liter vs. 1688 ± 908, and 3590 ± 1936 IU/ liter vs. 2945 ± 1803, respectively). In-hospital mortality was also not significantly different in the IABP versus control treatment group, (50% [7/14] vs. 44% [7/16]). Despite the failure of IABP therapy to reduce infarct size or improve mortality, these investigators concluded that "we remain convinced on the basis of pathophysiological principles, animal studies and clinical experience that counterpulsation has a role in the management of myocardial infarction." The second trial, by Flaherty and colleagues, studied 20 patients with acute MI and large thallium radionuclide defects presenting within 12 hours of acute MI symptom onset.[33] Patients without hypotension or frank cardiogenic shock were randomized to standard therapy versus standard therapy plus intravenous nitroglycerin with IABP counterpulsation. IABP therapy was administered for 4.6 ± 1.9 days. No beneficial effect on infarct expansion, LV function, survival or recurrent MI was evident for the nitroglycerin + IABP treatment strategy.

IABP Studies in the Reperfusion Era

Despite the absence of proven mortality benefit, IABP counterpulsation has become an accepted treatment strategy for cardiogenic shock in the reperfusion era. Multiple observational studies and retrospective analyses have demonstrated modest but significant improvements in survival with IABP counterpulsation. Cumulatively, these studies report 63% survival with IABP-treated cardiogenic shock. This survival figure compares favorably with historic estimates of approximately 80% mortality for cardiogenic shock, but should be interpreted cautiously because of the nonrandomized assignment of IABP therapy, retrospective analyses, and observational study designs. Selection bias of more healthy, salvageable patients and disproportionate use of other aggressive therapies (angiography, mechanical ventilation, and revascularization) largely explain these treatment outcomes as illustrated in Table 5 and the examples below.[12-14, 27, 34-48]

In most of these positive studies, patients benefit not just from IABP counterpulsation but also from more favorable baseline characteristics (younger age, later onset of shock, more favorable hemodynamics) and a far higher rate of angiography and revascularization. Bengston's review[45] of cardiogenic shock at Duke noted that IABP therapy was used in 99 of 200 patients. No in-hospital mortality difference was noted, as the mortality rate was 48% among IABP patients and 57% among those not so

Table 5.

IABP Counterpulsation in Acute Myocardial Infarction Related Cardiogenic Shock. Overall Mortality and Effect of Revascularization.

Reference	Year	N	Mortality N (%)	Mortality N (%) IABP + (−) Revasc	Mortality N (%) IABP + (+) Revasc
Dunkman[13]	1972	40	30 (75)	16/25 (84)	9/15 (60)
Leinbach[34]	1972	11	8 (73)	4/4 (100)	5/7 (71)
Scheidt[12]	1973	87	72 (83)	—	—
Willerson[14]	1975	23	21 (91)	18/19 (95)	3/4 (75)
Bardet[35]	1977	42	29 (69)	22/25 (88)	7/17 (41)
Beckman[36]	1977	40	32 (80)	22/29 (76)	10/11 (91)
Hagemeijer[37]	1977	17	8 (47)	8/17 (47)	
Jackson[38]	1977	23	18 (78)	16/21 (76)	2/2 (100)
Johnson[39]	1977	28	15 (54)	11/18 (66)	5/10 (50)
Forssell[40]	1979	15	14 (93)	14/15 (93)	
O'Rourke[41]	1979	74	49 (66)	11/18 (61)	38/56 (68)
DeWood[42]	1980	40	19 (47)	11/21 (52)	8/19 (42)
Pierri[43]	1980	47	29 (62)	12/13 (92)	27/34 (65)
Goldberger[44]	1986	20	16 (80)	16/19 (84)	1/1 (100)
Bengston[45]	1992	99	48 (48)	27/43 (63)	21/56 (37)
Waksman[46]	1993	55	29 (53)	—	—
Stomel[47]	1994	51	28 (55)	21/26 (81)	7/25 (28)
Anderson[27]	1997	62	30 (48)	14/30 (47)	16/32 (50)
Kovack[48]	1997	27	9 (33)	—	—
Total		**801**	**504 (63)**	**242/343 (71)**	**159/289 (55)**

IABP = intra-aortic balloon pump.

treated. Conversely, when surgical or percutaneous revascularization was used with IABP, the mortality rate was 38% versus 63% for IABP counter-pulsation alone (p < 0.01). In the SHOCK Registry (n = 173) compiled by Hochman et al., similar results were obtained.[49] Unadjusted mortality was significantly lower with the use of IABP than without IABP (57% vs. 72%, p = 0.04). IABP patients, however, were significantly younger and significantly more likely to undergo cardiac catheterization (88% vs. 30%) and subsequent revascularization procedures. After adjustment for cardiac catheterization status, there was no significant association between mortality and IABP use.

IABP Counterpulsation and Thrombolytic Therapy

Combined use of intravenous thrombolytic therapy (TT) and IABP counterpulsation in hypotensive acute MI patients has considerable pathophysiologic and antithrombotic appeal. Becker pointed out that thrombolytic efficacy in cardiogenic shock is decreased because of hemodynamic, metabolic, and mechanical factors that prevent achievement and maintenance of infarct-related artery patency.[50] Animal studies suggest that resistance to thrombolysis may be caused by inadequate coronary perfusion pressure and poor drug penetration into the nascent coronary clot. In a hypotensive canine acute MI model, Prewitt and colleagues demonstrated that the rate and extent of coronary thrombolysis were impaired with moderate hypotension, and that norepinephrine infusion could increase aortic perfusion pressure and improve thrombolysis.[51] Two years later, these same investigators demonstrated that IABP counterpulsation significantly improves the rate of thrombolysis by augmenting aortic diastolic pressure.[52] Gurbel et al. also investigated the effect of IABP counterpulsation on thrombolytic efficacy in a hypotensive canine acute MI model.[53] These investigators demonstrated that successful reperfusion occurred significantly earlier in hypotensive dogs treated with IABP plus alteplase versus alteplase alone, (13 ± 2 minutes vs. 39 ± 9 minutes, p = 0.02). Enhanced thrombolysis resulted in this study from augmented diastolic blood pressure and seemed to be unrelated to minimal changes in coronary blood flow. Thus, IABP therapy might improve infarct artery patency through greater delivery and penetration of thrombolytic drug into the thrombus. Therefore, cardiogenic shock outcomes might be improved with IABP plus thrombolysis if bleeding/ safety issues and systemic hemodynamic factors do not negate these advantages.

The combination of TT with IABP counterpulsation has been examined retrospectively in a number of observational studies and clinical trials. Most studies suggest that the IABP counterpulsation can safely be combined with TT.[54] In the Thrombolysis and Myocardial Infarction (TAMI) Trials, 85 of 810 (10.5%) patients with cardiogenic shock or impending cardiogenic shock following thrombolysis were treated with IABP counterpulsation.[55] In patients receiving IABP therapy, in-hospital mortality was 32% and vascular complications occurred in 12%. In cardiogenic shock patients treated with IABP, there was a significantly reduced incidence of reinfarction or reocclusion and a significant improvement in global and noninfarct zone functional recovery. The Randomized IABP Study Group prospectively investigated whether IABP counterpulsation would reduce the rate of reocclusion of the infarct-related artery after patency had been established.[56] Non-shock AMI patients (n = 182) following primary/rescue percutaneous transluminal coronary angioplasty (PTCA) or intracoronary lytic therapy were randomized to IABP counterpulsation for 48 hours versus standard care. Patients randomized to IABP counterpulsation had significantly less reocclusion of the infarct-related artery compared with control patients, (8% vs. 21%, p < 0.03). Although there was no significant mortality difference, there was a significantly lower composite event rate of death, stroke, reinfarction, or emergency revascularization in patients assigned to IABP therapy, (13% vs. 24%, p < 0.04). Kovack and colleagues explored whether IABP combined with thrombolysis improved survival in 335 cardiogenic shock patients treated at two Michigan community hospitals.[48] In this cohort, 46 AMI patients presented within 12 hours of AMI onset and received thrombolysis, including 27 patients (59%) who underwent IABP counterpulsation. Patients treated with IABP had a significantly greater cardiac index (2.0 vs. 1.5 L/min/m^2, p = 0.04), greater rate of transfer for revascularization (85% vs. 37%, p < 0.05), and higher overall hospital survival, (67% vs. 32%, p = 0.02).

Still, patients with cardiogenic shock at hospital admission have largely been excluded from the larger, multicenter thrombolytic trials during the past two decades.[57] In the Global Utilization of Streptokinase and Tissue Plasminogen Activator for Occluded Coronary Arteries (GUSTO-1) trial, cardiogenic shock was not an exclusion criterion. Cardiogenic shock occurred in 2972 patients (7.2%); 315 had shock on arrival and 2657 developed shock after hospital admission, resulting in 55% mortality at 30-day follow-up.[58] Placement of an IABP was significantly more frequent in patients with cardiogenic shock versus those without cardiogenic shock (25% vs. 2%, p < 0.001). Among cardiogenic shock patients, mortality in those patients who underwent angiography alone (34%), PTCA (34%), or coronary angioplasty bypass graft (CABG) (29%) was significantly improved compared with those who did not undergo any invasive procedure, (75%, all p < 0.001). Comparing treatment strategies and outcomes between regions, IABP insertion was performed more frequently for cardiogenic shock in the United States compared to other countries, (35% vs. 7%, p < 0.001).[59] Aggressive diagnostic and therapeutic procedures were also used more frequently in the United States including cardiac catheterization, PTCA and mechanical ventilation. Adjusted 30-day and 1-year mortality was significantly lower among patients treated in the United States than among those treated in other countries, (50% vs. 66%, and 56% vs. 70%, both p < 0.001). Increased survival was associated with revascularization procedures and treatment in the United States, while IABP therapy was not independently associated with mortality.

Anderson et al. specifically examined the use, complications, and outcomes associated with IABP counterpulsation in GUSTO-1 patients presenting at hospital admission with cardiogenic shock.[27] There were 68 (22%) IABP placements in 310 acute MI patients presenting with shock. Increased moderate bleeding episodes (47% vs. 12%, p < 0.0001), severe or life-threatening bleeding episodes (10% vs. 5%, p = 0.16), and need for red blood cell transfusion (66% vs. 13%, p < 0.0001) were noted in IABP patients. Despite increased bleeding events, there was a trend toward lower 30-day mortality in those patients treated with IABP versus no-IABP (47 % vs. 60 %, adjusted p = 0.11). The median time to death was significantly delayed in the IABP group vs. the no-IABP group (67 hours vs. 7.2 hours, p = 00002).

More recent observational data also suggest therapeutic efficacy for IABP counterpulsation in cardiogenic shock patients. In the United States National Registry of Myocardial Infarction 2, Barron and colleagues reported on the outcomes of 21,718 acute MI patients who presented with or developed cardiogenic shock.[60] Thirty-two percent (6993) received IABP counterpulsation. IABP use was associated with younger age and greater likelihood of receiving reperfusion therapy. Outcomes were compared separately for IABP use in patients receiving TT and primary angioplasty.

Compared to patients not receiving IABP therapy, IABP was associated with lower in-hospital mortality amongst TT-treated patients (49% vs. 69%, p < 0.001), but not patients undergoing primary angioplasty, (47% vs. 44%, p = ns). In the Should We Emergently Revascularize Occluded Coronaries for Cardiogenic Shock (SHOCK) Trial, IABP therapy was recommended in both the early revascularization and intensive medical therapy groups and was utilized in 86% of patients in both groups.[61] One-year survival analysis showed a nonsignificant treatment effect for IABP counterpulsation after adjustment for randomized treatment assignment and other mortality predictors, (Relative Risk, 0.71, p = 0.39)[62] Informative data concerning IABP counterpulsation and cardiogenic shock outcomes has also been reported from the larger SHOCK Trial Registry.[63] In an unadjusted analysis, cardiogenic shock patients selected for IABP had lower in-hospital mortality than those who did not receive IABP, (50% vs. 72%, p < 0.0001). Survival was further compared after dividing patients into four groups based on IABP and TT use. There was significantly different in-hospital mortality among patients treated with no TT/ no IABP, TT only, IABP only, and IABP + TT, (77% vs. 63% vs. 52% vs. 47%, respectively, p < 0.0001). Early (≤ 6 hours) versus later use of IABP did not significantly influence mortality. Revascularization rates were three-fold higher in patients receiving IABP therapy, and concomitant revascularization improved survival significantly in excess of IABP or TT effect.

Only one randomized controlled clinical trial of IABP counterpulsation in cardiogenic shock has been conducted in the reperfusion era. The Thrombolysis and Counterpulsation to Improve Cardiogenic Shock Survival (TACTICS) trial intended to randomize patients with ST elevation and acute MI complicated by cardiogenic shock, hypotension, or severe heart failure.[64] Eligible patients were randomized to TT alone versus TT plus IABP counterpulsation. Due to difficulties in randomizing critically ill patients, the TACTICS trial was able to enroll only 57 of an intended 500 patients. As a result, the study was grossly underpowered to detect a treatment difference between groups, and baseline characteristics were unevenly distributed between treatment groups. A higher proportion of patients with adverse features (anterior MI location, diabetes) were enrolled in the IABP group. At 6-month follow-up, patients treated with thrombolysis plus IABP had a nonsignificant 7.3% absolute and 18% relative reduction in mortality. Adjusted 6-month mortality was relatively reduced by 24%, (p = 0.23). TACTICS trial outcome and safety results are shown in Table 6.

IABP Counterpulsation Plus Revascularization for Acute MI-CS

The randomized control and observational trials of IABP counterpulsation along with thrombolysis for cardiogenic shock are summarized in Figure 2 and generally show improved survival which either does not achieve statistical significance, or is highly confounded by other therapies

Table 6.

Results of the Thrombolysis and Counterpulsation to Improve Shock Survival (TACTICS) Trial.[64]

	Thrombolysiš Alone N=27	Thrombolysis + IABP N=30	Adjusted* P Value
30-day Mortality	9 (33%)	8 (27%)	0.30
6-month Mortality	11 (41%)	10 (33%)	0.23
Severe Bleeding	0	1 (3%)	NS
Moderate Bleeding	7 (26%)	7 (23%)	NS

*Adjusted for baseline differences in mortality predictors (diabetes, anterior MI location, blood pressure, heart rate, etc). IABP = intra-aortic balloon pump.

(i.e., revascularization). More persuasive observational data demonstrate improved cardiogenic shock survival when IABP counterpulsation is followed by subsequent revascularization with either angioplasty or bypass surgery. In 1972, Dunkman contrasted cardiogenic shock patients treated with IABP alone versus similar patients treated with pre-/perioperative IABP plus bypass surgery.[13] In-hospital mortality was 84% (21/25) versus 60% (9/15) favoring IABP adjunctive therapy. In 1980, DeWood reported 42% in-hospital mortality among 19 cardiogenic shock patients treated

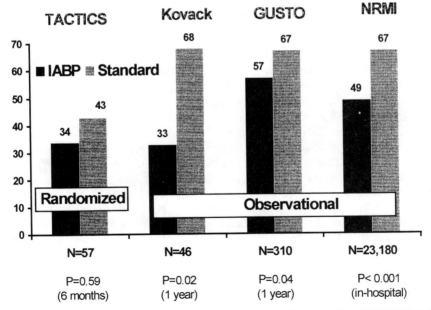

Figure 2. Mortality Results from Randomized and Observational IABP Trials. Figure compares mortality in IABP Counterpulsation (black columns) versus No IABP-Standard Therapy groups (gray columns) in selected randomized and observational studies of acute myocardial infarction related cardiogenic shock.

with IABP counterpulsation and early surgery versus 52% in 21 patients treated with IABP alone, p = ns).[42] In this study, survival benefit from surgery was largely confined to patients operated on within 16 hours of acute MI presentation. Hospital mortality in this early surgery + IABP subgroup was 25%.

IABP counterpulsation has been used in patients with cardiogenic shock to provide hemodynamic support during primary and rescue PTCA. Pooled data from several earlier trials showed PTCA reperfusion success rates of about 75% and overall hospital mortality of 46% in cardiogenic shock.[65] No randomized control study has specifically investigated whether IABP counterpulsation improves catheterization lab complications, outcomes, or survival in cardiogenic shock patients. Among 1490 primary PTCA patients, Brodie and colleagues reported that cardiogenic shock was the strongest predictor of adverse catheterization laboratory events – death, ventricular fibrillation, cardiac arrest, prolonged hypotension, (odds ratio 2.18, 95% CI 1.58 – 3.02).[66] In patients with cardiogenic shock (n = 119) treated with primary PTCA, IABP counterpulsation was used before the percutaneous intervention in 52% (62/119) of cases. IABP use was associated with fewer adverse events in the catheterization lab (14.5% vs. 35.1%, p = 0.009) including significant reductions in ventricular fibrillation (13% vs. 30%, p = 0.02) and cardiopulmonary arrest (6% vs. 22%, p = 0.01).

More recent randomized trial data from high-risk acute MI patients undergoing primary angioplasty casts some doubts on these favorable associations. In the Second Primary Angioplasty in Myocardial Infarction (PAMI-II) Trial, patients with acute MI were identified as high-risk based upon meeting one of the following criteria: (1) age > 70 years, (2) three-vessel coronary artery disease, (3) LV ejection fraction ≤ 45%, (4) saphenous vein graft occlusion, (5) persistent ventricular arrhythmias, or (6) suboptimal PTCA result.[28] Patients stratified as high risk were considered eligible for IABP randomization unless contraindicated because of peripheral vascular disease, aortic aneurysm, aortic valve insufficiency, or hemodynamic instability. Eligible high-risk patients were then randomized to 36-48 hours of IABP (n = 211) or traditional care (n = 226) with a primary composite endpoint of death, reinfarction, infarct-related artery reocclusion, stroke, or new-onset heart failure/sustained hypotension. There was no significant difference in the primary endpoint in patients treated prophylactically with an IABP versus those treated with traditional care (28.9% vs. 29.2%, p = 0.95). The IABP strategy reduced recurrent ischemia (13.3% vs. 19.6%, p = 0.08), and unscheduled repeat catheterization (7.6% vs. 13.3%, p = 0.05), but did not reduce infarct-artery reocclusion (6.7% vs. 5.5%, p = 0.64), reinfarction (6.2% vs. 8.0%, p = 0.46) or mortality (4.3% vs. 3.1%, p = 0.52). IABP assignment was associated with a higher incidence of stroke (2.4% vs. 0%, p = 0.03) and hemorrhagic complications (36.0% vs. 27.4%, p = 0.05).

Similar results were reported at a European tertiary center by van't Hof et al.[67] These investigators performed primary angioplasty in 238 high risk acute MI patients and randomized 118 to IABP and 120 to no IABP treatment with a primary endpoint of death, nonfatal reinfarction, stroke, or ejection fraction < 30% at 1-month follow-up. The primary endpoint was reached in 26% of patients in each group, (p = 0.94) with no significant difference in individual endpoints or secondary analysis of infarct size.

In both of these randomized trials, protocols specifically excluded patients with hemodynamic instability or cardiogenic shock and all patients underwent attempted revascularization. Thus, results may not extrapolate to cardiogenic shock patients treated in the community. The IABP can stabilize hemodynamic parameters, improve vital organ perfusion, and possibly enable more cardiogenic shock patients to receive revascularization therapy. More definitive, future randomized trials of IABP counterpulsation along with primary percutaneous revascularization in cardiogenic shock are unlikely to occur given prior difficulties of enrolling cardiogenic shock patients into trials and strong interventional cardiology biases.

Published Guidelines

The American College of Cardiology and American Heart Association most recently addressed IABP use in cardiogenic shock patients in the "Guidelines for the Management of Patients with Acute Myocardial Infarction" published in 1996.[2] Recommendations for the patient with cardiogenic shock were based on scientific evidence and expert panel opinion and classified as Class I (general agreement that a given procedure or treatment is beneficial, useful and effective), Class IIa (conflicting evidence, weight of evidence/opinion in favor of usefulness/efficacy), and Class IIb (conflicting evidence with usefulness/efficacy less well established by evidence/opinion). As shown in Table 7, IABP therapy was recommended as a Class I indication for patients with cardiogenic shock not quickly reversed with pharmacological therapy as a stabilizing measure for angiography and prompt revascularization, and in patients with mechanical post-MI complications such as acute mitral regurgitation or ventricular septal defect.

Conclusion

Despite the absence of positive, randomized-control trial data, IABP counterpulsation has become widely accepted therapy for cardiogenic shock. Supporting evidence consists largely of observational data associating IABP use and other aggressive therapies with improved cardiogenic shock survival. Such observational data are subject to patient selection bias and confounding rates of concomitant interventions. Conservatively, one can conclude that IABP therapy is not definitive therapy for cardiogenic shock, although it may limit the severity and duration of the shock state and its associated organ damage while patients await emergent and life-saving revascularization.

Table 7.

ACC/ AHA Guidelines for the Management of Patients with Acute Myocardial Infarction[2]

Recommendations for Intra-aortic Balloon Counterpulsation

Class I	
Evidence and/or general agreement that a given procedure or treatment is beneficial, useful, and effective	1. Cardiogenic shock not quickly reversed with pharmacological therapy as stabilizing measure for angiography and prompt revascularization
	2. Acute mitral regurgitation or ventricular septal defect complicating myocardial infarction as a stabilizing therapy for angiography and repair/ revascularization
	3. Recurrent intractable ventricular arrhythmias with hemodynamic instability
	4. Refractory post-MI angina as a bridge to angiography and revascularization
Class II a	
Conflicting evidence and/or a divergence of opinion about the usefulness/ efficacy of a procedure or treatment with weight of evidence/ opinion in favor of usefulness/ efficacy	1. Signs of hemodynamic instability, poor LV function, or persistent ischemia in patients with large areas of myocardium at risk
Class II b	
Conflicting evidence and/or a divergence of opinion about the usefulness/ efficacy of a procedure or treatment with usefulness/ efficacy less well established by evidence/ opinion	1. In patients with successful PTCA after failed thrombolysis or those with three-vessel coronary disease to prevent reocclusion
	2. In patients known to have large areas of myocardium at risk with or without active ischemia

ACC = American College of Cardiology; AHA = American Heart Association; LV = left ventricular; MI = myocardial infarction; PTCA = percutaneous transluminal coronary angioplasty.

References

1. Califf RM, Bengstson JR. Cardiogenic shock. *N Engl J Med* 1994; 330:1724-1730.
2. Ryan TJ, Anderson JL, Antman EM, et al. ACC/ AHA Guidelines for management of patients with acute myocardial infarction. *J Am Coll Cardiol* 1996; 28:1328-1428.
3. Mueller H, Ayres S, Giannelli S Jr., et al. Effect of isoproterenol, l-norepinephrine, and intraaortic counterpulsation on hemodynamics and myocardial metabolism in shock following acute myocardial infarction. *Circulation* 1972; 44:335-351.
4. Mahaffey KW, Kruse KR, Ohman EM. Perspectives on the use of intra-aortic balloon counterpulsation in the 1990s. In Topol EJ (ed); Textbook of Interventional Cardiology. Philadelphia, W.B. Saunders, 1996, pp 303-321.
5. Kantrowitz A, Kantrowitz A. Experimental augmentation of coronary flow by retardation of arterial pressure pulse. *Surgery* 1953; 34:678-687.

6. Harkin D. Assisted circulation. Third World Congress of Cardiology Meeting. Brussels, 1958.

7. Kantrowitz A, McKinnon WMP. The experimental use of the diaphragm as auxiliary myocardium. *Surg Forum* 1958; 9:266-268.

8. Moulopoulos SD, Topaz S, Kolff WJ. Diastolic balloon pumping with carbon dioxide in the aorta: A mechanical assistance to the failing circulation. *Am Heart J* 1962; 63:669-675.

9. Kantrowitz A, Tjonneland S, Freed PS, et al. Initial clinical experience with intraaortic balloon pumping in cardiogenic shock. *JAMA* 1968; 203:113-118.

10. Nanas JN, Olsen DB, Hamanaka Y, et al. Experience with a valveless, implantable abdominal aortic counterpulsating device. *Trans Am Soc Artif Intern Organs* 1984; 30:540-544.

11. Kern MJ, Aguirre FV, Tatineni S, et al. Enhanced coronary blood flow velocity during intraaortic balloon counterpulsation in critically ill patients. *J Am Coll Cardiol* 1993; 21:359-368.

12. Scheidt S, Wilner G, Mueller H, et al. Intra-aortic balloon counterpulsation in cardiogenic shock: Report of a cooperative clinical trial. *N Engl J Med* 1973; 288:979-984.

13. Dunkman WB, Leinbach RC, Buckley MI, et al. Clinical and hemodynamic results of intraaortic balloon pumping and surgery for cardiogenic shock. *Circulation* 1972; 47:465-477.

14. Willerson JT, Curry GC, Watson JT, et al. Intraaortic balloon counterpulsation in patients in cardiogenic shock, medically refractory left ventricular failure and/or recurrent ventricular tachycardia. *Am J Med* 1975; 58:183-191.

15. Mueller M, Ayres SM, Conklin EF, et al. The effects of intra-aortic counterpulsation on cardiac performance and metabolism in shock associated with acute myocardial infarction. *J Clin Invest* 1971; 50:1885-1900.

16. Gill CC, Wechsler AS, Newman GE, et al. Augmentation and redistribution of myocardial blood flow during acute ischemia by intra-aortic balloon pumping. *Ann Thorac Surg* 1973; 16:445-453.

17. Powell WJ Jr., Daggett WM, Magro AE, et al. Effects of intra-aortic balloon counterpulsation on cardiac performance, oxygen consumption, and coronary blood flow in dogs. *Circ Res* 1970; 26:753-764.

18. Port SC, Patel S, Schmidt DH. Effects of intra-aortic balloon counterpulsation on myocardial blood flow in patients with severe coronary artery disease. *J Am Coll Cardiol* 1984; 3:1367-1374.

19. Williams DO, Korr KS, Gewirtz H, et al. The effect of intra-aortic balloon counterpulsation on regional myocardial blood flow and oxygen consumption in the presence of coronary artery stenosis in patients with unstable angina. *Circulation* 1982; 66:593-597.

20. MacDonald RG, Hill JA, Feldman RL. Failure of intra-aortic balloon counterpulsation to augment distal coronary perfusion pressure during percutaneous transluminal coronary angioplasty. *Am J Cardiol* 1987; 59:359-361.

21. Goldberg MJ, Rubenfire M, Kantrowitz A, et al. Intra-aortic balloon pump insertion: A randomized study comparing percutaneous and surgical techniques. *J Am Coll Cardiol* 1987; 9:515-523.

22. Sanders KM, Stern TA. Management of delirium associated with the use of the intra-aortic balloon pump. *Am J Crit Care* 1993; 2:371-377.

23. McCabe JC, Abel RM, Subramanian VA, et al. Complications of intra-aortic balloon insertion and counterpulsation. *Circulation* 1978; 57:769-773.

24. Kantrowitz A, Wasfie T, Freed PS, et al. Intra-aortic balloon pumping 1967 through 1982: Analysis of complications in 733 patients. *Am J Cardiol* 1986; 57:976-983.

25. Alderman JD, Gabliani GI, McCabe CH, et al. Incidence and management of limb ischemia with percutaneous wire guided intraaortic balloon catheters. *J Am Coll Cardiol* 1987; 9:524-530.

26. Collier PE, Liebler GA, Park SB, et al. Is percutaneous insertion of the intra-aortic balloon pump through the femoral artery the safest technique? *J Vasc Surg* 1986; 3:629-634.

27. Anderson RD, Ohman EM, Holmes DR, et al. Use of intraaortic balloon counterpulsation in patients presenting with cardiogenic shock: Observations from the GUSTO-1 study. *J Am Coll Cardiol* 1997; 30:708-715.

28. Stone GW, Marsalese D, Brodie BR, et al. A prospective, randomized evaluation of prophylactic intraaortic balloon counterpulsation in high risk patients with acute myocardial infarction treated with primary angioplasty. *J Am Coll Cardiol* 1997; 29:1459-1467.

29. Nash IS, Lorell BH, Fishman BF, et al. A new technique for sheathless percutaneous intra-aortic balloon catheter insertion. *Cathet Cardiovasc Diag* 1991; 23:57-60.

30. Gottlieb SO, Brinker JA, Borkon MA, et al. Identification of patients at high risk for complications of intra-aortic balloon counterpulsation: A multivariate risk factor analysis. *Am J Cardiol* 1984; 53:1135-1139.

31. Wasfie T, Freed PS, Rubenfire M, et al. Risks associated with intra-aortic balloon pumping in patients with and without diabetes mellitus. *Am J Cardiol* 1988; 61:558-562.

32. O'Rourke MF, Norris RM, Campbell TJ, et al. Randomized controlled trial of intraaortic counterpulsation in early myocardial infarction with acute heart failure. *Am J Cardiol* 1981; 47:815-820.

33. Flaherty JT, Becker LC, Weiss JL, et al. Results of a randomized prospective trial of intra-aortic balloon counterpulsation and intravenous nitroglycerine in patients with acute myocardial infarction. *J Am Coll Cardiol* 1985; 6:434-446.

34. Leinbach RC, Dinsmore RE, Mundth ED, et al. Selective coronary and left ventricular cineangiography during intra-aortic balloon pumping for cardiogenic shock. *Circulation* 1972; 45:845-852.

35. Bardet J, Masquet C, Kahn JC, et al. Clinical and hemodynamic results of intra-aortic balloon counterpulsation and surgery for cardiogenic shock. *Am Heart J* 1977; 93:280-288.

36. Beckman CB, Geha AS, Hammond GL, et al. Results and complications of intra-aortic balloon counterpulsation. *Ann Thorac Surg* 1977; 24:550-559.

37. Hagemeijer F, Laid JD, Haalebos MP, et al. Effectiveness of intra-aortic balloon pumping without cardiac surgery for patients with severe heart failure secondary to recent myocardial infarction. *Am J Cardiol* 1977; 40:951-956.

38. Jackson G, Cullum P, Pastellopoulos A, et al. Intra-aortic balloon assistance in cardiogenic shock after myocardial infarction or cardiac surgery. *Br Heart J* 1977; 39:598-604.

39. Johnson SA, Scanlon PJ, Loeb HS, et al. Treatment of cardiogenic shock in myocardial infarction by intra-aortic balloon counterpulsation and surgery. *Am J Med* 1977; 62:687-692.

40. Forssell G, Nordlander R. Nyquist O, et al. Intra-aortic balloon pumping in the treatment of cardiogenic shock complicating acute myocardial infarction. *Acta Med Scand* 1979; 206:189-194.

41. O'Rourke MF, Norris RM, Chang VP. Arterial counterpulsation in severe refractory heart failure complicating acute myocardial infarction. *Br Heart J* 1979; 41:308-313.

42. DeWood MA, Notske RN, Hensley GR, et al. Intra-aortic balloon counterpulsation with and without reperfusion for myocardial infarction shock. *Circulation* 1980; 61:1105-1112.

43. Pierri MK, Zema M, Kligfield P, et al. Exercise tolerance in late survivors of balloon pumping and surgery for cardiogenic shock. *Circulation* 1980; 62(Suppl I):138-141.

44. Goldberger M, Tabak SW, Shah PK. Clinical experience with intra-aortic balloon counterpulsation in 112 consecutive patients. *Am Heart J* 1986; 111:497-502.

45. Bengston JR, Kaplan AJ, Pieper KS, et al. Prognosis in cardiogenic shock after acute myocardial infarction in the interventional era. *J Am Coll Cardiol* 1992;20:1482-1489.

46. Waksman R, Weiss AT, Gotsman MS, et al. Intra-aortic balloon counterpulsation improves survival in cardiogenic shock complicating acute myocardial infarction. *Eur Heart J* 1993; 14:71-74.

47. Stomel RJ, Rasak M, Bates ER. Treatment strategies for acute myocardial infarction complicated by cardiogenic shock in a community hospital. *Chest* 1994; 105:997-1002.

48. Kovack PJ, Rasak MA, Bates ER, et al. Thrombolysis plus aortic counterpulsation: Improved survival in patients who present to community hospitals with cardiogenic shock. *J Am Coll Cardiol* 1997; 29:1454-1458.

49. Hochman JS, Boland J, Sleeper LA, et al. Current spectrum of cardiogenic shock and effect of early revascularization on mortality: Results of an international registry. *Circulation* 1995; 91:873-881.

50. Becker RC. Hemodynamic, mechanical, and metabolic determinants of thrombolytic efficacy: A theoretic framework for assessing the limitations of thrombolysis in patients with cardiogenic shock. *Am Heart J* 1993; 125:919-928.

51. Prewitt RM, Gu S, Garber PJ, et al. Marked systemic hypotension depresses thrombolysis induced by intracoronary administration of recombinant tissue-type plasminogen activator. *J Am Coll Cardiol* 1992; 20:1626-1633.

52. Prewitt RM, Gu S, Schick U, et al. Intraaortic balloon counterpulsation enhances coronary thrombolysis induced by intravenous administration of a thrombolytic agent. *J Am Coll Cardiol* 1994; 23:794-798.

53. Gurbel PA, Anderson RD, MacCord CS, et al. Arterial diastolic pressure augmentation by intra-aortic balloon counterpulsation enhances the onset of coronary artery reperfusion by thrombolytic therapy. *Circulation* 1994; 89:361-365.

54. Silverman AJ, Williams AM, Wetmore RW, et al. Complications of intraaortic balloon counterpulsation insertion in patients with thrombolytic therapy from acute myocardial infarction. *J Invas Cardiol* 1991; 4:49-52.

55. Ohman EM, Califf RM, George BS et al. The use of intraaortic balloon pumping as an adjunct to reperfusion therapy in acute myocardial infarction. *Am Heart J* 1991; 121:895-901.

56. Ohman EM, George BS, White CJ, et al. Use of aortic counterpulsation to improve sustained coronary artery patency during acute myocardial infarction. *Circulation* 1994; 90:792-799.

57. Col NF, Gurwitz JH, Alpert JS, et al. Frequency of inclusion of patients with cardiogenic shock in trials of thrombolytic therapy. *Am J Cardiol* 1994; 73:149-157

58. Holmes DR, Bates ER, Kleiman NS, et al. Contemporary reperfusion therapy for cardiogenic shock: The GUSTO-I trial experience. *J Am Coll Cardiol* 1995; 26:668-674.

59. Holmes DR, Califf RM, Van de Werf F, et al. Difference in countries' use of resources and clinical outcome for patients with cardiogenic shock after myocardial infarction: Results from the GUSTO trial. *Lancet* 1997; 349:75-78.

60. Barron HV, Every NR, Parsons LS, et al. The use of intra-aortic balloon counterpulsation in patients with cardiogenic shock complicating acute myocardial infarction: Data from the National Registry of Myocardial Infarction 2. *Am Heart J* 2001; 141:933-939

61. Hochman JS, Sleeper LA, Webb JG, et al. Early revascularization in acute myocardial infarction complicated by cardiogenic shock. *N Engl J Med* 1999; 341:625-634.

62. French JK, Miller JK, Palmieri S, et al. Cardiogenic shock treated with thrombolytic therapy and intra-aortic balloon counterpulsation(abstract). *Circulation* 1999; 100(suppl): I-370.

63. Sanborn TA, Sleeper LA, Bates ER, et al. Impact of thrombolysis, intra-aortic balloon pump counterpulsation, and their combination in cardiogenic shock complicating acute myocardial infarction: A report from the SHOCK trial registry. *J Am Coll Cardiol* 2000; 36:1123-1129.

64. Ohman EM, Nannas J, Stomel RJ, et al. Thrombolysis and counterpulsation to improve cardiogenic shock survival (TACTICS): Results of a prospective randomized trial(abstract). *Circulation* 2000;102(suppl): II-600.

65. Stone GW. Primary PTCA in high risk patients with acute myocardial infarction. *J Invas Cardiol* 1997;(suppl. F):12F-21F.

66. Brodie BR, Studkey TD, Hansen C, et al. Intra-aortic balloon counterpulsation before primary percutaneous transluminal coronary angioplasty reduces catheterization laboratory events in high-risk patients with acute myocardial infarction. *Am J Cardiol* 1999; 84:18-23.

67. van't Hof AWJ, Liem AL, deBoer MJ, et al. A randomized comparison of intra-aortic balloon pumping after primary coronary angioplasty in high risk patients with acute myocardial infarction. *Eur Heart J* 1999; 20:659-665.

Chapter 6

Coronary Artery Bypass Grafting for Cardiogenic Shock

Verdi J. DiSesa, MD, Manisha A. Patel, MD, and Steven M. Hollenberg, MD

Introduction

Although there have been advances in the treatment of acute myocardial infarction (MI), complications such as cardiogenic shock still occur.[1] Cardiogenic shock in the setting of acute MI carries a very high morbidity and mortality, and, in hospitalized patients, is the most common cause of death.[2-6] These high mortality rates have changed very little when conservative management strategies are used.[1] For example, patients treated with thrombolytics have lower rates of development of cardiogenic shock, but once shock has been established, mortality rates remain unchanged with fibrinolytic therapy.[7] More aggressive application of invasive management in acute MI has tended to improve outcome. Invasive strategies such as angioplasty, coronary artery bypass grafting (CABG), infarctectomy, repair of free wall rupture and ventricular septal defect, and repair of mitral insufficiency have all been used.[8] Effective management of the subset of patients with cardiogenic shock requires a rapid, well-organized approach and appropriate application of high-risk therapies.[9,10] The optimal form of treatment continues to be a controversial issue.[11] The following discussion will attempt to elucidate the current role of CABG in the management of this challenging patient population.

Mechanisms of Cardiogenic Shock

Cardiogenic shock can be defined as circulatory failure resulting in inability of the heart to deliver sufficient oxygen to the peripheral tissues

From: Hollenberg SM, Bates ER. *Cardiogenic Shock.* Armonk, NY: Futura Publishing Co., Inc.; ©2002.

to meet metabolic demand, in spite of adequate volume status.[12,13] In this clinical situation, the diagnosis may be suggested by hypotension with systolic pressure below 90 mm Hg or values 30 mm Hg below baseline for more than 30 minutes, with oliguria, peripheral vasoconstriction with acrocyanosis, and mental status changes manifested as agitation or obtundation. Cardiac index less than 2.2 L/min/m^2, an elevated arteriovenous oxygen difference of more than 5.5 mL/dL, and pulmonary artery wedge pressure of more than 15 mm Hg confirm the diagnosis.

In the setting of acute MI, cardiogenic shock can be caused by various mechanisms.[6,12,14] Mechanical reasons include left ventricular (LV) muscle loss with pump failure, ventricular septal defect with left-to-right shunt, acute mitral regurgitation with elevated pulmonary venous pressures, or cardiac rupture resulting in pericardial tamponade, all of which clearly reduce LV function and cardiac output to levels inadequate for support of end-organ perfusion. In addition, right ventricular infarction can produce the same symptoms. The most prevalent cause of cardiogenic shock, however, is LV dysfunction, which will be the focus of this discussion.

Pathophysiology

In 1957, an experimental animal model of coronary occlusion by embolization clearly illustrated the relationship between infarction and cardiogenic shock, which occurred in one-sixth of animals.[15] Autopsy studies, first in animals and then in humans, demonstrated cardiogenic shock to be related to loss of 40% of ventricular myocardial function.[16,17] Hamarayan et al.[18] published a quantitative study of infarcted myocardium in 20 patients who died of cardiogenic shock, in which the total ventricular infarcted area ranged from 20% to 72% (mean 43%); more than 30% of the total LV mass was involved in all but one patient. This was confirmed in an autopsy study by Page et al.,[19] in which the ventricles of patients who died of MI, 20 with cardiogenic shock and 14 without, were studied. Histopathology determined that the group with cardiogenic shock lost 40% to 70% of LV tissue and those without shock, less than 30%. A similar study by Alonso et al.[20] in the same types of patients found comparable results, with mean LV damage of 51% in patients with cardiogenic shock versus 23% in those without shock.

Pathologic examination of the ischemic myocardium also shows a rim of tissue at the lateral margins of the infarct which undergoes necrosis after the acute event. Although this may not account for a significant amount of contractile tissue, revascularization and therefore salvage of stunned or jeopardized viable myocardium has been shown to play a role in limiting extension of the infarct to optimally preserve myocardial function.[12]

The clinical course of cardiogenic shock is one of progressive deterioration, if timely intervention is not made. The physiologic response begins with compensatory mechanisms involving sympathetic stimulation, the kidneys, and local vasoregulation. The first measurable changes include an autonomically induced increased heart rate and vasoconstriction accompanied by an increase in contractility of viable myocardium. This is coupled with activation of the renin-angiotensin system by decreased renal perfusion as well as by autonomic stimulation, leading to fluid retention and increased intravascular volume. An increase in antidiuretic hormone production also occurs in response to hypotension, which further accentuates fluid retention by the kidney. Selective vasoconstriction then redistributes this increased volume preferentially to key end-organs, such as the brain and heart. In spite of compensatory mechanisms, decreased coronary perfusion pressure further contributes to myocardial depression. Of course, this is accentuated in patients with multivessel coronary artery disease, where lower coronary perfusion pressure also decreases flow to both normal and infarcted areas, potentiating the ischemia and loss of contractile function. The progression of cardiac dysfunction eventually overwhelms the peripheral compensation and results in shock.[10,12]

IABP Support

In the early 1970s, counterpulsation was used in humans in the setting of cardiogenic shock. Dunkman et al.[17] studied 40 patients with MI and cardiogenic shock and documented that the intra-aortic balloon pump (IABP) produced beneficial hemodynamic effects at the time of initial placement, with peak improvement at 25 hours. The difficulty was found in successfully weaning patients from IABP and maintaining adequate hemodynamic status after removal of the device. Of the 40 enrolled patients, 25 were treated with IABP alone, and only four survived. Of the 15 who underwent CABG in addition to IABP, there were six survivors. In 1980, Subramanian et al.[21] investigated outcome in patients with cardiogenic shock following acute MI. Sixty-seven subjects were evaluated and treated with IABP counterpulsation, cardiac catheterization and cardiac surgery where appropriate. In eight, the IABP could not be placed, and all died within 12 hours of admission; another 12 were moribund and died within 2 hours. Of the 47 who underwent angiography, 34 were operated on, with six survivors. There was only one survivor out of the 13 who were not revascularized surgically.

Johnson et al.[22] studied 18 patients in shock from acute MI who were treated with IABP but without surgery and compared them to a second cohort of 19 patients who underwent surgical revascularization. The survival rates were comparable, 44% versus 42%, although the interval between infarction and surgery was highly variable, ranging from 2.5 hours up to 60 days. It became clear that the IABP, by decreasing afterload and increasing coronary perfusion, provided a means of temporary stabilization of these patients.[17,23,24] However, the inability to wean patients from the device led to further examination of the role of surgery.

Surgical Intervention

Early Reports

The early 1970s brought numerous accounts of salvage of patients in shock by submitting them for emergency CABG, in some cases combined with infarctectomy.[25-29] Resection of infarcts had been documented as beneficial in canine animal models. Glass et al.[28] studied 40 dogs in which coronary arteries were ligated, cardiac output measured until cardiac arrest or hemodynamics incompatible with life were documented, and then cardiopulmonary bypass was instituted and the infarct resected. There were 18 long-term survivors. Clinical application was quick to follow.

Najafi et al.[25] reported a series of 6 patients, all in cardiogenic shock, who underwent emergency resection of LV aneurysms and infarctectomy with only one operative mortality. Concurrently, Schimert et al.[26] reported operations on five groups of patients: those with localized LV akinesis requiring resection; infarct and papillary muscle dysfunction leading to infarct resection coupled with mitral valve replacement; anteroseptal infarct with ventricular septal defect requiring infarctectomy and defect closure; isolated papillary muscle rupture leading to mitral valve replacement; and early coronary occlusion requiring thrombectomy. They observed four deaths, three intraoperative and one at 48 hours postoperatively, out of a total of 24 patients. Review of the literature supported survival rates for surgically treated patients to be 60% to 70%.[17,23,29,30]

Scott et al.[31] analyzed 69 patients who received IABP support for cardiogenic shock in the setting of acute MI. Twenty-nine of these underwent surgical revascularization, with a survival rate of 59%. Bolooki's review[8] of published experience over a 20-year period indicated that 66% of patients survived after emergency revascularization for acute MI with shock.

DeWood et al.[32] studied 40 patients with shock due to acute MI. Twenty-one were treated with medical therapies including IABP, and 19 also underwent CABG. The in-hospital mortality rate was highest for the nonoperated group (52.4% vs. 42.1%). In addition, it was noted that the subset of patients who were revascularized within 16 hours had the lowest mortality.

Timing of Surgery

The timing of surgery, however, remained controversial. Hill et al.[33] studied patients with impending and acute MIs and found a lower mortality rate for those undergoing surgery prior to an acute infarct compared to those undergoing CABG during an acute ischemic event. It was proposed by some that operation within hours of the infarction was beneficial due to the response of the myocardium to restored perfusion, obviating the need for resection of infarcted tissue.[22,33-37] Others proposed that revascularization be delayed for 10-28 days to avoid reperfusion effects such as hemorrhagic necrosis and to allow demarcation of the infarct for subsequent resection.[29,38,39] Animal models of infarction and reperfusion were used to help resolve this issue.[35] Maroko et al.[34] used a canine model of left anterior descending artery occlusion followed by reperfusion after 3 hours. Animals were euthanized at 24 hours and histological confirmation of infarction was obtained. The control group, which did not undergo reperfusion, showed abnormal histological features in 97% of tissue, compared to only 43% in the group that underwent reperfusion.

With the salutory effects of myocardial reperfusion documented in animals, the clinical correlate was then further defined. The benefit of emergency revascularization in the setting of acute MI was studied by Cohn et al.,[37] who presented a series of eight such patients without operative or late deaths and with no significant complications. These findings were supported by Sustaita et al.[39] in a study of 20 patients undergoing emergency CABG for impending or acute MI with or without cardiogenic shock. The study documented 19 survivors, 16 of whom were free of angina. Johnson et al.[22] studied 37 patients with acute MI and shock, 18 treated with IABP alone, 19 treated with surgery. The time from infarct to surgery ranged from 2.5 hours to 60 days. There was a trend towards improved survival and better functional outcome for those patients undergoing early revascularization.

Therefore, further investigations were undertaken in the early 1980s to clarify the optimal timing of surgery. Subramanian et al.[21] followed patients with cardiogenic shock after acute MI who were treated with IABP stabilization and then emergency CABG and correction of mechanical problems such as ventricular septal defects and mitral insufficiency performed within 2-3 hours. Of note, akinetic segments were not bypassed to avoid producing reperfusion hemorrhagic necrosis. Sixteen of the 34 patients who were operated on survived to 22 months. This 47% survival rate was comparable to that found in several other surgical studies.[23,40]

Late Survival Rates

Late survival rates were further examined by DeWood et al.,[32] who compared patients treated with aortic counterpulsation and patients who underwent emergency surgical revascularization with placement of an IABP intraoperatively and continued for 48 hours postoperatively. Although there was no significant difference in early mortality (42% in medical vs. 52.4% in surgical patients) there was a divergence in long-term survival favoring those treated surgically (28.6% vs. 52.7%). Interestingly, among the surgical patients, the lowest mortality rate, 25%, was observed in those treated within 16 hours of the onset of infarction, whereas those operated on after 18 hours had a 71.4% mortality rate.

Alternatives to Surgical Reperfusion

Before 1980, surgery had been the only means of reperfusion. The development of fibrinolytic therapy and angioplasty offered the possibility of nonsurgical interventions which could produce reperfusion and effectively interrupt myocardial necrosis.[30,41,42] Fibrinolytics were shown to improve infarct artery patency in the Thrombolysis in Myocardial Infarction (TIMI) trial in 1985,[43] and to improve survival in MI in the Gruppo Italiano per lo Studio della Streptochinasi nell' Infarto Miocardico

(GISSI) trial in 1986,[44] and the International Study of Infarct Survival (ISIS-2) trial in 1988.[45] Fibrinolytics also were shown in several randomized trials to prevent the development of cardiogenic shock.[46,47] Despite these encouraging findings in patients presenting with acute MI, fibrinolytics alone did not decrease mortality significantly in the population with cardiogenic shock.[44,46-48]

Further work was undertaken to determine the effects of early aggressive treatment on survival. An analysis of the Global Utilization of Streptokinase and Tissue Plasminogen Activator for Occluded Coronary Arteries (GUSTO-I) trial examined patients with acute MI complicated by cardiogenic shock to ascertain the impact of early angiography, angioplasty, or surgery on survival.[11] Of the group treated with an aggressive strategy (n = 406), 63% underwent revascularization within 24 hours of angiography. Angioplasty was performed in 43%, CABG in 14%, and both procedures in 5%. Thirty-day mortality was significantly lower in the group undergoing aggressive early interventions (38% vs. 62%, p = 0.0001). This trend continued at 1 year (44.2% vs. 66.4% respectively, p = 0.001).[11]

The issue of whether catheter interventional or surgical reperfusion was more beneficial remained unclear. Phillips et al.[49] studied three groups of patients with evolving MI treated with streptokinase, streptokinase and angioplasty, and surgery. Analysis of those who developed shock, who accounted for 11%, revealed that 72% were treated surgically with a 38% mortality rate; the remainder were treated with combinations of fibrinolytics and angioplasty. Other studies compared patients in shock treated with fibrinolytics alone to patients who underwent placement of an IABP as well as revascularization either with angioplasty or CABG.[50] Revascularized patients, whether by interventional or surgical means, had a significantly increased survival, which was increased further by timely and aggressive intervention.[51]

Recent Reports

With the availability of fibrinolytics and angioplasty, surgery became relegated to those patients who had contraindications for these procedures or those who failed the initial interventional efforts, frequently because of the presence of severe multivessel disease. Given these selection criteria, it is not surprising that major surgical complication rates were high. Guyton et al.[52] found that 17 of 69 patients undergoing emergency CABG were in shock and that four required cardiopulmonary resuscitation. After operation, 94% needed inotropic drugs and 71% had ongoing IABP support. Twelve percent died in-hospital and major complications occurred in 47%. It should be noted that a 3-year survival of 88% was documented.

Santoro et al.[14] recently reviewed the major randomized trials that included surgery. They concluded that it was likely that the promising long-term results were attributable to the beneficial effects of reperfused sites remote from the infarct area improving compensatory function of noninfarcted myocardium, or to cardiopulmonary bypass, ventricular decompression, and administration of cardioplegic solutions reducing the injurious effects of reperfusion. Buckberg and colleagues[53] examined the optimal approach to myocardial protection during surgery for patients in cardiogenic shock. Their strategy included total vented bypass to prevent further damage from wall tension, gentle reperfusion to reduce postischemic edema, and a beating empty state period of 30 minutes following removal of the aortic cross clamp to avoid premature high energy demands on the myocardium. In addition, the largest areas of remote functioning muscle were grafted first to maximize protection of the LV mass responsible for maintaining the cardiac output.

Alternatives to Surgery

Alternatives such as emergency percutaneous cardiopulmonary bypass-supported high-risk angioplasty have been attempted.[54-56] In one such study,[54] eight patients in cardiogenic shock were placed on percutaneous cardiopulmonary bypass as a means to facilitate complex angioplasty. However, no comparisons were made to alternate means of stabilization such as IABP and no significant outcome data were generated. Although the procedure was less invasive and initial survival rates appeared promising, the studies to date have been unrandomized and underpowered and the technique has not gained wide acceptance.

Published series of patients undergoing surgery for cardiogenic shock have suggested lower mortality rates than for catheter interventional approaches. However, since all studies have been nonrandomized thus far, selection bias sets limitations on the interpretation of the data, and the optimal strategy is not well defined.[57]

An international registry was established from 1992-1993 to examine the spectrum of cardiogenic shock, the proportion of patients who were candidates for early revascularization, and the impact of early revascularization.[6] Two hundred thirty-one patients with shock complicating acute MI were registered, of which 58% underwent angiography. Fibrinolytics were administered to 42%, 26% went on to angioplasty, and 8% to bypass surgery. Overall mortality was 66%, 51% for those undergoing cardiac catheterization and 85% for those who did not. The mortality rate for patients undergoing revascularization was 51%. The heterogeneity of the patient population and the small number of patients undergoing coronary artery bypass for shock made it difficult to draw conclusions about the role of surgery. It was clear that employment of invasive strategies was increasing and was associated with improved survival but further randomized trials were needed to delineate the role of each treatment option.[12,58]

The SHOCK Trial

A step toward clarification of the role of surgery came with the Should We Emergently Revascularize Occluded Coronaries for Cardiogenic Shock

(SHOCK) investigation, a multicenter, randomized, unblinded trial that enrolled patients from 1993-1998.[59] Patients who presented within 36 hours of the development of cardiogenic shock in acute MI were randomized to emergency revascularization, with angiography within 6 hours of randomization, followed by angioplasty or CABG depending on coronary anatomy, or medical treatment using IABP and fibrinolytics where indicated. These patients underwent delayed revascularization if clinically warranted at a minimum of 54 hours after randomization. The primary endpoint was 30-day mortality. Secondary endpoints were 6- and 12-month mortality.[59]

This landmark study clarified many aspects of the pathophysiology and the optimal management of cardiogenic shock, including not only revascularization, but also the timing of shock after MI, resultant pulmonary congestion, associated ECG changes, incidence of diabetes, and occurrence of mechanical complications such as mitral insufficiency, ventricular septal defect, and free wall rupture. Of 1492 patients screened for inclusion in the study, 302 were randomized: 152 assigned to revascularization and 150 to medical therapy. The median time between onset of infarction and shock was 5.6 hours. The two treatment groups were comparable except that more patients in the medical group had undergone previous CABG (10% vs. 2%, p = 0.003). Of the patients assigned to revascularization, 64% underwent angioplasty and 36% had bypass surgery at a median of 14 hours after onset of infarction. Comparison of the surgical and angioplasty groups showed that surgical patients were more likely to have left main disease (40% vs. 14%, p < 0.001) and three-vessel disease (79% vs. 60%, p = 0.008).[59]

The 30-day mortality rates for the revascularization and medical treatment groups were 46.7% and 56.0% (p = 0.11).[59] In the revascularization group, 30-day mortality for the patients having angioplasty was 45.3% and 42.1% for those having surgery. Mortality at 6 months was lower in the revascularization group (50.3% vs. 63.1%, p = 0.027), a trend which continued at 12 months. Although there was no significant difference in mortality at 30 days, there was clearly a survival benefit from early revascularization observed at 6 months and beyond.[59,60]

Surgical Strategies

Myocardial Protection

Efforts toward reducing further perioperative myocardial damage are clearly important in the patient population with acute MI and cardiogenic shock. The composition and administration of cardioplegia plays a critical role and is directed towards producing prompt arrest and lowering the metabolic rate to lower energy demands, maintaining substrate availability for ongoing energy needs, and limiting reperfusion injury. Blood cardioplegia offers the advantage of an oxygenated solution and can be incorporated into an operative strategy such as that outlined by Buckberg et al.[61] for patients with cardiogenic shock. This begins with warm blood cardioplegia induction and uses substrate enrichment with glutamine and aspartate. The operative plan then involves grafting viable areas of myocardium first, since the infarcted muscle does not regain contractility immediately even if reperfused. Those arteries with the largest distribution are grafted first, progressing to those with smaller territories and finally the infarct artery. Multidose cold blood cardioplegia is given periodically throughout the procedure. Route of administration can be antegrade or retrograde and, in addition, should be given down the grafts. Finally, warm blood cardioplegia is given and the grafts are perfused while performing the proximal anastomoses. In addition to optimal cardioplegic protection, oxygen demands are minimized by keeping the left ventricle well decompressed, for example by using a superior pulmonary vein vent. An operative strategy such as this has been shown to result in faster recovery of left ventricular performance even in the setting of acute MI and cardiogenic shock.[61-63]

Off-Pump Surgery

CABG on a beating heart has been successfully performed in the emergency setting. Though experience is limited as yet, initial results by Hirose et al.[64] show a significantly shorter recovery period (11.5 vs. 21.8 ± 14.9 days) compared with patients undergoing conventional emergency CABG with cardiopulmonary bypass (CPB). Locker et al.[65] evaluated patients undergoing emergency CABG within 48 hours of acute MI, 37 operated on with CPB, 40 without. Forty-six percent of those on CPB and 38% of the off-pump patients were in cardiogenic shock. Results showed the mean number of grafts to be 3 in the CPB group and 1.9 in the off-pump group ($p < 0.0001$). Mortality was 24% in the CPB group and only 5% in the off-pump group, ($p = 0.015$). However, 6- to 66-month follow-up revealed late mortality of 0% in the CPB group and 22% in the off-pump group ($p < 0.0066$), recurrent angina of 0% versus 15% ($p = 0.04$), and reintervention rate of 0% versus 15% ($p=0.04$). Thus, off-pump CABG in the setting of cardiogenic shock is feasible, but appears to be best utilized only if a complete revascularization with good anastomoses can be performed.

Choice of Conduit

The long-term patency benefits of arterial grafts have been well established. However, in the emergency setting the choice of bypass conduit must take other factors into consideration, such as the length of time required for conduit harvesting and the stability of the patient. There are proponents of complete arterial revascularization in the emergency setting[66] who have had good results, with no late deaths or need for redo CABG. Conduits for complete arterial revascularization could be harvested with the patient on cardiopulmonary bypass if unstable, but this is unlikely to gain wide acceptance. The use of the internal mammary artery (IMA) itself in patients undergoing emergency CABG has not produced a higher in-hospital mortality[67] or a significant difference in outcome at 1 year.[68] The postoperative course for patients with IMA grafts and those with saphenous vein grafts was not found to be significantly different, with similar rates of reexploration, perioperative MI, wound infection, respiratory complications and stroke.[69] However, patients with IMA grafts had fewer cardiac deaths, (2.7% vs. 9.4%, p < 0.01).[69] No separate analysis of patients in cardiogenic shock has been performed. It would therefore seem justifiable to use the most conveniently obtained conduit (typically saphenous vein) for a patient in frank cardiogenic shock or to take the IMA down while on CPB if the patient is stable.

Perioperative Support

For the patient in cardiogenic shock, the merits of inotropic support and aortic counterpulsation in the perioperative period have already been well documented. Additional consideration should be given to the use of ventricular assist devices for post cardiotomy low output syndrome. In this setting, the intended duration of support would be a few days, as bridge to recovery.[70] A series by Noon et al. examined 141 patients with post cardiotomy failure. Fifty-four percent were successfully weaned from the assist device, however, only 22% survived to discharge.[71]

Conclusions

Reperfusion of ischemic myocardium in patients with acute MI and cardiogenic shock is related to the ultimate outcome. At present, it is clear that revascularization by interventional or surgical means achieves reperfusion more effectively than more conservative medical management. It is also evident that patients with acute MI and cardiogenic shock benefit from initial attempts at medical stabilization, including IABP if necessary, followed by catheter based interventions aimed at improving patency of the infarct-related artery. Emergency bypass surgery for patients in shock remains a high-risk endeavor, yet some patients cannot be adequately treated acutely without surgery. At the present state of our knowledge, bypass surgery appears to be most prudently applied to four sets of patients in shock: (1) patients with contraindications to fibrinolytics and angioplasty (2) patients whose infarct vessel cannot be opened by catheter-based interventions (3) patients with hemodynamic instability and ischemia despite medical and catheter-based therapies (4) patients with ongoing instability and coronary anatomy better suited to surgery such as left main or severe three-vessel disease. These conclusions are supported by the American College of Cardiology and American Heart Association guidelines for acute MI management.[72,73] Advances in surgical therapy now make this approach more feasible in properly selected patients. Since the benefits of early revascularization on myocardial salvage are different from the late effects on ventricular remodeling, the optimal timing of surgical revascularization procedures still needs clarification and will require further randomized clinical trials.

References

1. Goldberg RJ, Gore JM, Alpert JS, et al. Cardiogenic shock after acute myocardial infarction. Incidence and mortality from a community-wide perspective, 1975 to 1988. *N Engl J Med* 1991; 325:1117-1122.
2. Scheidt S, Ascheim R, Killip T. Shock after acute myocardial infarction. A clinical and hemodynamic profile. *Am J Cardiol* 1970; 26:556-564.
3. Killip T, Kimball JT. Treatment of myocardial infarction in a coronary care unit. A two year experience with 250 patients. *Am J Cardiol* 1967; 20:457-464.
4. Gunnar R, Loeb HS, Rahimtoola SH. Hemodynamic studies in shock with myocardial infarction. In: Gunnar RM, ed. Shock in Myocardial Infarction. New York: Grune and Stratton, 1974:113-127.
5. Brodie B, Stuckey T, Weintraub R, et al. Timing and mechanism of death after direct angioplasty for acute myocardial infarction. *Am Coll Cardiol* 1995; 25:295A-296A.
6. Hochman JS, Boland J, Sleeper LA, et al. Current spectrum of cardiogenic shock and effect of early revascularization on mortality. Results of an International Registry. *Circulation* 1995; 91:873-881.
7. Holmes DR, Jr., Bates ER, Kleiman NS, et al. Contemporary reperfusion therapy for cardiogenic shock: The GUSTO-I trial experience. *J Am Coll Cardiol* 1995; 26:668-674.
8. Bolooki H. Emergency cardiac procedures in patients in cardiogenic shock due to complications of coronary artery disease. *Circulation* 1989; 79:I137-I148.
9. Hollenberg SM, Kavinsky CJ, Parrillo JE. Cardiogenic shock. *Ann Intern Med* 1999; 131:47-59.
10. Califf RM, Bengtson JR. Cardiogenic shock. *N Engl J Med* 1994; 330:1724-1730.
11. Berger PB, Holmes DR, Jr., Stebbins AL, et al. Impact of an aggressive invasive catheterization and revascularization strategy on mortality in patients with cardiogenic shock in the Global Utilization of Streptokinase and Tissue Plasminogen Activator for Occluded Coronary Arteries (GUSTO-I) trial. An observational study. *Circulation* 1997; 96:122-127.
12. Barry WL, Sarembock IJ. Cardiogenic shock: Therapy and prevention. *Clin Cardiol* 1998; 21:72-80.
13. Dole WP, O'Rourke RA. Pathophysiology and management of cardiogenic shock. *Curr Probl Cardiol* 1983; 8:1-72.
14. Santoro GM, Buonamici P. Reperfusion therapy in cardiogenic shock complicating acute myocardial infarction. *Am Heart J* 1999; 138:S126-S131.
15. Agress C, Binder, JM. Cardiogenic Shock. *Am Heart J* 1957; 54:458-477.
16. Sugg WL, Webb WR, Ecker RR. Reduction of extent of myocardial infarction by counterpulsation. *Ann Thorac Surg* 1969; 7:310-316.
17. Dunkman WB, Leinbach RC, Buckley MJ, et al. Clinical and hemodynamic results of intraaortic balloon pumping and surgery for cardiogenic shock. *Circulation* 1972; 46:465-477.

18. Harnarayan C, Bennett MA, Pentecost BL, et al. Quantitative study of infarcted myocardium in cardiogenic shock. *Br Heart J* 1970; 32:728-732.

19. Page DL, Caulfield JB, Kaster JA, et al. Myocardial changes associated with cardiogenic shock. *N Engl J Med* 1971; 285:133-137.

20. Alonso DR, Scheidt S, Post M, et al. Pathophysiology of cardiogenic shock. Quantification of myocardial necrosis, clinical, pathologic and electrocardiographic correlations. *Circulation* 1973; 48:588-596.

21. Subramanian VA, Roberts AJ, Zema MJ, et al. Cardiogenic shock following acute myocardial infarction; late functional results after emergency cardiac surgery. *N Y State J Med* 1980; 80:947-952.

22. Johnson SA, Scanlon PJ, Loeb HS, et al. Treatment of cardiogenic shock in myocardial infarction by intraaortic balloon counterpulsation surgery. *Am J Med* 1977; 62:687-692.

23. Sanders CA, Buckley MJ, Leinbach RC, et al. Mechanical circulatory assistance. Current status and experience with combining circulatory assistance, emergency coronary angiography, and acute myocardial revascularization. *Circulation* 1972; 45:1292-1313.

24. Dilley RB, Ross J, Jr., Bernstein EF. Serial hemodynamics during intra-aortic balloon counterpulsation for cardiogenic shock. *Circulation* 1973; 48:III99-III104.

25. Najafi H, Hunter JA, Dye WS, et al. Emergency left ventricular aneurysmectomy for dying patients. *Ann Thorac Surg* 1970; 10:327-333.

26. Schimert G, Lajos TZ, Bunnell IL, et al. Operation for cardiac complications following myocardial infarction. *Surgery* 1970; 67:129-140.

27. Lillehei C, Lande AJ, Rassman WR, et al. Surgical managment of myocardial infarction. *Circulation* 1969; 39(suppl IV):315-335.

28. Glass BA, Carter RL, Albert HM, et al. Excision of myocardial infarcts. Experimental and clinical studies. *Arch Surg* 1968; 97:940-946.

29. Leinbach RC, Gold HK, Dinsomore RE, et al. The role of angiography in cardiogenic shock. *Circulation* 1973; 48:III95-III98.

30. DeWood MA, Spores J, Notske RN, et al. Medical and surgical management of myocardial infarction. *Am J Cardiol* 1979; 44:1356-1364.

31. Scott ML, Milam JR. Long term management of the intra aortic balloon pump dependent patient. *Angiology* 1983; 34:192-196.

32. DeWood MA, Notske RN, Hensley GR, et al. Intraaortic balloon counterpulsation with and without reperfusion for myocardial infarction shock. *Circulation* 1980; 61:1105-1112.

33. Hill JD, Kerth WJ, De Leval MR, et al. Myocardial infarction and preinfarction: Results of emergency myocardial revasularization. *J Cardiovasc Surg (Torino)* 1974; 15:205-208.

34. Maroko PR, Libby P, Ginks WR, et al. Coronary artery reperfusion. I. Early effects on local myocardial function and the extent of myocardial necrosis. *J Clin Invest* 1972; 51:2710-2716.

35. Ginks WR, Sybers HD, Maroko PR, et al. Coronary artery reperfusion. II. Reduction of myocardial infarct size at 1 week after the coronary occlusion. *J Clin Invest* 1972; 51:2717-2723.

36. Bresnahan GF, Roberts R, Shell WE, et al. Deleterious effects due to hemorrhage after myocardial reperfusion. *Am J Cardiol* 1974; 33:82-86.

37. Cohn LH, Gorlin R, Herman MV, et al. Aorto-coronary bypass for acute coronary occlusion. *J Thorac Cardiovasc Surg* 1972; 64:503-513.

38. Parmley WW, Chuck L, Kivowitz C, et al. In vitro length-tension relations of human ventricular aneurysms. Relation of stiffness to mechanical disadvantage. *Am J Cardiol* 1973; 32:889-894.

39. Sustaita H, Chatterjee K, Matloff JM, et al. Emergency bypass surgery in impending and complicated acute myocardial infarction. *Arch Surg* 1972; 105:30-35.

40. O'Rourke MF, Chang VP, Windsor HM, et al. Acute severe cardiac failure complicating myocardial infarction. Experience with 100 patients referred for consideration of mechanical left ventricular assistance. *Br Heart J* 1975; 37:169-181.

41. Phillips SJ, Kongtahworn C, Zeff RH, et al. Emergency coronary artery revascularization: A possible therapy for acute myocardial infarction. *Circulation* 1979; 60:241-246.

42. Phillips S, Zeff RH, Kongtahworn C. Emergency myocardial revascularization in acute myocardial infarction (abstract). *Asso Thorac Cardiovasc Surg Asia* 1976; 10:23.

43. TIMI Study Group. The thrombolysis in myocardial infarction (TIMI) trial. Phase I findings. *N Engl J Med* 1985; 312:932-936.

44. Gruppo Italiano per lo Studio Della Streptochinasi Nell'Infarto Miocardico (GISSI). Effectiveness of intravenous thrombolytic treatment in acute myocardial infarction. *Lancet* 1986; 2:397-402.

45. ISIS-2 Collaborative Group. Randomised trial of intravenous streptokinase, oral aspirin, both, or neither among 17 187 cases of suspected acute myocardial infarction: ISIS-2. *Lancet* 1988; 2:349-360.

46. AIMS Trial Study Group. Effect of intravenous APSAC on mortality after acute myocardial infarction: Preliminary report of a placebo-controlled clinical trial. *Lancet* 1988; 1:545-549.

47. Wilcox RG, von der Lippe G, Olsson CG, et al. Trial of tissue plasminogen activator for mortality reduction in acute myocardial infarction. Anglo-Scandinavian Study of Early Thrombolysis (ASSET). *Lancet* 1988; 2:525-530.

48. Yusuf S, Collins R, Peto R, et al. Intravenous and intracoronary fibrinolytic therapy in acute myocardial infarction: Overview of results on mortality, reinfarction and side- effects from 33 randomized controlled trials. *Eur Heart J* 1985; 6:556-585.

49. Phillips SJ, Kongtahworn C, Skinner JR, et al. Emergency coronary artery reperfusion: A choice therapy for evolving myocardial infarction. Results in 339 patients. *J Thorac Cardiovasc Surg* 1983; 86:679-688.

50. Stomel RJ, Rasak M, Bates ER. Treatment strategies for acute myocardial infarction complicated by cardiogenic shock in a community hospital. *Chest* 1994; 105:997-1002.

51. Berger PB, Tuttle RH, Holmes DR, Jr., et al. One-year survival among patients with acute myocardial infarction complicated by cardiogenic shock, and its relation to early revascularization: Results From the GUSTO-I Trial. *Circulation* 1999; 99:873-878.

52. Guyton RA, Arcidi JM, Jr., Langford DA, et al. Emergency coronary bypass for cardiogenic shock. *Circulation* 1987; 76:V22-27.

53. Beyersdorf F, Buckberg GD. Myocardial protection in patients with acute myocardial infarction and cardiogenic shock. *Semin Thorac Cardiovasc Surg* 1993; 5:151-161.

54. Shawl FA, Domanski MJ, Hernandez TJ, et al. Emergency percutaneous cardiopulmonary bypass support in cardiogenic shock from acute myocardial infarction. *Am J Cardiol* 1989; 64:967-970.

55. Shawl F, Domanski, MJ, Hernandez, TJ, et al. Percutaneous cardiopulmonary bypass to support high risk elective coronary angioplasty. *J Am Coll Cardiol* 1989; 13:160A.

56. Vogel RA, Tommaso CL, Gundry SR. Initial experience with coronary angioplasty and aortic valvuloplasty using elective semipercutaneous cardiopulmonary support. *Am J Cardiol* 1988; 62:811-813.

57. Domanski MJ, Topol EJ. Cardiogenic shock: Current understandings and future research directions. *Am J Cardiol* 1994; 74:724-726.

58. Dzavik V, Burton JR, Kee C, et al. Changing practice patterns in the management of acute myocardial infarction complicated by cardiogenic shock: Elderly compared with younger patients. *Can J Cardiol* 1998; 14:923-930.

59. Hochman JS, Sleeper LA, Webb JG, et al. Early revascularization in acute myocardial infarction complicated by cardiogenic shock. *N Engl J Med* 1999; 341:625-634.

60. Hochman JS, Sleeper LA, White HD, et al. One-year survival following early revascularization for cardiogenic shock. *JAMA* 2001; 285:190-192.

61. Buckberg G, Marelli, D. Myocardial protection. In: Kaiser L, Kron IL, Spray, TL (eds). Mastery of Cardiothoracic Surgery. Philadelphia: Lippincott-Raven, 1998.

62. Allen B, Buckberg GD. Myocardial protection managment during adult cardiac operations. In: Baue A, Geha, AS, Hammond, GI et al., (eds). Thoracic and Cardiovascular Surgery. New York: Appleton and Lange, 1995.

63. Rosenkranz ER, Buckberg GD, Laks H, et al. Warm induction of cardioplegia with glutamate-enriched blood in coronary patients with cardiogenic shock who are dependent on inotropic drugs and intra-aortic balloon support. *J Thorac Cardiovasc Surg* 1983; 86:507-518.

64. Hirose H, Amano A, Yoshida S, et al. Emergency off-pump coronary artery bypass grafting under a beating- heart. *Ann Thorac Cardiovasc Surg* 1999; 5:304-309.

65. Locker C, Shapira I, Paz Y, et al. Emergency myocardial revascularization for acute myocardial infarction: Survival benefits of avoiding cardiopulmonary bypass. *Eur J Cardiothorac Surg* 2000; 17:234-238.

66. Nishida H, Tomizawa Y, Endo M, et al. [Complete arterial revascularization in emergency CABG]. *Kyobu Geka* 1999; 52:688-692.

67. Yamagishi I, Sakurada T, Abe T. Emergency coronary artery bypass grafting after acute myocardial infarction. What influences early postoperative mortality? *Ann Thorac Cardiovasc Surg* 1998; 4:28-33.

68. Nollert G, Amend J, Reichart B. Use of the internal mammary artery as a graft in emergency coronary artery bypass grafting after failed PTCA. *Thorac Cardiovasc Surg* 1995; 43:142-147.

69. Zapolanski A, Pliam MB, Bronstein MH, et al. Arterial conduits in emergency coronary artery surgery. *J Card Surg* 1995; 10:32-39.

70. Tjan TD, Schmid C, Deng MC, et al. Evolving short-term and long-term mechanical assist for cardiac-failure -- a decade of experience in Munster. *Thorac Cardiovasc Surg* 1999; 47 Suppl 2:294-297.

71. Noon GP, Lafuente JA, Irwin S. Acute and temporary ventricular support with BioMedicus centrifugal pump. *Ann Thorac Surg* 1999; 68:650-654.

72. Ryan TJ, Anderson JL, Antman EM, et al. ACC/AHA guidelines for the management of patients with acute myocardial infarction. A report of the American College of Cardiology/American Heart Association Task Force on Practice Guidelines. *J Am Coll Cardiol* 1996; 28:1328-1428.

73. Ryan TJ, Antman EM, Brooks NH, et al. 1999 update: ACC/AHA Guidelines for the Management of Patients With Acute Myocardial Infarction: Executive Summary and Recommendations: A report of the American College of Cardiology/American Heart Association Task Force on Practice Guidelines (Committee on Management of Acute Myocardial Infarction). *Circulation* 1999; 100:1016-1030.

Chapter 7

Percutaneous Coronary Intervention in Cardiogenic Shock

Sandeep Nathan, MD and Lloyd W. Klein, MD

Introduction

Cardiogenic shock is a clinical syndrome characterized by severely depressed circulatory function with profound physiologic and metabolic derangements. Although it has been widely recognized for nearly a century as a feared complication of an acute or recent myocardial infarction (MI), the incidence of cardiogenic shock has changed little over this time, even though the incidence of many other major cardiovascular diagnoses, including acute MI, has continued to decline.[1-3] Moreover, the mortality rate remains unacceptably high, in the range of 40% to 80% in the 1990s, despite significant advances in both the understanding and treatment of ischemic heart disease. In fact, there is some evidence to suggest that in-hospital mortality actually rose slightly during this time period. In the Worcester Heart Attack study, which followed 4762 patients admitted to community medical centers with acute MI, mortality for cardiogenic shock was 74% in 1975, but rose to 82% at the end of the study period in 1988.[4]

Restoration of Thrombolysis in Myocardial Infarction (TIMI) grade III (i.e. angiographically normal) flow is attainable in greater than 90% of patients undergoing primary (direct) percutaneous transluminal coronary angioplasty (PTCA), in contrast to the 50% to 60% TIMI grade III flow rates achieved with thrombolytic therapy in eligible patients.[5-7] Of the available therapies for acute MI complicated by cardiogenic shock, expeditious reestablishment of flow in the infarct-related vessel via mechanical means should afford the greatest benefit. This theoretic benefit has been seen fairly consistently in observational and registry studies spanning

From: Hollenberg SM, Bates ER. *Cardiogenic Shock.* Armonk, NY: Futura Publishing Co., Inc.; ©2002.

nearly two decades, but only recently has it been tested in randomized clinical trials.

Historical Perspective

Over the past 25 years, PTCA has evolved from the technically difficult and somewhat cumbersome procedure initially performed by Andreas Gruentzig and colleagues, to encompass a family of sophisticated, interrelated technologies, referred to collectively as percutaneous coronary intervention (PCI). The historic first procedure, performed September 16, 1977 on a 38-year-old patient with a high-grade proximal left anterior descending artery (LAD) coronary stenosis and severe angina, was a resounding success. Despite the technical challenges associated with the bulky fixed-wire balloon apparatus and stiff Teflon guide catheters of the day, normal antegrade coronary flow was reestablished, with relief of the patient's angina and durable results even at 10-year angiographic follow-up. From these humble roots, the worldwide use of PCI has since grown exponentially, with more than 600,000 procedures performed in 1999 and proven utility in an ever-expanding range of clinical scenarios including unstable coronary syndromes and cardiogenic shock.[8]

Percutaneous coronary intervention in the setting of acute MI was first performed in November 1980 by Drs. Geoffrey Hartzler and Barry Rutherford at the Mid America Heart Institute in Kansas City, Missouri.[8] Although existing and emerging data also supported the use of intracoronary thrombolytic infusions and emergent coronary artery bypass grafting as potential strategies for myocardial salvage during acute MI, the initial success and low complication rate associated with percutaneous revascularization led to the adoption of this approach by Hartzler's group as the exclusive mode of infarct intervention at their center. O'Keefe et al. later recognized in the subgroup analysis of the initial 1000-patient Mid America experience that the observed mortality of 44% in the subset of 79 patients presenting with cardiogenic shock, represented an approximate 50% relative reduction in the mortality seen with intravenous thrombolytic therapy or conservative medical management.[9]

Before long, many other centers also adopted primary PTCA in a similar capacity or as a provisional strategy, as in thrombolytic-ineligible patients. Proponents believed that the high overall success rate and speed with which recanalization could typically be accomplished in experienced centers made primary PTCA a particularly attractive option for the treatment of high-risk patient subsets. However, data to support these contentions were as yet unavailable in the early 1980s.

Clinical Studies of PCI in Cardiogenic Shock

Although numerous trials of PCI in acute MI have yielded post-hoc analyses of small subsets of patients with cardiogenic shock, the main body of data directly addressing the utility of mechanical revascularization in cardiogenic shock may be organized into three groups: observational studies, registry data, and multicenter randomized trials.

Observational Studies

To date, there have been over 30 case series or observational studies addressing this issue, involving nearly 1300 patients.[9-31] The mean in-hospital mortality in patients undergoing successful percutaneous revascularization of the infarct-related vessel across these series was approximately 45% (see Table 1).[1,5,32] While this figure represents a dramatic improvement over historical mortality estimates of 80% to 90%, these data should be regarded with caution for several reasons. Given the non-randomized nature of these studies, a significant element of selection bias may have contributed to these favorable results. It is likely that emergent coronary intervention was deferred in certain patients who were inherently higher risk by way of advanced age, comorbid medical conditions, and a higher degree of instability at the time of presentation. It is also important to consider the subgroup of patients who died prior to arrival in the cardiac catheterization laboratory and were therefore excluded altogether from the analyses. The fact that reported mortality ranged widely from 14% to 78% in these studies lends further support to the view that uncontrolled patient-related or procedural factors, as well as small patient numbers, may have impacted significantly on overall outcome.[9-31,33] A review by Barry and Sarembock of nine observational studies spanning the years 1988 to 1995 revealed overall mortality to be 55% in 587 cardiogenic shock patients.[32] A total of 324 patients from this group underwent attempted PTCA with an average success rate of 73% (range 54%-89%). Among this subset of patients, the average in-hospital mortality was 37%. Failed PTCA conferred a mortality rate of 79%, which was similar to the mortality of patients in whom PTCA was not attempted (83%). While these data do not definitively prove the superiority of PTCA over supportive therapy alone, it is clear that persistent occlusion of the infarct-related vessel post-PTCA attempt does result in extremely high mortality rates. This finding is corroborated by the Duke database, which found that patency of the infarct-related vessel was an independent predictor of survival with better long-term prognostic value than age, peak creatine phosphokinase (CPK) elevation or ejection fraction.[19]

Of the published observational studies, only two series to date have examined the efficacy of early percutaneous revascularization in consecutive, unselected patients in patients presenting with MI and cardiogenic shock. It is interesting to note that, although consecutive enrollment presumably mitigated some of the confounding variables discussed above, these two studies yielded fairly disparate results.[22,31] In 1994, Himbert, et al. reported on 25 consecutive patients presenting early in the course of cardiogenic shock, of whom 18 patients underwent emergent PTCA with a mean time to treatment of 271 ± 106 minutes.[26] Percutaneous intervention was successful in 16 (89%) of patients; however, 14 (78%) of the 18 patients subsequently died before discharge from the hospital. This

Table 1.

Summary of Selected Observational Studies of Percutaneous Coronary Intervention (PCI) in Cardiogenic Shock

Author	Year	Shock patients undergoing PCI	Successful PCI (%)	Overall PCI mortality (%)	Successful PCI mortality (%)	Unsuccessful PCI mortality (%)
O'Neill[33]	1985	27	89	30	25	67
Heuser[10]	1986	10	60	30	17	75
Disler[11]	1987	7	71	57	40	100
Landin[12]	1988	34	79	41	30	86
Laramee[13]	1988	39	86	41	NR	NR
Lee[14]	1988	24	54	50	23	82
Verna[15]	1989	7	100	14	14	—
Meyer[17]	1990	25	88	47	41	100
Lee[18]	1991	69	71	45	31	80
Bengston[19]	1992	44	84	43	38	71
Gacioch[20]	1992	48	73	45	39	93
Hibbard[22]	1992	45	62	44	29	71
Moosvi[23]	1992	38	78	NR	44	92
Yamamoto[24]	1992	26	76	62	44	90
Seydoux[25]	1992	21	85	43	33	100
Himbert[26]	1994	18	89	78	81	50
Morrison[27]	1995	17	71	53	33	100
Eltchaninoff[28]	1995	33	75	36	24	75
Antoniucci[29]	1998	66	94	26	21	100
Calton[30]	1999	18	79	28	21	50
Perez-Castellano[31]	1999	65	72	71	62	94

NR = not reported; PCI = percutaneous coronary intervention.

series was limited, however, by the fact that 15 of 25 patients had prior cardiopulmonary resuscitation (CPR) for more than 15 minutes, suggesting that some may not have been salvageable by any means. Four years later, Antoniucci et al. published results of a series of 66 consecutive patients in cardiogenic shock, all of whom underwent primary PTCA with a mean time to treatment of 216 ± 90 minutes.[29] Procedural success was 94%, with in-hospital mortality noted to be 26% overall and 21% in the subset of patients with successful PTCA result. It has been suggested that the reduced time to reperfusion may have impacted favorably on mortality. Another important consideration when comparing these two series is use of provisional infarct-artery stenting in 47% of patients in the latter study, a strategy which has been demonstrated to reduce the incidence of abrupt vessel closure and minimize the risk of recurrent ischemic insults in the infarct artery territory.[29,34] A thorough discussion of the role of stenting may be found in Chapter 9. It is important to note that, as catheter-based interventional technologies and adjunctive therapies continue to evolve and become incorporated into clinical practice to varying degrees, the effect of these secular trends may further confound the direct comparison of such observational study results with one another.

Registry Data

In the past 10 years, a number of publications have reported on data gathered through a total of eight multicenter registries of acute MI including over 33,000 patients with cardiogenic shock (see Table 2).[4,34-45] The earliest of these, the Worcester Heart Attack study, was a large community-based registry which evaluated temporal trends in cardiogenic shock in 9076 patients admitted with a diagnosis of acute MI to 16 hospitals in the vicinity of Worcester, MA, between 1975 and 1997.[4,35] There was no significant variability in the adjusted risk of developing cardiogenic shock over the 23-year study period, with an overall incidence of 7.1%. Although patients admitted in later years experienced the same risk of developing cardiogenic shock as patients seen in the early years of the study, unadjusted analysis of the small number of shock patients undergoing revascularization procedures did suggest that a higher proportion of these patients survived to hospital discharge than did those managed conservatively.

A later population-based registry, the Californian study, also found a mortality benefit from early revascularization in a cohort of 1122 shock patients, representing 1.8% of the 63,964 acute MIs treated in the state of California in 1994.[36] While equal proportions of shock and nonshock patients underwent cardiac catheterization (37% and 35%, respectively), more shock patients underwent percutaneous revascularization (23% vs. 17%, p = 0.001) or CABG (12% vs. 9%, p = 0.001). Patients undergoing PTCA or CABG on either the day of admission or the day after were grouped together as a single patient set in the accompanying analysis of early revascularization. Univariate analysis found that early revasculari-

Table 2.

Summary of Registry Data of Percutaneous Coronary Intervention (PCI) in Cardiogenic Shock

Study	Years of registry	Shock patients undergoing PCI	PCI Success (%)	Unrevascularized mortality (%)	Revascularized mortality (%)	Successful PCI mortality (%)	Unsuccessful PCI mortality (%)
SHOCK$_R$[42]	1991–93	55	69	79	51	61	73
SMASH$_R$[47]	1992–96	30	90	74	50	NR	NR
Californian[36]	1994	259	NR	68	33	NR	NR
NRMI–2[41]	1994–97	5,493	NR	69	54	NR	NR
MITRA[44,45]	1994–97	81	NR	73	52	NR	NR
Ajani, et al.[43]	1995–99	46	63	—	37	10	82

NR = not reported. Of note, some studies grouped the minority of patients undergoing emergent CABG together with those revascularized via PCI.

zation conferred a significant in-hospital survival advantage. In-hospital mortality was reduced from 68% to 32% (p = 0.001) with an odds ratio of 0.20 (p = 0.0001). The revascularized patients were, however, significantly younger, and more likely to be male, nondiabetics without a prior history of PTCA or bypass surgery, suggesting therefore an element of selection bias. Also confounding the generalizability of these data was the grouping of PTCA and CABG patients together without clear delineation of the considerations driving the decision of one revascularization strategy versus the other. Moreover, both the 1.8% incidence of cardiogenic shock (1.8% as opposed to the more commonly cited range of 7%-20%) and the usage of thrombolytics (17% of patients with and 12% of patients without cardiogenic shock) were considerably lower than in other published series.[1,2,5,36]

Several important contributions were provided by the substudy analysis of the large randomized Global Utilization of Streptokinase and Tissue Plasminogen Activator (t-PA) for Occluded Coronary Arteries (GUSTO-1) trial.[37-39,46] The GUSTO-1 trial primarily evaluated the efficacy of various fibrinolytic and antithrombotic regimens in acute MI. Additionally this trial yielded important information regarding the development of cardiogenic shock following the administration of fibrinolytics, as well as the short- and long-term prognosis of shock patients undergoing early revascularization. A total of 42,021 patients presenting with ST-elevation MI within 6 hours of onset of symptoms were randomized to one of four thrombolytic strategies: streptokinase with subcutaneous or intravenous heparin, accelerated t-PA with intravenous heparin, or combined streptokinase and t-PA plus intravenous heparin. There were no specific protocol requirements determining use of coronary angiography or mechanical revascularization, both of which were at the discretion of the treating physician. Patients meeting the prospectively defined criteria for cardiogenic shock (n = 2972) comprised 7.2% of the total study population, with the minority of patients (11%) initially presenting in shock and the remaining 89% developing shock later during their hospital course. Analysis of 30-day and 1-year outcomes was performed after dividing patients into an "aggressive strategy" treatment arm with coronary angiography within 24 hours of onset of shock (n = 406) and a "conservative" management arm (n = 1794).[37,38] The shock cohort was more likely than the nonshock cohort to be older, of female gender, with a history of diabetes mellitus and prior MI, have an anterior infarction, and also had a longer time to administration of thrombolytic therapy. The minority of shock patients (n = 406, 18.5%) underwent early coronary angiography with fewer patients still (n = 255, 11.6%) undergoing revascularization within 24 hours of angiography. Of this latter group, PTCA was performed in 175 patients, coronary artery bypass graft surgery in 36 patients, and both procedures in 22 patients. Despite the exclusion of 155 patients who died within 1 hour of shock onset (whose default inclusion in the "conservative" limb would have resulted in considerable skew of the data in favor of "aggressive" therapy), early angiography was associated with improved clinical outcomes, with 30-day mortality reduced from 61% to 38% (p = 0.001). Additionally, a successful angioplasty result, defined as residual stenosis less than 50% (n = 175, 75% of PTCA patients), was strongly linked to survival (35% mortality vs. 55% in unsuccessful PTCA, p = 0.007). The relationship persisted on subsequent analyses that excluded patients who died within 3 and 6 hours following the development of shock. Closer examination of the conservative and aggressive treatment cohorts does, however, reveal significant disparities in baseline characteristics that may partially account for the improved survival in the latter group. Patients who received "aggressive" management were younger, with a lower incidence of prior MI and had received initial treatment more quickly, suggesting that operator bias may have contributed to the selection of a "healthier" population for the early invasive approach.

The GUSTO-1 shock substudy yielded several other important findings that have since been corroborated in other series. The early survival advantage seen in the subset selected for angiography and revascularization was still present at 1-year follow-up, independent of differences in baseline variables (92% vs. 85% 1-year survival, p = 0.0001). The development of shock conferred a significant mortality risk over uncomplicated MI. The greatest risk of death was within the first 30 days, with 88% of shock patients who survived to 30 days still alive at 1 year.[38] It may be inferred from these data that following thrombolysis, early angiography and revascularization may be beneficial in a younger, somewhat lower risk subgroup of shock patients with demonstrable short- and long-term survival benefit, when deemed eligible for such a strategy by the primary physician.

The single largest registry of cardiogenic shock patients, derived from the National Registry of Myocardial Infarction-2 (NRMI-2), similarly supported the association between revascularization and survival. NRMI-2 followed a total of 26,280 shock patients, representing 6.2% of the 426,253 cases of acute MI gathered in 1662 participating United States medical centers between 1994 and 1997.[40,41] Although shock patients were less likely to undergo cardiac catheterization than non-shock patients (37.4% vs. 49.0%, p < 0.001), improved short-term survival was noted in those who then underwent revascularization during the reference hospitalization, either via PTCA (12.8% mortality vs. 43.9%, p < 0.001) or CABG (6.5% vs. 23.9%, p < 0.001). These data complement the GUSTO-1 substudy data and are important not only because of the sheer number of patients from whom these values are derived, but also because NRMI-2 was a national cross-sectional study felt to more closely represent general clinical practice than carefully selected trial populations.[37,38,40,41] Attendant with the breadth of this study, however, is an unquantifiable element of heterogeneity with regard to the diagnostic criteria used and the general approach to management of shock across the numerous sites involved.

Hochman et al. reported on a smaller but prospectively collected series of cardiogenic shock patients for the multicenter SHOCK (Should We Emergently Revascularize Occluded Coronary Arteries for Cardiogenic Shock) Registry, which preceded the randomized SHOCK trial discussed below.[42] Nineteen United States and international centers registered 251 consecutive patients diagnosed with cardiogenic shock. As seen in other series, patients selected for cardiac catheterization were significantly younger than those who were not. Patients selected for early revascularization with PTCA or CABG evidenced lower mortality than those deemed ineligible. Interestingly, however, a mortality benefit was demonstrated in those who underwent cardiac catheterization versus those who did not (51% vs. 85%, p < 0.0001) even when revascularization was not performed (58%). The difference in mortality odds ratio remained significant even after adjustment for age, thrombolytic therapy, MI location, and ECG findings (4.76 vs. 5.49, p < 0.0001). This finding may potentially be ascribable to selection bias on the basis of comorbid conditions and severity of disease. No patient characteristics could be identified to predict survival in those undergoing early revascularization, although the small number of patients in this registry likely precluded the detection of any differences.[42]

Randomized Trials (See Chapter 8)

Two decades of nonrandomized investigations have largely upheld the relative benefit of early invasive therapies in cardiogenic shock, but attempts to confirm these findings through randomized trials have been both time-consuming and difficult. In fact, several promising multicenter studies were abandoned shortly after being proposed. At the time of this writing, there are no large investigations planned for the foreseeable future.[1,2] We are therefore left with data from two small randomized studies: the (Swiss) Multicenter Trial of Angioplasty for Shock - (S)MASH and the SHOCK trial.[47-49] These trials are considered in detail in Chapter 8.

Patient Selection and Technical Considerations

Observational and trial data both underscore the critical importance of careful patient selection when considering revascularization for cardiogenic shock, and the question of which shock patients will predictably benefit from early invasive therapies has not yet been settled. One-year follow-up from the SHOCK trial only provides a partial answer in identification of age < 75 years as a clinically significant characteristic.[49] It is clear that other unspecified variables have been factored into patient selection in the numerous observational studies that have shown more robust mortality reduction with revascularization than is demonstrable in the SHOCK or SMASH trials.[1,2,5,32,48,49] The interpretation of observational studies and registries should be approached with caution due to inconsistencies in the criteria for cardiogenic shock utilized and potential disparities between patient groups drawn from different centers, as described with GUSTO-1.[5,38,39,50] Additionally, many patients reported to have undergone early revascularization did so in the context of thrombolytic failure, i.e., "rescue angioplasty," which should be distinguished from primary coronary intervention. Similarly, there may be differences in background or supportive therapies, independent of revascularization status. This is apparent in the GUSTO-1 substudy, in which 74.6% of patients undergoing aggressive invasive therapy received IABP support versus only 7.9% of conservatively managed patients.[37]

Given the available data and the discussed limitations, several key considerations should guide the decision to pursue an early invasive strategy with percutaneous revascularization. Foremost is the demonstration of viable myocardium in jeopardy or ongoing ischemia, likely to be alleviated by intervention. In this regard, evolution of electrocardiographic changes and continued anginal symptoms may aid in rapid bedside assessment. The likelihood of a substantial degree of myocardial salvage diminishes with increasing time from onset of shock.[1-3,5,6,32,34,50,51] This observation has led some authors to suggest a 10- to 12-hour window for intervention rather than the 18-hour cutoff utilized by the SHOCK trial investigators. Most studies uphold the SHOCK trial finding that early intervention is of greater benefit in younger patients (< 75 years of age) and in those with fewer comorbidities. Other factors likely to influence the overall outcome of percutaneous intervention are the severity, distribution and diffuseness of coronary artery disease and degree of baseline left ventricular (LV) impairment.[50] The latter concern relates to the fact that patients with previously compromised LV function, either due to prior MI or normal age-related myocyte attrition, are less likely to tolerate further decrement in myocardial pump function. Importantly, these individuals may be expected to return to a lower level of function than those with previously normal ejection fraction, even after successful intervention.

It has been proposed that assessment of myocardial reserve may also serve an important discriminatory function.[2,52] Excluding malignant ventricular arrhythmias and mechanical complications, progressive pump failure with refractory hypotension is the cause of death in most shock patients. It therefore follows that the status of cardiac reserve may convey important prognostic information. Tan et al. have demonstrated in a small, unselected series of cardiogenic shock patients that if resting cardiac power output (flow output × arterial pressure) is less than 0.4 watts after optimizing intracardiac filling pressures, indicative of critically depressed LV function, mortality was 100% on medical therapy alone.[52] This was also found to be true of patients with higher resting values who were unable to increase their output to > 1.0 watts with maximal inotropic stimulation (dobutamine 40 mcg/kg/min).[52] These indices may identify a patient subset in whom the exceedingly high mortality rate with conservative management mandates the use of aggressive interventions, but will require validation in larger cohorts of patients. Further investigation in this area is warranted as a comprehensive predictive model incorporating all discussed parameters is as yet lacking. At present, however, age and time to intervention remain most predictive of success with early invasive therapy. Per the 1999 revision to the American College of Cardiology/American Heart Association acute MI treatment guidelines, PCI is designated a Class I recommendation for the treatment of cardiogenic shock in patients who are within 36 hours of an acute ST-elevation (Q-wave or new left bundle branch block) MI, are younger than 75 years old, and in whom revascularization can be performed within 18 hours of onset of shock.[53]

While issues related to intra-aortic balloon pump (IABP) counterpulsation are discussed in detail in Chapter 5, it is pertinent to the current discussion to note that IABP remains a useful adjunct to intervention for cardiogenic shock by augmenting diastolic coronary flow, decreasing afterload, and improving systemic perfusion.[1,2,5,32] Although balloon counterpulsation has not been demonstrated to significantly improve coronary perfusion distal to a flow-limiting stenosis, it is useful in this capacity following lesion modification via coronary intervention. While consistent mortality benefit is difficult to demonstrate, IABP use is believed to decrease reocclusion in the infarct artery, and may help maintain normal or near-normal flow through noninfarct related coronary beds in the face of systemic hypotension. This, in turn, may aid in stabilizing the spiral of worsening ischemia with progressive myocardial dysfunction and hypotension.[2,5,32]

In a small number of experienced centers, supported coronary intervention using percutaneous cardiopulmonary support (CPS) may be available for prophylactic use in extremely high-risk patients, or as a salvage maneuver when complete hemodynamic collapse is imminent.[6,7,32,54] Successful use of CPS not only requires skilled operators, perfusionists and experienced support staff, but also insertion of large bore (18-20 Fr) arterial and venous cannulae by which blood is withdrawn, passed through a membrane oxygenator, warmed and circulated. In addition, high levels of systemic anticoagulation must be maintained throughout. The advantage of CPS over IABP is that it provides complete circulatory support during PCI with cardiac output of up to 5 L/min, independent of native cardiac output or underlying cardiac rhythm. Use of CPS for supported PCI in patients with ejection fraction < 25%, target vessel supplying > 50% of the viable myocardium, or both, was evaluated in the National Registry of Elective Cardiopulmonary Bypass Supported Angioplasty.[7,54] Mortality was significantly reduced in patients treated prophylactically with CPS, although this benefit was at the cost of increased complications in this group (versus those treated on a standby basis). Cardiopulmonary support has also been demonstrated to be feasible in the context of unstable angina and severely impaired LV function. It should be noted, however, that the nonpulsatile flow provided by CPS may precipitate a "coronary steal" effect in vulnerable segments, further exacerbating myocardial dysfunction. Furthermore, extended use of CPS has been associated with activation of platelets and the coagulation cascade and vascular sequelae. This technology is best utilized for short-term support in a highly selected patient population, with clear clinical endpoints and shock likely to be reversed by coronary intervention.

PCI Failure and Microvascular Injury

While the safety and success of PCI has improved greatly since its inception, the rate of successful procedural outcomes in the context of cardiogenic shock still remains well below that of elective intervention, or even infarct angioplasty in the absence of shock. A survey of the literature suggests that PCI for cardiogenic shock is successful 70% to 80% of the time versus > 90% success rates associated with elective intervention.[2,7,19,37,48] Patients who have failed PCI must be considered for IABP and emergent CABG, or possibly LV assist device as a bridge to cardiac transplantation.

Another pertinent issue is that of defining procedural success. The SHOCK trial investigators used the criteria of 50% or less residual stenosis in the infarct-related vessel, with improvement of 20% or greater in the severity of stenosis and TIMI grade 2 or 3 flow.[48,49] As clear differences in clinical outcome are known to exist between TIMI grade 2 versus TIMI grade 3 flow post-intervention, a more rigorous definition of procedural success would not be unreasonable. While stricter criteria may improve further the observed survival rate in those patients achieving TIMI grade 3 flow, procedural success rates (77% in the SHOCK trial) would be considerably lower.

Restoration of myocardial perfusion depends not only on relief of the flow-limiting epicardial coronary stenoses, but also on preservation of microvascular integrity in the myocardial territory subtended by the infarct-related artery.[1,7,55-57] Even short periods of coronary occlusion result in myocyte necrosis with progressive occlusion of the capillaries with cellular debris. Microembolization of thrombus and atheromatous material may compound this process.[55] Other putative mechanisms of microvascular injury include interstitial edema and free radical-mediated endothelial injury.[1,55,56] Resultant loss of microvascular integrity is believed to be the physiologic basis of the "no-reflow phenomenon" (TIMI grade 0-1) or "slow flow" (TIMI grade 2) in the vessel on angiography.[7,57] Importantly, these processes may exist even in the face of angiographically "normal" flow. Additionally, it has been demonstrated that microvascular injury may continue to progress for several hours following reperfusion. Abnormal perfusion even with TIMI grade 3 flow translates into impaired systolic performance of the left ventricle and major adverse cardiac events in the postinfarction period. Treatment of microvascular injury remains the subject of controversy. Exclusion of flow-limiting coronary dissection and treatment of superimposed coronary vasospasm are imperative. Bolus intracoronary administration of calcium channel antagonists such as verapamil has been widely endorsed, however hypotension may preclude their use in the setting of cardiogenic shock.[1,7,55-57] Adenosine and nitroprusside are other options. Various distal embolization protection devices are currently under investigation and may prove useful in the future, particularly in vein graft intervention and in lesions manifesting a large thrombus burden. The use of glycoprotein IIb/IIIa receptor antagonists in this context is reasonable but demonstration of their efficacy will require further study.

Summary

Cardiogenic shock complicates approximately 7% to 10% of all cases of myocardial infarction and has been associated with a 70% to 80% in-hospital mortality rate. Percutaneous coronary intervention has theoretic benefits based on pathophysiologic observations, and numerous observational studies have reported robust benefit with use of PCI in cardiogenic shock with a pooled in-hospital mortality rate of 45%. These data need to be interpreted with some caution due to potential selection bias. Data from GUSTO-1 have shown, however, that in patients selected for early angiography and revascularization, early survival advantage persisted at 1-year follow-up, independent of differences in baseline variables. In addition to younger age, important clinical variables involved in the selection of patients for percutaneous intervention include confirmation of myocardial viability or continuing ischemia, time to intervention, distribution and severity of coronary artery disease and degree of baseline LV impairment. Aggressive medical management with inotropes, pressors, IABP and ventilatory support, as appropriate, should comprise background therapy for all patients. Careful consideration of these factors and the overall medical condition of the patient should guide the use of invasive therapies for cardiogenic shock.

References

1. Davies CH. Revascularization for cardiogenic shock. *QJM* 2001; 94:57-67.

2. Williams SG, Wright DJ, Tan LB. Management of cardiogenic shock complicating acute myocardial infarction: Towards evidence based medical practice. *Heart* 2000; 83:621-626.

3. White HD. Cardiogenic shock: A more aggressive approach is now warranted. *Eur Heart J* 2000; 21:1897-1901.

4. Goldberg RJ, Samad NA, Yarzebski J, et al. Temporal trends in cardiogenic shock complicating acute myocardial infarction. *N Engl J Med* 1999; 340:1162-1168.

5. Hollenberg SM, Kavinsky CJ, Parrillo JE. Cardiogenic shock. *Ann Intern Med* 1999; 131:47-59.

6. Webb JG. Interventional management of cardiogenic shock. *Can J Cardiol* 1998; 14:233-244.

7. Ellis SG, Holmes DR. Strategic Approaches in Coronary Intervention. New York: Lippincott Williams and Wilkins, 2000.

8. King SB, 3rd. The development of interventional cardiology. *J Am Coll Cardiol* 1998; 31:64B-88B.

9. O'Keefe JH, Jr., Bailey WL, Rutherford BD, et al. Primary angioplasty for acute myocardial infarction in 1,000 consecutive patients. Results in an unselected population and high-risk subgroups. *Am J Cardiol* 1993; 72:107G-115G.

10. Heuser RR, Maddoux GL, Ramo BW, et al. Coronary angioplasty in the treatment of cardiogenic shock: The therapy of choice (abstract). *J Am Coll Cardiol* 1986; 7:219A.

11. Disler L, Haitas B, Benjamin J, et al. Cardiogenic shock in evolving myocardial infarction: Treatment by angioplasty and streptokinase. *Heart Lung* 1993; 16:649-652.

12. Landin RJ, Rothbaum DA, Linnemeier TJ, et al. Hospital mortality of patients undergoing emergency angioplasty for acute myocardial infarction: Relation-

ship of mortality to cardiogenic shock and unsuccessful angioplasty (abstract). *Circulation* 1988; 78 (Suppl II):II-9.

13. Laramee LA, Rutherford BD, Ligon RW, et al. Coronary angioplasty for cardiogenic shock following myocardial infarction (abstract). *Circulation* 1988; 78 (Suppl II):II-634.

14. Lee L, Bates ER, Pitt B, et al. Percutaneous transluminal coronary angioplasty improves survival in acute myocardial infarction complicated by cardiogenic shock. *Circulation* 1988; 78:1345-1351.

15. Verna E, Repetto S, Boscarini M, et al. Emergency coronary angioplasty in patients with severe left ventricular dysfunction or cardiogenic shock after acute myocardial infarction. *Eur Heart J* 1989; 10:958-966.

16. Shawl FA, Domanski MJ, Hernandez TJ, et al. Emergency percutaneous cardiopulmonary bypass support in cardiogenic shock from acute myocardial infarction. *Am J Cardiol* 1989; 64:967-970.

17. Meyer P, Blanc P, Baudouy M, et al. [Treatment of primary cardiogenic shock by coronary transluminal angioplasty during the acute phase of myocardial infarction]. *Arch Mal Coeur Vaiss* 1990; 83:329-334.

18. Lee L, Erbel R, Brown TM, et al. Multicenter registry of angioplasty therapy of cardiogenic shock: Initial and long-term survival. *J Am Coll Cardiol* 1991; 17:599-603.

19. Bengtson JR, Kaplan AJ, Pieper KS, et al. Prognosis in cardiogenic shock after acute myocardial infarction in the interventional era. *J Am Coll Cardiol* 1992; 20:1482-1489.

20. Gacioch GM, Ellis SG, Lee L, et al. Cardiogenic shock complicating acute myocardial infarction: The use of coronary angioplasty and the integration of the new support devices into patient management. *J Am Coll Cardiol* 1992; 19:647-653.

21. O'Neill WW. Angioplasty therapy of cardiogenic shock: Are randomized trials necessary? *J Am Coll Cardiol* 1992; 19:915-917.

22. Hibbard MD, Holmes DR, Jr., Bailey KR, et al. Percutaneous transluminal coronary angioplasty in patients with cardiogenic shock. *J Am Coll Cardiol* 1992; 19:639-646.

23. Moosvi AR, Khaja F, Villanueva L, et al. Early revascularization improves survival in cardiogenic shock complicating acute myocardial infarction. *J Am Coll Cardiol* 1992; 19:907-914.

24. Yamamoto H, Hayashi Y, Oka Y, et al. Efficacy of percutaneous transluminal coronary angioplasty in patients with acute myocardial infarction complicated by cardiogenic shock. *Jpn Circ J* 1992; 56:815-821.

25. Seydoux C, Goy JJ, Beuret P, et al. Effectiveness of percutaneous transluminal coronary angioplasty in cardiogenic shock during acute myocardial infarction. *Am J Cardiol* 1992; 69:968-969.

26. Himbert D, Juliard JM, Steg PG, et al. Limits of reperfusion therapy for immediate cardiogenic shock complicating acute myocardial infarction. *Am J Cardiol* 1994; 74:492-494.

27. Morrison D, Crowley ST, Bies R, et al. Systolic blood pressure response to percutaneous transluminal coronary angioplasty for cardiogenic shock. *Am J Cardiol* 1995; 76:313-314.

28. Eltchaninoff H, Simpfendorfer C, Franco I, et al. Early and 1-year survival rates in acute myocardial infarction complicated by cardiogenic shock: A retrospective study comparing coronary angioplasty with medical treatment. *Am Heart J* 1995; 130:459-464.

29. Antoniucci D, Valenti R, Santoro GM, et al. Systematic direct angioplasty and stent-supported direct angioplasty therapy for cardiogenic shock complicating acute myocardial infarction: In-hospital and long-term survival. *J Am Coll Cardiol* 1998; 31:294-300.

30. Calton R, Jaison PM, David T. Primary angioplasty for cardiogenic shock complicating acute myocardial infarction. *Indian Heart J* 1999; 51:47-54.

31. Perez-Castellano N, Garcia E, Serrano JA, et al. Efficacy of invasive strategy for the management of acute myocardial infarction complicated by cardiogenic shock. *Am J Cardiol* 1999; 83:989-993.

32. Barry WL, Sarembock IJ. Cardiogenic shock: Therapy and prevention. *Clin Cardiol* 1998; 21:72-80.

33. O'Neill W, Erbel R, Laufer N, et al. Coronary angioplasty therapy of cardiogenic shock complicating acute myocardial infarction (abstract). *Circulation* 1985; 72(Suppl II):309.

34. Santoro GM, Buonamici P. Reperfusion therapy in cardiogenic shock complicating acute myocardial infarction. *Am Heart J* 1999; 138:S126-131.

35. Goldberg RJ, Gore JM, Alpert JS, et al. Cardiogenic shock after acute myocardial infarction. Incidence and mortality from a community-wide perspective, 1975 to 1988. *N Engl J Med* 1991; 325:1117-1122.

36. Edep ME, Brown DL. Effect of early revascularization on mortality from cardiogenic shock complicating acute myocardial infarction in California. *Am J Cardiol* 2000; 85:1185-1188.

37. Berger PB, Holmes DR, Jr., Stebbins AL, et al. Impact of an aggressive invasive catheterization and revascularization strategy on mortality in patients with cardiogenic shock in the Global Utilization of Streptokinase and Tissue Plasminogen Activator for Occluded Coronary Arteries (GUSTO-I) trial. An observational study. *Circulation* 1997; 96:122-127.

38. Berger PB, Tuttle RH, Holmes DR, Jr., et al. One-year survival among patients with acute myocardial infarction complicated by cardiogenic shock, and its relation to early revascularization: Results from the GUSTO-I trial. *Circulation* 1999; 99:873-878.

39. Holmes DR, Jr., Califf RM, Van de Werf F, et al. Difference in countries' use of resources and clinical outcome for patients with cardiogenic shock after myocardial infarction: Results from the GUSTO trial. *Lancet* 1997; 349:75-78.

40. Rogers WJ, Canto JG, Lambrew CT, et al. Temporal trends in the treatment of over 1.5 million patients with myocardial infarction in the US from 1990 through 1999: The National Registry of Myocardial Infarction 1, 2 and 3. *J Am Coll Cardiol* 2000; 36:2056-2063.

41. Goldberg RJ, Gore JM, Thompson CA, et al. Recent magnitude of and temporal trends (1994-1997) in the incidence and hospital death rates of cardiogenic shock complicating acute myocardial infarction: The second national registry of myocardial infarction. *Am Heart J* 2001; 141:65-72.

42. Hochman JS, Boland J, Sleeper LA, et al. Current spectrum of cardiogenic shock and effect of early revascularization on mortality. Results of an International Registry. *Circulation* 1995; 91:873-881.

43. Ajani AE, Maruff P, Warren R, et al. Impact of early percutaneous coronary intervention on short- and long- term outcomes in patients with cardiogenic shock after acute myocardial infarction. *Am J Cardiol* 2001; 87:633-635.

44. Gitt AK, Schiele R, Seidl K, et al. Influence of recanalisation therapy on prognosis of cardiogenic shock in acute myocardial infarction in unselected patients of the MITRA-Study (abstract). *J Am Coll Cardiol* 1999; 33:375A.

45. Zahn R, Schiele R, Schneider S, et al. Decreasing hospital mortality between 1994 and 1998 in patients with acute myocardial infarction treated with primary angioplasty but not in patients treated with intravenous thrombolysis. Results from the pooled data of the Maximal Individual Therapy in Acute Myocardial Infarction (MITRA) Registry and the Myocardial Infarction Registry (MIR). *J Am Coll Cardiol* 2000; 36:2064-2071.

46. Holmes DR, Jr., Bates ER, Kleiman NS, et al. Contemporary reperfusion therapy for cardiogenic shock: The GUSTO-I trial experience. The GUSTO-I Investigators. Global Utilization of Streptokinase and Tissue Plasminogen Activator for Occluded Coronary Arteries. *J Am Coll Cardiol* 1995; 26:668-674.

47. Urban P, Stauffer JC, Bleed D, et al. A randomized evaluation of early revascularization to treat shock complicating acute myocardial infarction. The (Swiss) Multicenter Trial of Angioplasty for Shock-(S)MASH. *Eur Heart J* 1999; 20:1030-1038.

48. Hochman JS, Sleeper LA, Webb JG, et al. Early revascularization in acute myocardial infarction complicated by cardiogenic shock. *N Engl J Med* 1999; 341:625-634.

49. Hochman JS, Sleeper LA, White HD, et al. One-year survival following early revascularization for cardiogenic shock. *JAMA* 2001; 285:190-192.

50. Klein LW. Optimal therapy for cardiogenic shock: The emerging role of coronary angioplasty. *J Am Coll Cardiol* 1992; 19:654-656.

51. Hasdai D, Topol EJ, Califf RM, et al. Cardiogenic shock complicating acute coronary syndromes. *Lancet* 2000; 356:749-756.

52. Tan LB, Littler WA. Measurement of cardiac reserve in cardiogenic shock: Implications for prognosis and management. *Br Heart J* 1990; 64:121-128.

53. Ryan TJ, Antman EM, Brooks NH, et al. 1999 update: ACC/AHA Guidelines for the Management of Patients With Acute Myocardial Infarction: Executive Summary and Recommendations: A report of the American College of Cardiology/American Heart Association Task Force on Practice Guidelines (Committee on Management of Acute Myocardial Infarction). *Circulation* 1999; 100:1016-1030.

54. Shawl FA, Quyyumi AA, Bajaj S, et al. Percutaneous cardiopulmonary bypass-supported coronary angioplasty in patients with unstable angina pectoris or myocardial infarction and a left ventricular ejection fraction ≥ 25%. *Am J Cardiol* 1996; 77:14-19.

55. Agati L. Microvascular integrity after reperfusion therapy. *Am Heart J* 1999; 138:S76-78.

56. Ambrosio G, Tritto I. Reperfusion injury: Experimental evidence and clinical implications. *Am Heart J* 1999; 138:S69-75.

57. Safian RD, Freed MS. The Manual of Interventional Cardiology. New York: Physicians" Press, 2001.

Chapter 8

Randomized Trials of Revascularization Therapy for Cardiogenic Shock

*Philip M. Urban, MD and
Jean-Christophe Stauffer, MD*

Introduction

Scope of the Problem

Cardiogenic shock occurs in about 7% of all patients admitted to hospital for acute myocardial infarction (MI).[1] About half present with established cardiogenic shock at the time of hospital admission, and the other half develop shock at a later stage, usually within the first 24-48 hours following admission.[2] Hospital mortality is high, and has been reported to vary between 50% and 80%.[1-4] Non-randomized retrospective series, available for over 30 years, have documented a favorable outcome associated with coronary revascularization.[4-6] As early as the late 1960s and early 1970s, coronary artery bypass surgery was shown to be associated with a survival rate of more than 50%,[5] and in the 1980s and 1990s, similar figures were reported for percutaneous coronary intervention (PCI).[6] Despite these encouraging results, it remained difficult to determine the exact benefit of revascularization from data in which a powerful selection bias probably existed. Not only were the patients selected to undergo the procedure, but they also had to survive the initial coronary angiogram and have coronary anatomy suitable for revascularization. In support of the concept that selection bias probably played a major role in most retrospective series, it should be noted that two separate groups[7,8] reported an improved outcome in those patients selected to undergo coronary angiography, whether revascularization was carried out or not.

From: Hollenberg SM, Bates ER. *Cardiogenic Shock.* Armonk, NY: Futura Publishing Co., Inc.; ©2002.

The logic of emergent revascularization for patients in cardiogenic shock remained compelling, however. Nearly all retrospective trials had shown that failed PCI was associated with a far worse prognosis than successful revascularization,[6] and, more importantly, several randomized, controlled trials in the 1990s clearly documented the benefit of direct PCI for patients with acute MI without shock.[9] In the PAMI trial,[10] it was also shown that patients at higher risk benefited most from PCI when compared to thrombolysis. It was in this context that two separate randomized, controlled trials[11,12] were launched in the early 1990s to evaluate the impact of emergent revascularization for cardiogenic shock. Without any initial awareness that a parallel effort was ongoing, both groups of investigators focused on the evaluation of immediate revascularization for patients with early cardiogenic shock complicating myocardial infarction. Only patients with primary pump failure were included. The SHOCK (SHould we emergently revascularize Occluded Coronary arteries for cardiogenic shocK) trial was powered to detect a 20%, and the SMASH (Swiss Multicenter trial of Angioplasty SHock) trial a 30%, absolute mortality reduction at 30 days. Both these figures were based upon the data available from retrospective series.[6] In this chapter, we will discuss both trials, the results of which have now been published.[11-13] The SHOCK trial was successfully completed, and has documented a major impact of emergent coronary revascularization on mortality for cardiogenic shock. Unfortunately, the SMASH trial had to be terminated prematurely because of major problems with patient recruitment. It does serve, however, as a valid and independent confirmation of the SHOCK trial results.

Specific Problems of Randomized, Controlled Trials for Cardiogenic Shock

A major paradox is immediately apparent. On the one hand, cardiogenic shock is associated with very high early mortality rates, and represents a pressing clinical question. It can thus be seen as an "ideal" problem to approach with a small randomized, controlled trial with hard endpoints and a short follow-up period. However, with baseline mortality rates in the 70% range, there are some major ethical considerations to ponder. Patients, relatives, and physicians are reluctant to let chance play a role in the decision making. The stakes are so high that individual convictions, case to case individual assessment, and patients' preference do (and should) play a critical role in the choices that are made.

The issue of consent is also a difficult one. Precious minutes can theoretically be lost if a fully informed consent is to be obtained in all cases. Patients' mentation is often not adequate, and even the family or relatives, when available, are generally under major stress and may be unable to understand the issue fully. This situation may require specific adjustments: in the SHOCK trial,[12] while 28 of the 30 participating centers (93%) obtained written informed consent from all patients or their surrogate, two centers (7%) received approval from their institutional review boards to follow a NIH-FDA specified procedure for exemption from informed consent.[14] In the SMASH trial,[11] obtaining written informed consent was recommended in all cases, but could be dispensed with "if the patient's condition made it necessary."

The Context

In the early 1990s, several European centers declined to participate in the SMASH trial because it was felt that it would not be ethical to undertake early invasive evaluation in such extremely ill patients. The situation changed rapidly during the following years, however, after publication of several encouraging studies documenting the superiority of PCI over thrombolysis for acute MI without cardiogenic shock.[9] Unfortunately, this did not improve patient recruitment into the SMASH trial, since many centers then felt that it had become unethical *not* to proceed to early evaluation and revascularization. In order to assess the perception of the situation in every day clinical practice, we undertook a survey of all fellows of the European Society of Cardiology in September 1998, prior to the publication of the results from both the SHOCK and the SMASH trials. We obtained an answer from 247 physicians. Although 110 (44.5%) thought that PCI was very useful in the treatment of cardiogenic shock, 123 (49.8%) found it probably useful, and only 14 (5.7%) thought that it was not useful. Several reasons for not using emergent revascularization in cardiogenic shock patients were given (Figure 1). It was in this complex

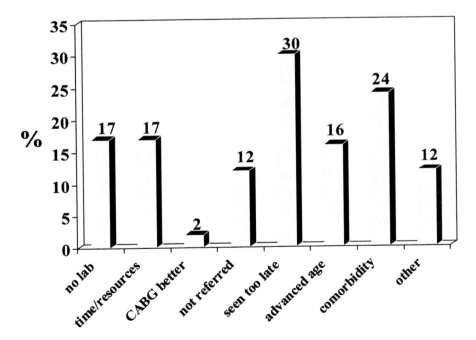

Figure 1. Reasons given for not proceeding with PCI for patients in cardiogenic shock. Results of a 1998 poll of 247 Fellows of the European Society of Cardiology.

and challenging setting that both the SHOCK and the SMASH trials were undertaken.

Design of the Trials

Although neither the SHOCK nor the SMASH investigators were aware that another trial was being set up at the time of designing their own project, both trials addressed the problem in a nearly identical manner. The major inclusion and exclusion criteria are listed in Table 1. Both trials chose 30-day, all-cause mortality on an intention to treat basis as the primary endpoint. Both trials further chose to assess 1-year mortality as a secondary endpoint.

Baseline Characteristics

The patients that were included in both trials were quite similar, and the median delay between the appearance of chest pain and shock onset was in the range of 2.5 to 6.2 hours (Table 2).

Intervention

In the SHOCK trial, the treatments actually given to the revascularization and the medical therapy arms of the study were as follows: cardiopulmonary resuscitation for ventricular tachycardia or ventricular fibrillation before randomization, 32.7% versus 23.9%; thrombolytic therapy, 49.3% versus 63.3%; inotropes or vasopressors, 99.3% versus 98.6%; intra-

Table 1.

Criteria for Inclusion/Exclusion, SHOCK and SMASH Trials

Inclusion criteria	SHOCK	SMASH
Cause of cardiogenic shock	pump failure	pump failure
Systolic blood pressure (mm Hg)	< 90 or requiring inotropes	< 90 despite inotropes
Maximum time from symptom onset to randomization (hours)	< 36+12	< 48
Cardiac index (L/min/m²)	< 2.2	< 2.2
Pulmonary capillary wedge pressure (mm Hg)	> 15	> 15
Exclusion criteria:		
MR, VSD, pericardial tamponade	Yes	Yes
Severe noncardiac disease	Yes	Yes
Unsuitable for revascularization	Yes	Yes
Age limit	No	No

MR = mitral regurgitation; VSD = ventricular septal defect.

Table 2.

	Baseline Characteristics at Inclusion	
	SHOCK	SMASH
Age (years)	66±10	65±9
Male gender (%)	68	67
Diabetes (%)	31	18
Prior heart failure (%)	6	25
Anterior MI (%)	60	45
Median time (hours) from chest pain to shock onset	5.0 (2.2–12.0)(invasive) 6.2 (2.4–15.5) (medical treatment)	2.5 (0.0–27.0)(invasive) 5.0 (0.0–45.0) (medical treatment)
CPR, VT, or VF prior to randomization (%)	33	28
Heart rate (bpm)	103 ± 22 (invasive) 100 ± 23 (med. treatment)	101 ± 30 (invasive) 105 ± 30 (med. treatment)
Systolic BP (mm Hg)	89 ± 23 (invasive) 87 ± 17 (med. treatment)	77 ± 10 (invasive) 78 ± 13 (med. treatment)

CPR = cardiopulmonary resuscitation; MI = myocardial infarction; VF = ventricular fibrillation; VT = ventricular tachycardia.

aortic balloon pump (IABP) counterpulsation, 86.2% versus 86.0%; pulmonary artery catheterization, 93.4% versus 96.0%; left ventricular (LV) assist device, 3.6% versus 0.9%; heart transplantation, 2.0% versus 0.7%; coronary angiography, 96.7% versus 66.7%; PCI, 54.6% versus 14%; coronary artery bypass grafting, 37.5% versus 11.3%; and PCI or coronary bypass grafting, 86.8% versus 25.3%. Overall compliance with the protocol was excellent: 97% of the patients assigned to revascularization underwent early coronary angiography and 87% underwent revascularization. Of the 20 patients assigned to revascularization who did not undergo a revascularization procedure, five died before coronary angiography could be performed. In the group assigned to medical therapy, the rate of crossover was only 2.7%, representing revascularization attempts less than 54 hours after randomization. Figures were similar in the SMASH trial, with 94% of the patients in the invasive group undergoing early angiography and 87% of them being revascularized. The interventions carried out in both the SHOCK and SMASH trials are illustrated in Figures 2, 3, and 4.

Results of the Trials

The SHOCK trial documented a nonsignificant trend favoring invasive treatment with the primary endpoint of 30-day mortality. There was a 46.7% mortality rate with invasive treatment and a 56.0% mortality rate with the medical approach. The absolute difference was thus 9.3%, with a 95% confidence interval (CI) for the difference of −20.5% to 1.9%

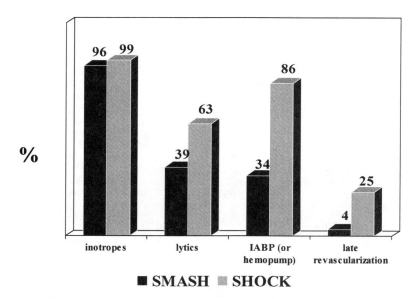

Figure 2. Interventions in the noninvasive groups of the SHOCK and SMASH trials (index hospital admission only). IABP = intra-aortic balloon pump.

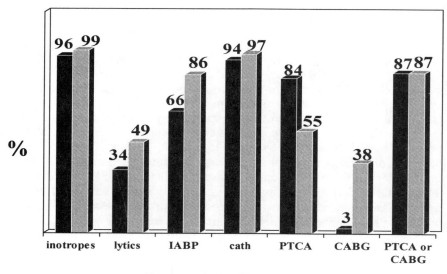

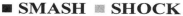

Figure 3. Interventions in the invasive groups of the SHOCK and SMASH trials (index hospital admission only). CABG = coronary artery bypass grafting; IABP = intra-aortic balloon pump; PTCA = percutaneous transluminal coronary angioplasty.

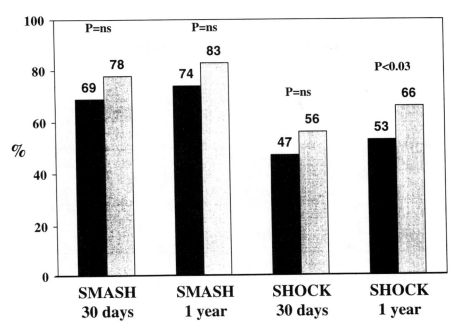

Figure 4. All cause mortality at 30 days (primary endpoint) and at 1 year for the SHOCK and SMASH trials.

(p = 0.11). However, after a follow-up of 1 year, the mortality rate had changed to 53% versus 66% respectively, an absolute difference in survival of 13.2% (95% CI of 2.2 – 24.1%, p = 0.025).

In the SMASH trial, a similar trend in 30-day absolute mortality reduction of 9% was observed (69% mortality in the invasive group vs. 78% in the medically manage group, RR = 0.88, 95% CI = 0.6-1.2, p = ns). These results are shown in Figure 4.

Although both trials were statistically negative concerning the primary endpoint of mortality at 30 days, the very positive results of the SHOCK trial after 1 year clearly indicate a major survival benefit following an early invasive approach for cardiogenic shock complicating acute myocardial infarction. Just as an early hazard has been shown to be associated with thrombolytic treatment,[15] it is very likely that there is a component of acute risk associated with early coronary angiography and revascularization in patients with cardiogenic shock.

Another important consideration to keep in mind when analyzing the results of both the SHOCK and the SMASH trials is that rather than truly assessing the isolated benefit of revascularization, both trials evaluated a therapeutic strategy. In addition to revascularization, the strategy also included the use of intravenous inotropic agents (99% in SHOCK and 96% in SMASH), thrombolytic therapy (49% in SHOCK, 34% in SMASH), and IABP counterpulsation (86% in SHOCK, 66% in SMASH). Also, despite initial apprehension that patient transfer for revascularization would be associated with an increased hazard, this was not shown to be the case in the SHOCK trial, where 55% of patients included were transferred from another hospital, prior to randomization. Results for transferred patients did not differ from those who were not transferred.

Differences and Similarities Between the SHOCK and SMASH Trials

The data from the SHOCK trial are the most definitive, and were used as a basis to modify the ACC/AHA guidelines that now recommend early revascularization for patients aged less than 75 years with cardiogenic shock within 36 hours of acute MI. However, several points of interest can be addressed by comparing the SMASH and SHOCK trials.

Although the SMASH trial was never completed, the data do seem to confirm that the absolute benefit at 30 days is within the range of nine lives saved per 100 patients treated, and this benefit is identical to that observed in the SHOCK trial. Furthermore, the SMASH trial data would suggest that this trend persists at 1-year follow-up (Figure 4). Both trials show a relatively low additional mortality rate beyond 30 days (5% mortality in both arms of the SMASH trial, 6% and 10% respectively in the invasive and medical arms of the SHOCK trial).

The higher mortality in both arms of the SMASH trial is also of interest. Most probably, this relates to a more severe definition of cardiogenic shock, requiring hypotension below systolic blood pressure of 90 mm Hg to persist despite administration of volume and inotropes as needed (Table 1). This was felt to be necessary because invasive measurement of left heart-filling pressures and cardiac output was not required prior to inclusion. In retrospect, this definition was probably too strict, and contributed to difficulties in patient recruitment. It also contributed to define a very high-risk cardiogenic shock population.

Other factors may have contributed to a higher mortality rate in the SMASH trial. These include a lower use of thrombolysis and IABP counterpulsation, in the medical arm in particular, as well as a markedly lower use of bypass surgery in the invasive group. Since the SHOCK trial data have clearly documented a similar survival benefit for selected patients undergoing surgery rather than PCI, despite having a higher incidence of diabetes and more severe coronary artery disease, it is quite possible that emergent bypass surgery was underutilized in the SMASH trial.

Recommendations

When the results of both the SHOCK and SMASH trials are put into perspective with results from other randomized, controlled trials of patients with acute MI (Figure 5), a critical point becomes apparent: while the *relative* risk reduction is moderate at 0.72 (95% CI, 0.54-0.95) for the SHOCK trial and 0.88 (95% CI, 0.60-1.20) for the SMASH trial, the *absolute* benefit is important, with a trend suggesting nine lives saved for 100 patients treated at 30 days in both trials, and a significant benefit at 1

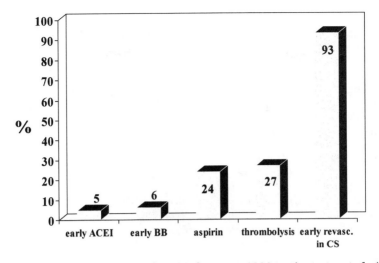

Figure 5. Number of lives saved at 30 days per 1000 patients treated. ACEI = angiotensin converting enzyme inhibitor; BB = beta blocker; CS = cardiogenic shock.

year in the SHOCK trial, with 13.2 lives saved for 100 patients treated. This latter figure corresponds to a number needed to treat (NNT) of 7.6, possibly the lowest figure ever observed in a randomized, controlled trial of cardiovascular disease. This justifies the formidable cost and logistics of emergent revascularization for cardiogenic shock patients.

We can only concur with the conclusion from the SHOCK trial:[13-14] "early revascularization improves one-year survival when shock complicates acute myocardial infarction." We recommend rapid transfer of patients, particularly those less than 75 years, to tertiary care hospitals for urgent coronary angiography and revascularization."

References

1. Goldberg RJ, Samad NA, Yarzebski J, et al. Temporal trends in cardiogenic shock complicating acute myocardial infarction. *N Engl J Med* 1999; 340:1162-1168.
2. Hasdai D, Califf RM, Thompson TD, et al. Predictors of cardiogenic shock after thrombolytic therapy for acute myocardial infarction. *J Am Coll Cardiol* 2000; 35:136-143.
3. Hochman JS, Buller CE, Sleeper LA, et al. Cardiogenic shock complicating acute myocardial infarction-Etiology, management and outcome: A report from the SHOCK trial registry. *J Am Coll Cardiol* 2000; 36:1063-1070.
4. Califf RM, Bengtson JR. Cardiogenic shock. *N Engl J Med* 1994; 330:1724-1730.
5. Pirwitz MJ, Hillis LD. Emergency coronary artery bypass surgery for acute myocardial infarction. *Cor Art Dis* 1994; 5:385-391.
6. Hollenberg SM, Kavinsky CJ, Parrillo JE. Cardiogenic shock. *Ann Int Med* 1999; 131:47-59.

7. Hochman JS, Boland J, Sleeper LA, et al. Current spectrum of cardiogenic shock and effect of early revascularization on mortality. Results of an international registry. SHOCK Registry Investigators. *Circulation* 1995; 91:873-881.
8. Berger PB, Holmes DR, Stebbins AL, et al. Impact of an aggressive invasive catheterization and revascularization strategy on mortality in patients with cardiogenic shock in the Global Utilisation of Streptokinase and Tissue plasminogen activator for Occluded coronary arteries (GUSTO-I) trial. *Circulation* 1997; 96:122-127.
9. Weaver WD, Simes J, Betriu A, et al. Comparison of primary coronary angioplasty and intravenous thrombolytic therapy for acute myocardial infarction. *JAMA* 1997; 278:2093-2098.
10. Stone GW. Predictors of in-hospital and 6-month outcome after acute myocardial infarction in the reperfusion era: The primary angioplasty in myocardial infarction (PAMI) trial. *J Am Coll Cardiol* 1995; 25:370-377.
11. Urban P, Stauffer JC, Khatchatrian N, et al. A randomized evaluation of early revascularization to treat shock complicating acute myocardial infarction. The (Swiss) Multicenter Trial of Angioplasty SHock - (S)MASH. *Eur Heart J* 1999; 20:1030-1038.
12. Hochman JS, Sleeper LA, Webb JG, et al. Early revascularization in acute myocardial infarction complicated by cardiogenic shock. *N Engl J Med* 1999; 341:625-634.
13. Hochman JS, Sleeper LA, White HD, et al. One year survival following early revascularization for cardiogenic shock. *JAMA* 2001; 285:190-192.
14. Hochman JS, Sleeper LA, Godfrey E, et al. Should we emergently revascularize occluded coronary arteries for cardiogenic shock: An international randomized trial of emergency PTCA/CABG – trial design. *Am Heart J* 1999; 137:313-321.
15. Fibrinolytic Therapy Trialists (FTT) Collaborative Group. Indications for fibrinolytic therapy in suspected acute myocardial infarction: Collaborative overview of early mortality and major morbidity results from all randomised trials of more than 1000 patients. *Lancet* 1994; 343:311-322.

Chapter 9

Stenting and Other New Developments in Interventional Therapy for Cardiogenic Shock

David Antoniucci, MD

Introduction

For many years, an acute myocardial infarction (MI), with or without shock, was considered an absolute contraindication to coronary stenting. The thrombotic milieu of an ulcerated coronary plaque complicated by thrombotic occlusion, in conjunction with the need for aggressive anticoagulation regimens, were felt to be associated with a prohibitive risk of stent thrombosis and bleeding complications. The practice of high-pressure balloon inflation for stent implantation, along with effective antiplatelet regimens and the omission of aggressive anticoagulation treatment, has now dramatically reduced both stent thrombosis and bleeding complications.

The first reported case of coronary stent implantation in the setting of cardiogenic shock complicating acute MI was published in 1991. Cannon et al.[1] described a patient who had bailout stenting for cardiogenic shock complicating acute occlusion of the right coronary artery. A balloon-expandable coil stent (Cook stent) was implanted for marked vessel recoil after coronary angioplasty, followed by prolonged intracoronary infusion of urokinase for 18 hours. Clinical and angiographic follow-up at 6 months showed satisfactory results, without any evidence of stent thrombosis or restenosis.

In 1996, four small observational studies showed that in the setting of acute MI, provisional coronary stenting was feasible, optimized the acute angiographic result, and improved clinical outcomes; only a minority of patients in these studies had cardiogenic shock.[2-5] In 1998, the Florence

From: Hollenberg SM, Bates ER. *Cardiogenic Shock*. Armonk, NY: Futura Publishing Co., Inc.; ©2002.

investigators showed in a series of 66 patients with cardiogenic shock complicating acute MI that a strategy of provisional coronary stenting improved the procedural success rate to 94%, and that this high success rate was associated with an overall mortality rate of 29%.[6] In this series, 47% of the patients had infarct-artery stenting for a poor or suboptimal angiographic result after angioplasty. Patients with a stented infarct-artery had a better event-free survival rate compared to patients who underwent angioplasty alone (70% vs. 40%, p = 0.026).

Since that time, there has been an explosion of information regarding optimal stenting techniques and a corresponding increase in the use of stents. The role of stenting for acute MI and for cardiogenic shock in particular is evolving at a rapid pace.

Rationale for the Use of Coronary Stenting in Acute Myocardial Infarction Complicated by Cardiogenic Shock

Pathophysiologic considerations and trial data support the use of mechanical revascularization for patients with cardiogenic shock caused by MI. Primary angioplasty has been shown to be superior to thrombolytic therapy in restoring normal coronary blood flow after infarction, with lower rates of recurrent ischemia, reinfarction, stroke, and death.[7-9]

Primary angioplasty in this setting does have its limitations, however. As a consequence of early reocclusion or renarrowing, patients with successful primary coronary angioplasty may have early recurrent ischemia. This may be due in part to the proclivity of infarct artery lesions to develop intimal tears after angioplasty in the setting of acute MI. The subsequent exposure of atherosclerotic plaque components, along with abnormalities of flow profiles, may explain restenosis or renarrowing in the acute phase.[10] A suboptimal angiographic result after successful primary coronary angioplasty is a strong predictor of early adverse events.[11] Optimization of the angiographic result using a coronary stent increases lumen size and minimizes the effects of dissections, which may reduce shear forces and platelet deposition.

Late restenosis or reocclusion may occur in more than 50% of patients after balloon angioplasty.[10] Abnormal flow profiles may also contribute to unfavorable vascular remodeling in the late phase after angioplasty. Optimization of the initial angiographic result, that is, achieving the largest achievable vessel diameter, is assumed to be inversely related to the risk of late restenosis or reocclusion.[12]

Thus, the postulated mechanisms of the benefit of stenting in acute MI are the achievement of an initial optimal angiographic result and the correction of any residual dissection by stenting in order to decrease the incidence of recurrent ischemia, and the clinical events related to recurrent ischemia, such as fatal and nonfatal reinfarction, and angina.

Randomized studies comparing primary stenting with primary coronary angioplasty in acute MI have not demonstrated a benefit of primary stenting in terms of decreased mortality, but they have shown a significant reduction in nonfatal reinfarction and repeat target vessel revascularization for recurrent angina.[13] These trials excluded patients with cardiogenic shock, and it is important to point out that most patients with recurrent ischemia experience only angina or nonfatal reinfarction, while death as a consequence of recurrent ischemia accounts for only a minority of deaths. The large majority of deaths after successful coronary angioplasty are due to refractory cardiogenic shock despite a patent infarct artery.[14,15] Thus, the expected benefit of stenting in terms of reduction of mortality is limited only to patients with a large area at risk or severe left ventricular (LV) dysfunction.

In patients with cardiogenic shock, the reocclusion of the infarct artery may be catastrophic, and as previously noted, stenting may reduce the incidence of reocclusion. For this reason, the rationale for the empirical use of stents in cardiogenic shock might be considered stronger than the one accepted for patients without cardiogenic shock.

On the other hand, it is mandatory to identify the factors which, in the setting of cardiogenic shock, may offset the potential benefit of stenting or even increase the risk of target vessel failure or deterioration of flow after stent implantation. These factors are not limited to the generic anatomical conditions associated with an increased risk of early and late in-stent restenosis or reocclusion, (such as small vessels, or long lesions that need multiple stent implantation), but include also the thrombotic burden, the stent design and material, the stent implantation technique, and the coronary perfusion pressure. All these factors may have a strong impact on the risk of stent thrombosis and of microvessel embolization, which result in a decreased effectiveness of reperfusion.

Clinical Studies of Coronary Stenting in Acute Myocardial Infarction Complicated by Cardiogenic Shock

Several observational studies have confirmed the efficacy of coronary stenting in the setting of acute MI complicated by cardiogenic shock. Neumann et al.[16] reported the results of coronary stenting in a series of 14 patients with cardiogenic shock. Multiple stent implantation was performed in most cases, and in all cases the procedure was successful. The in-hospital mortality rate was 29%. Webb et al.,[17] in a series of 15 patients with cardiogenic shock who underwent coronary stenting, reported a 73% survival rate after a follow-up of 10 ± 8 months. Carlos et al.[18] reported the results of percutaneous mechanical intervention in 39 patients with cardiogenic shock, 10 of whom had coronary stent implantation. In this series, there was a trend toward decreased mortality in stent patients as compared to patients who underwent coronary angioplasty alone or angioplasty with atherectomy (10% vs. 48.3%, p = 0.08).

Fabbiocchi et al.[19] performed coronary stenting in a series of 18 patients with cardiogenic shock. The in-hospital mortality rate was 28%. In a retrospective analysis including 177 patients with cardogenic shock,[20] a strategy of provisional stenting resulted in improved procedural success rate (85% vs. 66%), and decreased reocclusion (8% vs. 29%) and mortality rates (29% vs. 46%) as compared to coronary angioplasty alone.

A positive effect of coronary stenting on procedural success was demonstrated in the randomized SHOCK trial.[21] This trial, which enrolled 302 patients over a period of 6 years, compared an early revascularization strategy with an initial conservative strategy in patients with cardiogenic shock complicating acute MI. In this study, the primary success rate of coronary intervention remained very low until the last 2 years of enrollment, with only 58% of patients achieving TIMI grade 3 flow after the procedure. This poor result may potentially be explained, at least in part, by the limited use of stents in the first 4 years of enrollment (no stents were used in 1993–1994, 14% in 1995–1996). In 1997 and 1998 stents were used in 76% of treated cases, and TIMI grade 3 flow was achieved in 68% of patients. However, the number of patients treated was small, and a subgroup analysis of patients enrolled in the last 2 years of the study (45 patients), did not show significant differences in mortality between stent patients (n = 34; mortality 35%) and patients who underwent balloon angioplasty alone (n = 11; mortality 45%). As expected, successful angioplasty resulted in decreased mortality compared to the rate of death in patients with an unsuccessful procedure (38% vs. 79%).

The positive interaction between infarct-artery stenting and survival in patients with cardiogenic shock was revealed in a German registry of MIs.[22] Between 1994 and 1998 a total of 4552 patients underwent primary coronary angioplasty in 72 centers within 24 hours after symptom onset; clinical and procedural data of these patients were entered into the registry. Acute MI was complicated by cardiogenic shock in 671 patients (15%). The procedural success rate in patients with cardiogenic shock was 85%, with a final TIMI grade 3 flow in 76% of patients, and TIMI grade 2 flow in another 9%. The overall mortality was 47%, and mortality was lower in patients with stenting (41%) compared to coronary angioplasty alone (52%, p = 0.0006). The incidence of TIMI grade 3 flow was higher in patients with stent implantation, explaining the significantly lower mortality compared to coronary angioplasty. However, this study was retrospective, and the coronary angioplasty alone group included all patients who had unsuccessful guidewire crossing of the occlusion, which introduced a negative selection bias.

The NCN (National Cardiovascular Network) investigators examined the in-hospital outcomes of patients with cardiogenic shock undergoing percutaneous intervention or coronary artery surgery at 19 centers in the first 6 months of 1998.[23] This study included 130 patients who underwent emergent percutaneous coronary intervention. Infarct artery stenting was performed in 72% of the cases. The in-hospital mortality was 34%. A multivariate analysis revealed that patients in whom stent placement was not performed had a significantly higher risk of death (odds ratio 4.0, 95% CI 1.68–9.49).

Kastrati et al.[24] reported the clinical outcome of 519 consecutive patients with acute MI who underwent infarct artery stenting. Cardiogenic shock was present in 43 patients (8%). In this series, stent placement failed in 4 patients. The 1-month mortality rate was 33% among patients with cardiogenic shock and successful stent implantation. Multivariate analysis showed that overlapping stenting (hazard ratio [HR] 2.13, CI 1.16–3.91), and residual dissection (HR 2.83, CI 1.53–5.21) were predictors of an adverse outcome at 30 days.

In the last few years, several randomized studies comparing elective infarct-artery stenting with coronary angioplasty alone, or coronary angioplasty and provisional stenting, have shown the superiority of elective stenting, mainly in terms of decreased incidence of nonfatal reinfarction and of the need for repeat target vessel revascularization, while there were no benefits in terms of decreased mortality.[3,13,25–27] However, most of these randomized trials excluded patients with cardiogenic shock, and as a consequence, it is uncertain if a strategy of provisional stenting is comparable or superior to a strategy of systematic stenting in this setting.

Technical Aspects

Stent Implantation Techniques

In patients with thrombus-containing lesions, particularly in the setting of acute MI, stent placement and expansion at high-pressure may be followed by a no-reflow phenomenon. This is usually manifested by worsening of chest pain associated with marked ST-segment elevation and hemodynamic deterioration. Obviously, failure of microvascular reperfusion may be catastrophic in the setting of cardiogenic shock. In the Stent-PAMI trial,[13] which excluded patients with cardiogenic shock, infarct artery stenting was associated with a trend toward a lower incidence of TIMI grade 3 flow at the end of the procedure, and increased mortality as compared to angioplasty alone. The negative effect on distal flow may be the result of microvascular dysfunction mediated by spasm, oxygen-free radical injury, neutrophil activation and plugging, local edema, or macro- and microembolization of the disrupted plaque and thrombus. There is evidence that embolization in the microvasculature after catheter-based interventions is extremely common, and that such embolization can result in impairment of myocardial perfusion even when epicardial flow is restored by mechanical intervention.[28,29] It is likely that the pathological substrate of acute MI, including an already disrupted atherosclerotic plaque with superimposed thrombosis, may potentiate the atherosclerotic-platelet embolization promoted by stenting. It has been hypothesized that conventional stenting technique, utilizing single or multiple high-pressure balloon inflations after stent deployment, may promote the embolization of atherosclerotic debris and thrombotic material extruded through the struts during initial stent expansion.[13]

Some studies have suggested that direct stenting without predilation and without high-pressure inflation after stent deployment could be expected to reduce embolization of plaque constituents and the incidence of the no-reflow phenomenon, thereby increasing perfusion and myocardial salvage in patients with acute MI.[30-34] Potential disadvantages of the direct stenting technique are embolization promoted during target lesion crossing attempt, stent loss, and incomplete balloon and stent expansion in a "hard" calcified lesion. Enhanced designs of second generation stents and delivery systems, as well as the enhanced crimping techniques, seem to overcome these potential limitations, while few lesions in the setting of acute MI are not dilatable.

However, a substantial percentage of patients with acute MI complicated by cardiogenic shock have anatomic characteristics that are currently considered unfavorable for direct stenting. These include diffuse disease, multiple focal lesions within the infarct artery, and heavy calcification that may prevent complete and uniform expansion of the stent. Unfortunately, the risk of the no-reflow phenomenon is high in this patient group, since the diffuse coronary atherosclerotic disease is a risk factor for microvascular embolization.[35-37] Nevertheless, there is no doubt that the increased vessel wall injury resulting from conventional stenting techniques that include repeat balloon dilations may be also considered a dominant risk factor for embolization. Paradoxically, the advantage of direct stenting in reduction of embolization could be expected to be superior in unfavorable anatomical settings, such as long lesions or multiple lesions within the infarct artery, currently considered to confer a higher potential for embolization.

Despite uncertainty regarding the indications and benefits, direct stenting should be considered in patients with cardiogenic shock and angiographic evidence of a large thrombus burden, particularly if thrombectomy devices are not available, since conventional balloon angioplasty or stenting are invariably associated with large embolization and myocardial flow disruption. A realistic approach in most patients with cardiogenic shock may be to consider a relatively less invasive stenting technique that includes a low-pressure predilation, and delivery and expansion of the stent with a single balloon inflation avoiding very high pressure (> 16 atmospheres).

Coronary Stenting in Multivessel Disease

Coronary stenting allows rapid and effective multivessel revascularization in the emergent scenario of cardiogenic shock in a patient with multivessel disease. Revascularization of ischemic, but noninfarcted, myocardium is of crucial importance, as the mechanical capacity of noninfarct remote zones is critical for maintaining cardiac output. There is, therefore, a strong rationale for treating severe coronary stenoses outside the infarct zone early in the acute phase of cardiogenic shock. Treatment may be more effective before the downward spiral of end-organ hypoperfusion leads to irreversible organ dysfunction. It is possible that patients with cardiogenic shock and severe multivessel disease may derive the greatest benefit from multivessel stenting, but this remains to be tested in clinical trials.

Coronary Stenting in Left Main Disease

Two early case series including 6 and 16 patients, respectively, reported disappointing results of emergency percutaneous interventions in left main disease complicated by shock.[38,39] This scenario has changed dramatically with the use of stents. The ULTIMA (Unprotected Left Main Trunk Intervention Multi-center Assessment) Registry, a prospective, multicenter, international registry of interventions on 277 patients with unprotected left main disease, included clinical and procedural data on 40 patients who underwent emergency percutaneous left main intervention for acute MI.[40] Left main stenting was performed in 17 patients (40%), while 23 patients underwent angioplasty alone. The angiographic success rate was 88%, and in-hospital coronary bypass surgery was needed for seven patients, six on an emergent basis. Overall in-hospital mortality was 55%, with a trend toward lower rates of in-hospital death and coronary surgery for patients undergoing primary stenting. The 1-month survival rate was 53% in the stent group and 35% in the angioplasty alone group (p = 0.18), while the freedom from death or coronary surgery was 42% and 17%, respectively (p = 0.047). The 1-year survival rate was 53% for the stented left main patients and 35% for the patients undergoing angioplasty alone. It is important to point out that in this registry the stent group appeared to have a greater amount of myocardium at risk, manifested by a higher myocardial jeopardy score.

Coronary Stenting In Right Ventricular Infarction

Isolated right ventricular infarction is a rare occurrence, but this condition may be associated with a severe low output state and shock that may be unresponsive to fluid administration, inotropic agents, and intra-aortic balloon pumping. Involvement of the right ventricle in inferior MI, however, is relatively frequent and is associated with a poor prognosis. Percutaneous recanalization of the occluded right coronary artery has a strong impact on mortality in patients with right ventricular infarction. A key study using direct angioplasty showed that restoration of normal flow in right ventricular branches resulted in dramatic recovery of right ventricular function and a mortality rate of only 2%, whereas unsuccessful reperfusion of the right ventricle was associated with persistent hemodynamic compromise and a mortality rate of 58%.[41]

Stenting of the right coronary artery using multiple stent implantation or long stents for diffuse disease may be complicated by occlusion of right ventricular branches. In this case, attempted recanalization of at least one major branch through the stent struts may be warranted in order to avoid refractory right ventricular dysfunction and shock.

Coronary Stenting in Cardiogenic Shock without ST-Segment Elevation

From an interventional viewpoint, the procedural scenario of patients with cardiogenic shock complicating acute MI without ST-segment elevation may be quite different from that with ST-segment elevation.

The GUSTO investigators analyzed the clinical and angiographic characteristics of patients with acute ischemic syndromes with and without ST-segment elevation.[42] Out of the 12,073 patients enrolled in the GUSTO-IIb trial, 373 patients developed cardiogenic shock, 200 without ST-segment elevation, and 173 with ST-segment elevation. Patients without ST-segment elevation were older, had diabetes mellitus and three-vessel disease more frequently, but had less TIMI grade 0 flow at angiography. Shock development occurred considerably later in patients without ST-segment elevation (median time 76.2 hours after study entry vs. 9.6 hours in patients with ST-segment elevation), and more frequently in the setting of recurrent ischemia or recurrent infarction. Only a minority of patients without ST-segment elevation underwent mechanical revascularization (21 patients underwent coronary angioplasty, and 51 had coronary surgery). Multivariate analysis showed a strong trend toward reduced mortality with percutaneous intervention (HR 0.68, 95% CI 0.45-1.00, p = 0.052), while coronary surgery was independently associated with increased mortality (HR 2.03, 95% CI 1.42-2.92, p < 0.001).

In interventional practice, patients with cardiogenic shock without ST-segment elevation are technically challenging because of the presence of more extensive coronary disease, more vascular comorbidities, and the frequent inability to identify the infarct artery (in the GUSTO-IIb cohort the infarct-related artery location was unknown in 24% of patients without ST-segment elevation, while the infarct artery could be identified in all patients with ST-segment elevation).[42] On the other hand, the more progressive development of shock in this subset of patients provides a larger time window for intervention.

Multivessel stenting in this scenario may be considered as a first treatment option, since this would allow complete revascularization with a high procedural success rate.

Coronary Stenting in the Elderly

As a part of the aging process, coronary arteries are prone to dilation, tortuosity, and calcification. These pathophysiologic alterations, in addition to a higher prevalence of other extracardiac comorbidities, have contributed to the lower success rate of primary angioplasty and higher mortality for elderly patients with acute MI complicated by cardiogenic shock as compared to younger patients. However, data from the National Cardiovascular Network Registry suggest that the use of stents might have dramatically improved the clinical outcome in the elderly.[43] In a series of 103 octogenarians with cardiogenic shock registered from 1994 through 1997, stent use increased from 6% to 66%. The overall mortality rate in this series of patients was 31% (95% CI 22-40%).

Adjunctive Therapies

Mechanical Reduction of Thrombus Burden

Several mechanical devices for native coronary thrombus lysis and aspiration are available commercially (TEC, InterVentional Technologies,

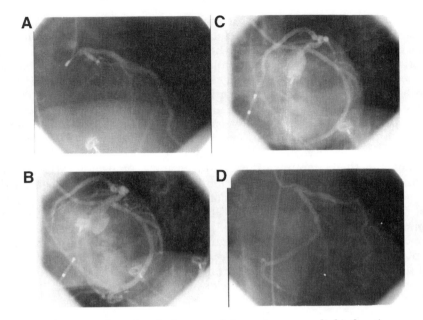

Figure 1. Integrated mechanical approach in acute myocardial infarction complicated by cardiogenic shock. **A:** Acute occlusion of a dominant circumflex artery;
subocclusive diffuse massive thrombosis. **B:** After thrombectomy a normal flow
was restored, and no angiographic evidence of thrombosis remained, only a mild
eccentric stenosis (13%) at the first portion of the circumflex artery. **C:** After direct
stenting. **D:** The 6-month scheduled angiography showing an optimal result.

Inc, San Diego, CA; AngioJet, Possis Medical Inc., Minneapolis, MN;
Acolysis, Angiosonics Inc., Morrissville, NC; X-SIZER, EndiCOR Medical,
San Clemente, CA). Their use in the setting of cardiogenic shock should
be considered in patients with angiographic evidence of massive coronary
thrombosis. Desirable features in such devices include the ability to track
the guidewire to navigate in native coronary vessels, minimization of
trauma to the vessel wall, and the ability to aspirate thrombotic debris
before antegrade crossing of the occlusion and to continue during retrieval,
so as to minimize the risk of embolization. (Figure 1).

Several emboli entrapment devices are currently under investigation.
However, their potential benefit may be limited in the native coronary
circulation, since these devices do not provide antiembolic protection of
the branches of the infarct artery. Further limitations may occur in acute
MI with total occlusion, since initial recanalization may shower debris
before the device can be deployed.

Glycoprotein IIb/IIIa Inhibitors

The first four cases of the use of abciximab in conjunction with coronary stenting in patients with cardiogenic shock were reported in 1996.[44]
In the last years, glycoprotein IIb/IIIa inhibitors have been used mostly

in selected patients considered at higher risk for stent thrombosis, so it is not possible to draw firm conclusions about their potential role as a routine adjunctive therapy in patients with cardiogenic shock undergoing stent implantation. However, available clinical data from randomized and observational studies strongly support the hypothesis that IIb/IIIa inhibitors in combination with stenting may benefit patients with cardiogenic shock.

The PURSUIT (Platelet Glycoprotein IIb/IIIa in Unstable Angina: Receptor Suppression Using Integrilin Therapy) trial is the first controlled clinical experience with the use of IIb/IIIa inhibitors in patients with cardiogenic shock complicating acute coronary syndromes without ST-segment elevation.[45] Of the 237 patients in this trial who developed cardiogenic shock, 117 (49.4%) received eptifibatide. In the multivariate analysis, randomization to eptifibatide did not affect the occurrence of cardiogenic shock (OR 0.95, CI 0.72–1.25, p = 0.71). However, randomization to eptifibatide reduced 30-day mortality among all cardiogenic shock patients (58.5% vs. 73.5%) and among cardiogenic shock patients with either MI (69% vs. 85%) or unstable angina (48% vs. 58%). In the multivariate analysis, eptifibatide reduced the odds of 30-day death by 48.9% (OR 0.51, 95% CI 0.28–0.94, p = 0.03).

The CADILLAC trial enrolled 2082 patients and compared four revascularization strategies in acute MI: coronary angioplasty alone, coronary angioplasty plus abciximab, stenting alone, and stenting plus abciximab.[46] At 6 months, no clinical benefit of abciximab could be demonstrated in patients who underwent coronary stenting (the incidence of the composite clinical endpoint of death, MI, target vessel revascularization was 10.9% in the stent alone arm, and 10.8% in the stent plus abciximab arm) . However, it is important to point out that the enrolled population was relatively young (mean age, 59 years) and at low risk, which resulted in low event rates. Patients with cardiogenic shock were excluded, and thus the applicability of the results to this population, or even to patients with large infarctions, is uncertain.

No benefit of abciximab could be demonstrated in the SHOCK trial comparing emergency revascularization with initial conservative therapy in 302 patients with cardiogenic shock.[21] Use of stents and IIb/IIIa inhibitors was relatively low, however. Of the patients receiving angioplasty in the emergency revascularization arm, only 35.7% were stented, while IIb/IIIa inhibitors were used in 41.7%. The rate of stent use for any lesion was 0% in 1993-1994, 19% in 1995-1996, and 74% in 1997-1998; the rate of use of IIb/IIIa inhibitors was 0% in 1993-1994, 27% in 1995-1996, and 59% in 1997-1998. Among the 45 patients assigned to emergency revascularization who underwent angioplasty in 1997 or 1998, 19 received both a stent and platelet glycoprotein IIb/IIIa receptor antagonist, and 15 received a stent only; the respective mortality rates were 37% and 33%. This small number of patients precludes firm conclusions regarding a potential benefit of IIb/IIIa inhibitors in conjunction with coronary stenting in patients with cardiogenic shock.

An observational study of 725 consecutive patients with MI undergoing primary percutaneous intervention from 1995 to 1999 identified 105 with cardiogenic shock and found that the use of stenting and abciximab reduced the incidence of death, MI or target vessel revascularization.[47] Among the 105 patients with cardiogenic shock, there were 37 deaths (35%), 17 repeat target vessel revascularization (16%), and 6 nonfatal reinfarctions (6%). Overall, death, reinfarction, and repeat target vessel revascularization occurred in 52 patients (50%). Major adverse events were less likely to occur in cardiogenic shock patients with stent use (37% vs. 60%), and abciximab use (33% vs. 60%). In a multivariate logistic regression analysis, the combination of abciximab and stenting was an independent predictor of the risk of 1-month major adverse events (OR 0.12; 95% CI 0.03–0.44; p = 0.001).

The benefit of abciximab in conjunction with coronary stenting in patients with and without cardiogenic shock was demonstrated in a retrospective analysis from Florence, based on a series of 561 consecutive patients with acute MI who underwent emergency percutaneous intervention between January 1999 and October 2000 (personal communication). The combination of abciximab and stenting was used in 325 patients, while 179 patients had stenting alone, 23 coronary angioplasty plus abciximab, and 34 coronary angioplasty alone. There were 59 patients with cardiogenic shock (10%); 35 patients had coronary stenting plus abciximab, and 24 underwent stenting alone (p = 0.636). Overall, the 1-month mortality was 4% in the abciximab group, and 12% in the remaining patients (p < 0.001). In the subgroup of patients with shock, the 1-month mortality was lower in patients who had received abciximab compared to the remaining patients (17% and 46%, respectively; p = 0.02). In a multivariate analysis , the use of abciximab resulted in lower 1-month mortality (OR 0.25, 95% CI 0.08-0.81, p = 0.022).

References

1. Cannon AD, Roubin GS, Macander PJ, et al. Intracoronary stenting as an adjunct to angioplasty in acute myocardial infarction. *J Invasive Cardiol* 1991; 3:255-258.

2. Garcia-Cantu E, Spaulding C, Corcos T, et al. Stent implantation in acute myocardial infarction. *Am J Cardiol* 1996; 77:451-454.

3. Rodriguez A, Bernardi V, Fernandez M, et al. In-hospital and late results of coronary stents versus conventional balloon angioplasty in acute myocardial infarction (GRAMI trial). Gianturco-Roubin in Acute Myocardial Infarction. *Am J Cardiol* 1998; 81:1286-1291.

4. Antoniucci D, Valenti R, Buonamici P, et al. Direct angioplasty and stenting of the infarct-related artery in acute myocardial infarction. *Am J Cardiol* 1996; 78:568-571.

5. Saito S, Hosokawa FG, Kim K, et al. Primary stent implantation without coumadin in acute myocardial infarction. *J Am Coll Cardiol* 1996; 28:74-81.

6. Antoniucci D, Valenti R, Santoro GM, et al. Systematic direct angioplasty and stent-supported direct angioplasty therapy for cardiogenic shock complicating acute myocardial infarction: In-hospital and long-term survival. *J Am Coll Cardiol* 1998; 31:294-300.

7. Grines CL, Browne KF, Marco J, et al. A comparison of immediate angioplasty with thrombolytic therapy for acute myocardial infarction. *N Engl J Med* 1993; 328:673-679.

8. GUSTO Angiographic Investigators. The effects of tissue plasminogen activator, streptokinase, or both on coronary-artery patency, ventricular function, and survival after acute myocardial infarction. *N Engl J Med* 1993; 329:1615-1622.

9. Zijlstra F, de Boer MJ, Hoorntje JC, et al. A comparison of immediate coronary angioplasty with intravenous streptokinase in acute myocardial infarction. *N Engl J Med* 1993; 328:680-684.

10. Brodie BR, Grines CL, Ivanhoe R, et al. Six-month clinical and angiographic follow-up after direct angioplasty for acute myocardial infarction. Final results from the Primary Angioplasty Registry. *Circulation* 1994; 90:156-162.

11. Stone GW, Marsalese D, Brodie BR, et al. A prospective, randomized evaluation of prophylactic intraaortic balloon counterpulsation in high risk patients with acute myocardial infarction treated with primary angioplasty. Second Primary Angioplasty in Myocardial Infarction (PAMI-II) Trial Investigators. *J Am Coll Cardiol* 1997; 29:1459-1467.

12. Foley DP, Melkert R, Serruys PW. Influence of coronary vessel size on renarrowing process and late angiographic outcome after successful balloon angioplasty. *Circulation* 1994; 90:1239-1251.

13. Grines CL, Cox DA, Stone GW, et al. Coronary angioplasty with or without stent implantation for acute myocardial infarction. Stent Primary Angioplasty in Myocardial Infarction Study Group. *N Engl J Med* 1999; 341:1949-1956.

14. Brodie BR, Stuckey TD, Hansen CJ, et al. Timing and mechanism of death determined clinically after primary angioplasty for acute myocardial infarction. *Am J Cardiol* 1997; 79:1586-1591.

15. Stone GW, Grines CL, Browne KF, et al. Implications of recurrent ischemia after reperfusion therapy in acute myocardial infarction: A comparison of thrombolytic therapy and primary angioplasty. *J Am Coll Cardiol* 1995; 26:66-72.

16. Neumann FJ, Walter H, Richardt G, et al. Coronary Palmaz-Schatz stent implantation in acute myocardial infarction. *Heart* 1996; 75:121-126.

17. Webb JG, Carere RG, Hilton JD, et al. Usefulness of coronary stenting for cardiogenic shock. *Am J Cardiol* 1997; 79:81-84.

18. Carlos BD, Linsday J, Pinnow EE, et al. New device intervention in cardiogenic shock (abstract). *J Am Coll Cardiol* 1997; 29:460A.

19. Fabbiocchi F, Bartorelli AL, Montorsi P, et al. Elective coronary stent implantation in cardiogenic shock complicating acute myocardial infarction: In-hospital and six-month clinical and angiographic results. *Catheter Cardiovasc Interv* 2000; 50:384-389.

20. Nakagawa Y, Hamasaki N, Kimura T, et al. Stent implantation in acute myocardial infarction is more beneficial in patients with cardiogenic shock than those without (abstract). *J Am Coll Cardiol* 1998; 31:232A.

21. Hochman JS, Sleeper LA, Webb JG, et al. Early revascularization in acute myocardial infarction complicated by cardiogenic shock. SHOCK Investigators. Should We Emergently Revascularize Occluded Coronaries for Cardiogenic Shock. *N Engl J Med* 1999; 341:625-634.

22. Zeymer U, Vogt A, Niederer W, et al. Primary PTCA with and without stent implantation in 671 patients with acute myocardial infarction complicated by cardiogenic shock. Results of the ALKK Primary-PTCA Registry (abstract). *J Am Coll Cardiol* 2000; 35:363A.

23. Mahoney EM, Thompson TD, Veledar E, et al. In-hospital mortality for patients with cardiogenic shock undergoing PTCA and CABG in 1998: Results from the National Cardiovascular Network (NCN) (abstract). *J Am Coll Cardiol* 2000; 35:351A.

24. Kastrati A, Pache J, Dirschinger J, et al. Primary intracoronary stenting in acute myocardial infarction: Long- term clinical and angiographic follow-up and risk factor analysis. *Am Heart J* 2000; 139:208-216.

25. Antoniucci D, Santoro GM, Bolognese L, et al. A clinical trial comparing primary stenting of the infarct-related artery with optimal primary angioplasty for acute myocardial infarction: Results from the Florence Randomized Elective Stenting in Acute Coronary Occlusions (FRESCO) trial. *J Am Coll Cardiol* 1998; 31:1234-1239.

26. Suryapranata H, van't Hof AW, Hoorntje JC, et al. Randomized comparison of coronary stenting with balloon angioplasty in selected patients with acute myocardial infarction. *Circulation* 1998; 97:2502-2505.

27. Saito S, Hosokawa G, Tanaka S, et al. Primary stent implantation is superior to balloon angioplasty in acute myocardial infarction: Final results of the primary angioplasty versus stent implantation in acute myocardial infarction (PASTA) trial. PASTA Trial Investigators. *Catheter Cardiovasc Interv* 1999; 48:262-268.

28. Topol EJ, Yadav JS. Recognition of the importance of embolization in atherosclerotic vascular disease. *Circulation* 2000; 101:570-580.

29. Ito H, Maruyama A, Iwakura K, et al. Clinical implications of the "no reflow" phenomenon. A predictor of complications and left ventricular remodeling in reperfused anterior wall myocardial infarction. *Circulation* 1996; 93:223-228.

30. Hamon M, Richardeau Y, Lecluse E, et al. Direct coronary stenting without balloon predilation in acute coronary syndromes. *Am Heart J* 1999; 138:55-59.

31. Herz I, Assali A, Solodky A, et al. Coronary stent deployment without predilation in acute myocardial infarction: A feasible, safe, and effective technique. *Angiology* 1999; 50:901-908.

32. Chan AW, Carere RG, Solankhi N, et al. Coronary stenting without predilatation in a broad spectrum of clinical and angiographic situations. *J Invasive Cardiol* 2000; 12:75-79.

33. Wilson SH, Berger PB, Mathew V, et al. Immediate and late outcomes after direct stent implantation without balloon predilation. *J Am Coll Cardiol* 2000; 35:937-943.

34. Moschi G, Migliorini A, Moir KJ, et al. Direct stenting without predilation in acute myocardial infarction (abstract). *Eur Heart J* 2000; 21:525.

35. Abbo KM, Dooris M, Glazier S, et al. Features and outcome of no-reflow after percutaneous coronary intervention. *Am J Cardiol* 1995; 75:778-782.

36. Abdelmeguid AE, Topol EJ, Whitlow PL, et al. Significance of mild transient release of creatine kinase-MB fraction after percutaneous coronary interventions. *Circulation* 1996; 94:1528-1536.

37. Califf RM, Abdelmeguid AE, Kuntz RE, et al. Myonecrosis after revascularization procedures. *J Am Coll Cardiol* 1998; 31:241-251.

38. Chauhan A, Zubaid M, Ricci DR, et al. Left main intervention revisited: Early and late outcome of PTCA and stenting. *Cathet Cardiovasc Diagn* 1997; 41:21-29.

39. Quigley RL, Milano CA, Smith LR, et al. Prognosis and management of anterolateral myocardial infarction in patients with severe left main disease and

cardiogenic shock. The left main shock syndrome. *Circulation* 1993; 88:II65-70.

40. Marso SP, Steg G, Plokker T, et al. Catheter-based reperfusion of unprotected left main stenosis during an acute myocardial infarction (the ULTIMA experience). Unprotected Left Main Trunk Intervention Multi-center Assessment. *Am J Cardiol* 1999; 83:1513-1517.

41. Bowers TR, O'Neill WW, Grines C, et al. Effect of reperfusion on biventricular function and survival after right ventricular infarction. *N Engl J Med* 1998; 338:933-940.

42. Holmes DR, Berger PB, Hochman JS, et al. Cardiogenic shock in patients with acute ischemic syndromes with and without ST-segment elevation. *Circulation* 1999; 100:2067-2073.

43. Batchelor WB, Anstrom KJ, Muhlbaier LH, et al. Contemporary outcome trends in the elderly undergoing percutaneous coronary interventions: Results in 7,472 octogenarians. National Cardiovascular Network Collaboration. *J Am Coll Cardiol* 2000; 36:723-730.

44. Schultz RD, Heuser RR, Hatler C, et al. Use of c7E3 Fab in conjunction with primary coronary stenting for acute myocardial infarctions complicated by cardiogenic shock. *Cathet Cardiovasc Diagn* 1996; 39:143-148.

45. Hasdai D, Kitt MM, Harrington RA, et al. Impact of platelet glycoprotein IIb/IIIa blockade on outcome of cardiogenic shock among patients with acute coronary syndromes without persistent ST-segment elevation (abstract). *Circulation* 1999; 100:I-433.

46. Stone GW. CADILLAC: A 4 arm prospective multicenter randomized trial of PTCA vs stenting with and without glycoprotein IIb/IIIa blockade in patients with acute myocardial infarction, 12th TCT Symposium, Washington, DC, 2000.

47. Giri S, Kiernan FJ, Mitchel JF, et al. Synergistic interaction between intracoronary stenting and IIb/IIIa inhibition for improving clinical outcomes in primary angioplasty for cardiogenic shock (abstract). *Circulation* 2000; 100:I-380.

Part III.

Other Considerations.

Chapter 10

Right Ventricular Infarction

Zoran S. Nedeljkovic, MD and Thomas J. Ryan, MD

"[The heart] *is an exceedingly strong muscle – 'muscle' in the sense not of 'tendon' but of compressed mass of flesh. It contains in one circumference two separate cavities, one here, the other there. These cavities are quite dissimilar: the one on the right side lies face downwards, fitting closely against the other. By 'right' I mean of course the right of the left side, since it is on the left side that the whole heart has its seat. Furthermore this chamber is very spacious, and much more hollow than the other. It does not extend to the extremity of the heart, but leaves the apex solid, being as it were stitched on outside.*"

—Hippocrates ca. 260 B.C

Introduction

Cardiogenic shock represents one of the most devastating complications of acute myocardial infarction (MI). It typically results from rapid deterioration of myocardial systolic function leading to systemic hypotension, organ hypoperfusion, and ultimately tissue hypoxia. Left untreated, shock invariably results in multiorgan failure and death. Shock represents a well-described complication of left ventricular (LV) ischemia and infarction, however it is also an important consequence of ischemia and infarction of the right ventricle. As will be discussed, right ventricular ischemia (RVI) is more common than right ventricular myocardial infarction (RVMI) and represents a potentially reversible form of right ventricular dysfunction that shares similar clinical features with RVMI. This chapter will review the pathophysiologic, clinical, and hemodynamic features of RVI and RVMI, and emphasize the key components of early recognition and management. Recent advances, particularly in the area of reperfusion strategies, will also be addressed.

From: Hollenberg SM, Bates ER. *Cardiogenic Shock*. Armonk, NY: Futura Publishing Co., Inc.; ©2002.

Historical Perspective

Although first described in 1930,[1] infarction of the right ventricle was not initially appreciated as a clinical entity with specific hemodynamic consequences. The fall in cardiac output and circulatory failure seen with acute MI was generally attributed to predominant ischemic injury of the left ventricle. Early work by Starr and associates demonstrated minimal or no increase in peripheral venous pressures, nor any significant change in cardiac output, despite extensive isolated mechanical damage to the right ventricle in open-chest dogs.[2] Experimental work by Bakos[3] involving severe damage to the canine right ventricle by electrocautery similarly demonstrated no significant increase in systemic venous or pulmonary arterial pressures. He suggested that the right ventricle continued to function as a passive pumping chamber through energy transmitted from actively contracting LV muscle bands, thereby maintaining RV output and normal systemic venous and pulmonary arterial pressures.[3] Alternatively, Kagan proposed that the maintenance of adequate right ventricular stroke output in the face of severe and extensive damage of its outer walls was due to a subsidiary contractile mechanism by the interventricular septum.[4] Fontan and co-workers were able to effectively bypass the right ventricle through the creation of a direct cavo-pulmonary anastamosis in a 12-year-old cyanotic child with tricuspid atresia.[5] This, as well as other successful techniques of atrio-pulmonary bypass in the correction of congenital heart disease, further questioned the importance of the right ventricle in the maintenance of a normal circulation.[6] Thus for many years, investigators viewed the right ventricle simply as a passive conduit for blood returning from the systemic veins, rather than an active pumping chamber.

During the early 1970s, the balloon-tipped pulmonary artery flotation catheter gained widespread popularity in the management of patients with acute MI. Central hemodynamic monitoring in the closed-chested model of patients with acute MI allowed identification of individuals with unsuspected volume depletion or significant LV dysfunction. Similarly, it proved helpful in monitoring a variety of hemodynamic parameters in response to selected therapy. As so often happens with the introduction of new technology, a previously unrecognized entity was described.[7] Cohn et al. originally reported the findings of RVMI among patients undergoing routine hemodynamic monitoring for acute MI.[8] The finding of (1) disproportionately elevated right-sided filling pressures, (2) near normal left-sided filling pressures, and (3) low cardiac output with apparently preserved LV function, constituted the classic hemodynamic profile of predominant RVMI (or ischemia).

Prevalence

Right ventricular ischemia is usually accompanied by some degree of LV ischemia or infarction. The overall prevalence of RVI and RVMI varies among different series, depending on which invasive or noninvasive indicators are used for the diagnosis.[9-16] Nonetheless, RVMI has been recognized to occur more frequently with certain subsets of LV ischemia and infarction, particularly those involving the inferior-posterior wall and posterior interventricular septum.[9-13]

In a large early series, Isner and Roberts examined 236 necropsy heart specimens from patients with recent MI and observed that RVMI occurred exclusively in hearts with posterior (inferior) LV infarction.[9] Of the 139 heart specimens with transmural inferior wall infarctions, 33 (24%) were also found to have RVMI. These data should be interpreted cautiously as they represent nonsurvivors, likely patients with more extensive ischemic injury. Additionally, this represents a pathologic study of true infarction and hence may have been an underestimate of the actual prevalence of ischemia. Most other series cite the incidence of RVI as approximately one-third of all inferior MIs.[9-18]

The subclinical prevalence of RV ischemia with inferior infarction may in fact be higher. Using radionuclide imaging techniques, Wackers et al. showed RV involvement in 24 of 64 patients (37.5%) with acute inferior MI.[13] As none of these patients exhibited the classic signs of right-sided failure, they concluded that RV involvement was relatively frequent in inferior infarctions, yet not necessarily associated with severe pump failure and hemodynamic compromise.

Right ventricular infarction can also be seen in association with anterior LV infarction, although much less frequently. In a postmortem study of 97 patients with anterior MI, Cabin et al. found that anterior biventricular necrosis was present in 13 of these patients (10%).[14] This was felt to result from ischemic injury to both anterior ventricular walls, which share a common blood supply. Isolated RVMI is exceedingly rare and poses a diagnostic challenge in the absence of signs of LV infarction.[15,16]

Anatomy

The principal cause of ischemia and subsequent infarction of the right ventricle is acute thrombotic occlusion of a coronary artery. Accordingly, understanding the anatomy of the coronary circulation with respect to the territories supplied by its branches can help identify common infarct-related arteries. It is generally believed that patients with inferior infarctions complicated by RVI have right coronary artery (RCA) occlusions, proximal to the takeoff of branches that supply the anterior and lateral wall of the right ventricle. However, based on pathologic series, the posterior wall of the right ventricle is most frequently involved, almost always concomitant with infarction of the posterior LV wall.[9,10] Thus, the association of RVI with inferior LV infarction arises from their common blood supply, namely the infero-posterior coronary circulation.

Coronary dominance refers to the artery which gives rise to (1) the posterior descending artery (PDA) which courses in the posterior interventricular groove and supplies branches to the interventricular septum, and (2) the posterolateral branches (PLB) which supply the inferior and lateral portions of the left ventricle. In 85% of the population, this anatomic

---

Table 1.

**Potential Theories to Explain
the Relative Infrequency of Right Ventricular Infarction**

---

1. RV has more favorable oxygen supply-demand ratio than LV
   Low resistance pulmonary arterial circuit
   Lower systolic pressure
   Generates less wall tension, Law of LaPlace
   $$T \propto (P \times r)/h \; *$$
   Smaller RV muscle mass
2. Coronary blood flow during both systole and diastole
3. Collateral circulation from the left coronary system
4. Direct intra-cavitary oxygen diffusion

---

* The Law of LaPlace relates wall tension (T) to pressure (P), radius (r), and wall thickness (h). LV = left ventricle; RV = right ventricle.

territory is supplied by the RCA, and explains why this artery is the most common culprit vessel associated with inferior LV and RVI. Less commonly, RVI can be seen with proximal occlusion of the left circumflex artery when this vessel gives rise to the posterior descending artery and posterolateral branches that supply the infero-posterior territory (left-dominant pattern).

Generally, larger infarcts are associated with proximal coronary occlusions, where more myocardium is at risk. It thus may seem somewhat surprising that the incidence of RVI with inferior LV infarction is relatively uncommon (i.e., only approximately one-third of all cases). Several theories have been proposed as to what renders the right ventricle relatively more resistant to irreversible ischemia and infarction (Table 1). First, the right ventricle has a more favorable balance between its myocardial oxygen supply and demand compared to the left ventricle, and is mechanically suited to operate against the relatively low impedance pulmonary circuit. As a consequence of the lower impedance to systolic flow, the right ventricle has to generate less pressure than the left ventricle, although both chambers deliver the same total cardiac output. As a result, the right ventricle generates less wall tension in accordance with LaPlace's Law and is roughly one-sixth the mass of the left. Wall tension and total muscle mass are among the major determinants of myocardial oxygen demand. Second, although the left ventricle receives most of its blood supply during diastole, the pattern of blood flow to the right ventricle is phasic, occurring throughout the cardiac cycle. As demonstrated in an elegant canine study by Hess, this appears to be due to lower intramyocardial compressive forces generated during systole by the right ventricle compared to the left.[19] As a result, RV subendocardial layers are relatively better perfused in comparison to the left ventricle, due to lower intramyocardial impedance. Third, extensive collateralization of blood to the right ventricle from the left-sided coronary circulation may develop as a result of recurrent ischemia, as has been recently proposed by Shikari et al.[20] These investigators retrospectively examined the association of preinfarction angina with RVMI in patients who had presented with acute inferior MI. They found that the presence of preinfarction angina was an independent predictor of the absence of RVMI. The patients with preinfarction angina were noted to have developed more extensive collateral vessels than those without angina, which may have been an explanation for the lower incidence of RVMI.[20] Indeed, repeated episodes of ischemia can lead to preconditioning and collateral formation, which subsequently protects myocardium from future infarction (ischemic preconditioning). Finally, due to the relatively thinner wall of the right ventricle, there is likely a more significant contribution from direct intracavitary diffusion of oxygen and better perfusion of subendocardial layers. Each of these factors may potentially protect the right ventricle from infarction and more importantly, increase the likelihood of reversal of ischemia. These features suggest that RV dysfunction in the setting of inferior LV infarction may represent stunned myocardium as a result of ischemia that has not progressed to complete infarction.[11,12]

Pathophysiology

The classic clinical features of RVI include hypotension, systemic venous congestion, and the absence of pulmonary congestion. Much progress has been made over the last several years in understanding the pathophysiology of RVI, especially with regard to alterations in systolic and diastolic properties of *both* chambers. Central to this understanding is the close relationship of both the left and right ventricle through the shared interventricular septum and the presence of an intact pericardium.

Acute MI and infarction typically results from disruption of a vulnerable atherosclerotic plaque. This subsequently leads to thrombus formation and near total or total occlusion of the coronary artery. As myocardial ischemia represents an imbalance between oxygen supply and demand, coronary occlusion can critically reduce oxygen supply and lead to tissue infarction. As already described, RVI typically results from occlusion of the right coronary artery proximal to the RV (marginal) branches.

The primary event in acute RVI is RV chamber enlargement due to impaired myocyte relaxation, depressed contractility, and impaired ventricular emptying, which leads to elevated right-sided volume and pressure. Clinically, this is manifest as elevated jugular venous pressure, neck vein distention, and peripheral venous congestion (positive hepatojugular reflux, hepatomegaly, and peripheral edema). Stretch of the right ventricle within the constraints of the pericardium further limits myocardial distensibility and may also contribute to elevated right-sided filling pressures. Decreased RV chamber compliance may also result directly from ischemia, independent of chamber dilatation and pericardial constraint. In the case of the right ventricle, it is likely that stretch within the constraints of an intact pericardium, coupled with increased chamber stiffness, contributes to elevated right-sided filling pressures and peripheral congestion seen with RVI. As a result, ischemia leads not only to a fall in the systolic (forward stroke volume) and diastolic performance (chamber stiffness) of the right ventricle, but also a *geometric* and conformational change (chamber enlargement). In turn, this impacts on the contralateral ventricle through the shared interventricular septum altering both its *diastolic* and *systolic* properties, a concept termed ventricular interdependence.[21-24]

Reduced LV diastolic filling (preload) appears to be at least one important mechanism in the genesis of the low-output state of RVI. Right ventricular ischemia and infarction can lead to low cardiac output by directly reducing LV filling secondary to depressed RV contractility. As demonstrated by Goldstein and colleagues in dogs with experimentally induced RVMI, volume loading led to improvements in RV output and augmented systemic output by increasing LV filling.[25] A second mechanism of impaired LV filling results from ischemia-induced acute RV dilatation and elevation of intrapericardial pressure.[26] The pericardium is a relatively stiff fibro-elastic sac enclosing a space in which small changes in volume lead to disproportionately larger changes in intrapericardial pressure. Elevated intrapericardial pressure in turn leads to equalization of diastolic pressures in the right and left ventricles. In another experimental series of RVMI, Goldstein et al. emphasized the role of elevated intrapericardial pressure by demonstrating improvement in cardiac output following pericardiectomy in dogs.[26] Following RVMI, volume loading led to an increase in LV end diastolic pressure (LVEDP) from 7 to 12 mm Hg. This was associated with a small increase in cardiac output. Following pericardiectomy, the mean LVEDP fell to 11 mm Hg, yet cardiac output and LV volumes were *higher* than in the animals with an intact pericardium. This is due to the fact that the LV pressure (which is responsible for its distention and filling) is diminished with high intrapericardial pressures. Pericardiectomy serves to relieve high intrapericardial pressures and can lead to improvements in systemic cardiac output in RVMI. This further underscores the importance of the intact pericardium. Thus, optimizing LV filling by pericardiectomy or volume loading can lead to improvements in cardiac output.

Finally, an increase in RV pressure and volume, coupled with the constraining effects of the pericardium, causes the interventricular septum to shift from its normal shape and position to a more flattened configuration, which may in fact bulge into the LV cavity (Figure 1).[27] This reversed septal curvature (reverse Bernheim effect) compromises LV diastolic filling by increasing stiffness, reducing chamber compliance, and raising filling pressures. These factors all contribute to a fall in LV diastolic volume, reduced cardiac output, and systemic hypotension without evident depression of LV systolic function. However, in humans, optimizing LV filling alone does not always lead to hemodynamic improvement (see below).

Right ventricular contractile performance has been difficult to quantify by conventional methods, as its complex geometry and shape make accurate volume measurements difficult. The RV free wall, septum, and left ventricle all contribute to RV stroke output. As previously mentioned, the right ventricle is anatomically and physiologically suited to operate against the relatively low-pressure pulmonary arterial circuit. Hence, conventional load-dependent indices of contractile function of the left

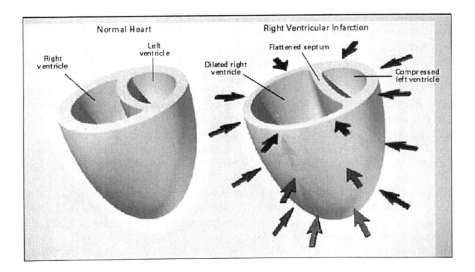

Figure 1. Pathophysiology of right ventricular infarction. Acute right ventricular dilatation coupled with pericardial restraining forces causes reversal of normal septal curvature and compression of left ventricular filling. (N Engl J Med 1998; 338:978-980. Reproduced with Permission. *Copyright ¤1998 Massachusetts Medical Society. All rights reserved.*)

ventricle (i.e., dP/dt) cannot be applied to the right ventricle because of differences in loading conditions (preload and afterload) between the two ventricles.[23,28] Pressure-volume analysis is derived from the simultaneous relation between ventricular volume and pressure during the cardiac cycle. It is useful in distinguishing between changes due to loading conditions from active and passive myocardial properties. Load-independent parameters of contractile performance (i.e., end-systolic pressure volume relation) have been shown to be similar between the right and left ventricles.[29,30] In other words, the instantaneous pressure-volume relationship demonstrated in both ventricles is indeed linear.

It has recently been appreciated that geometric alterations in the orientation of the interventricular septum in response to acute RVI impacts not only LV diastolic function, but LV systolic function as well. In an experimentally induced model of RVI in pigs, Brooks and associates demonstrated that alterations in septal curvature significantly impacted on LV contractile performance independently of the effects of LV inferior wall ischemia or diastolic filling (preload).[24] Systolic function was assessed by pressure-volume analysis, which has the advantage of being load-independent and thus is not affected by changes in preload. The two indices of LV systolic function derived were the slope of the end-systolic pressure-volume relation (LV ESPVR) and that of the stroke work-end diastolic volume (EDV) relation (preload-recruitable stroke work, PRSW). Changes in LV compliance with acute ischemia and RV dilatation were demonstrated by increases in LVEDP as well as an increase in the slope of the LV end diastolic pressure-volume relation (LV EDPVR). When the pericardium was subsequently opened, these changes were not seen. This was consistent with prior observations that in the presence of an intact pericardium, RV ischemia decreases LV compliance and impairs its diastolic filling properties. However, RCA occlusion was also shown to impair LV systolic function as evidenced by a decline in the slopes of both the PRSW and LV ESPVR. Both pericardiotomy and dobutamine infusion partially reversed these changes. Therefore, the *position* of the interventricular septum appears to play a crucial role in both LV diastolic and systolic performance through distortions in LV cavity geometry.

Previous reports emphasized the contribution of the left ventricle, through the shared interventricular septum, in augmenting RV performance when there is damage to the RV free wall.[21] It has been proposed that alterations in the alignment of the septal fibers, secondary to RV ischemia, diminish the LV contribution to RV systolic performance (LV systolic interaction).[22] The clinical implication of this finding is that efforts to restore the normal position and curvature of the interventricular septum in response to ischemia can improve the mechanical efficiency of biventricular systolic contraction. This may also serve as an explanation of why volume loading alone may produce variable results and may not improve overall circulatory function.[22] Thus, the determinants of RV stroke output lie not only in the pressure generated in the right ventricle itself (free wall and septum) but by the LV contribution as well.

Clinical Features

The clinical diagnosis of RVMI is made when there are signs of RV dysfunction in the setting of acute inferior LV infarction. Clinicians should be able to perform a focused history and physical examination and interpret key data from the ECG and other noninvasive studies to be able to accurately diagnose RV infarction and to institute appropriate therapy within the first 30 minutes of presentation.

Physical Examination

The classic triad of hypotension, clear lung fields, and elevated jugular venous pressure (JVP) is a specific but not sensitive finding in RV infarction. In 1983, Dell'Italia prospectively studied 53 consecutive patients with inferior wall infarctions to determine the sensitivity and specificity of physical findings in the diagnosis of RV infarction.[31] Patients presenting with inferior MI (based on history, ECG, and cardiac-specific enzyme elevations) were all evaluated before therapy was instituted and 1-2 hours before hemodynamic assessment. Eight of the 53 patients had hemodynamic characteristics consistent with RVMI (15%). There was no significant difference in the presence of pulmonary rales, a third or fourth heart sound, or mitral or tricuspid regurgitation, between the two groups. Statistically significant differences between the two groups were found with respect to the presence of elevated JVP (> 8 cm H_2O), clear lung fields, and the presence of Kussmaul's venous sign (defined as an inspiratory rise in JVP). The presence of an elevated JVP was seen in 7 of the 8 patients with RVI and in 14 of the 45 without RVI, making it a relatively sensitive (88%) but not specific (69%) sign. Both an elevated JVP and clear lung fields were present in 4 of the 8 patients with RVI and in 8 of the 45 without RVI, which did not prove to be sensitive (50%) but was fairly specific (82%) for RVI. Similarly, the presence of all three clinical findings was not very sensitive (25%), but reached a higher specificity (96%).

Interestingly, Kussmaul's sign was present in all eight patients with hemodynamically proven RVI and in none of the 45 patients without, yielding a dramatic 100% sensitivity and specificity. Furthermore, the presence of both Kussmaul's sign and elevated JVP had a sensitivity of 88% and specificity of 100%. Importantly, patients with other potential causes of RV dysfunction were excluded from this series. Patients with known constrictive pericardial disease, pericardial tamponade, congestive heart failure, pulmonary embolus, chronic obstructive lung disease, and cor pulmonale were not included in this study. It is postulated that Kussmaul's venous sign results from the relative noncompliance of the acutely ischemic, dilated right ventricle and the constraining effects of the pericardium, leading to an inspiratory fall in the rate of superior vena cava flow and a rise in the jugular venous pressure.

Hemodynamic Assessment

The clinical syndrome of RV infarction consists of a low cardiac output, disproportionately elevated right-heart (RA) compared to left-heart (pulmonary capillary wedge, or PCW) filling pressures, and equalization of diastolic pressures between the left and right ventricle.[32] As previously mentioned, right heart catheterization in the setting of acute MI led to the initial recognition of the unique hemodynamic profile of RVMI. In 1974, Cohn and co-workers[8] studied 78 patients with acute MI and identified 6 patients in whom RV filling pressures were equal to or greater (mean 20 mm Hg) than LV filling pressures (mean 16 mm Hg). Five of these patients had inferior wall infarction; all were hypotensive and five were in shock; all had signs of systemic venous congestion without pulmonary congestion; and four were in complete heart block. Two patients (both with shock) died and RVMI was documented at autopsy. Of the remaining four patients, three were in shock and were treated with dextran infusion to raise the LVEDP above 20 mm Hg. This represented the first antemortem clinical diagnosis of RVMI.

Although elevated RV filling pressures disproportionate to LV filling pressures represents the classic hemodynamic profile of RVI, false negative cases have been reported. Dell'Italia demonstrated that hemodynamic findings can be unmasked by volume loading in an additional 20% of patients that do not initially present with classic signs of RVI.[33] In 1981, Lopez-Sendon and others tested various hemodynamic signs to determine which were the most sensitive and specific in diagnosing RVI.[34] One reliable finding was that of RA pressure greater than 10 mm Hg, and greater than or within 5 mm Hg of the PCW pressure. This can be expressed alternatively as a ratio of the RA to the PCW as being > 0.8. A second finding is that of a severe noncompliant RA waveform pattern ("M" or "W" wave form with steep *y* descent) in patients with normal sinus rhythm (Figure 2). The presence of both signs had the highest specificity (97%-100%) and sensitivity (82%).[34]

Patients with RVMI can demonstrate a variety of RA pressure waveform morphologies, which can provide useful information regarding the compensatory status of the RA in maximizing RV preload. The "M" waveform pattern is characterized by a low *a* (atrial) wave amplitude, while the "W" form is characterized by a high *a* wave amplitude. Patients demonstrating the RA "W" pattern have been shown to have higher peak RV pressures, better cardiac output, better response to volume infusion and inotropes, and less frequently require revascularization for shock, when compared with patients with the "M" pattern.[21] Therefore, the amplitude of the *a* wave is an important indicator of RA function and thus an important determinant of hemodynamic stability (Figure 2).

Right ventricular dysfunction causes impaired right-heart filling throughout diastole. This is indicated by elevated RV filling pressures, the characteristic RV dip and plateau waveform, and equalization of diastolic filling pressures between the RA, RV, and PCW. This pattern results from the combination of ischemia-induced myocardial stiffness, altered compliance, and the restraining effects of the pericardium. As previously

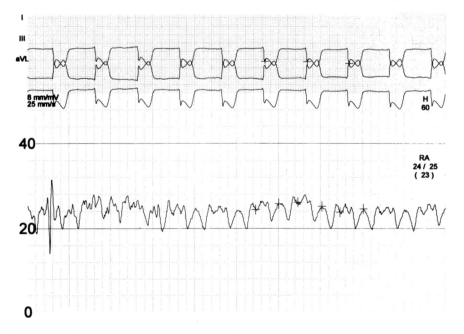

Figure 2. Right atrial pressure tracing during acute right ventricular infarction. Mean right atrial pressure is elevated (23 mm Hg) with very steep *x* and *y* descents demonstrating the characteristic "M" or "W" configuration. The nadir of the *y* descent corresponds to the abrupt cessation of early diastolic ventricular filling.

noted, ischemia and infarction lead to RV dilatation, elevated intrapericardial pressure, and reversal of the normal septal curvature. Filling pressures are elevated early and abruptly rise and plateau through the remainder of diastole, as there is increased impedance to filling due to elevated intrapericardial pressure and pericardial restraint (Figure 3).

Understanding the hemodynamic profile of RVI can be useful in distinguishing this entity from other forms of pericardial heart disease. Lorell and co-workers described 12 patients with the clinical diagnosis of RVI, four of whom were incorrectly diagnosed as having cardiac tamponade before the clinical features of RVI were appreciated.[35] Careful retrospective examination of the hemodynamic data identified features that are useful in distinguishing cardiac tamponade from RV dysfunction secondary to ischemia and infarction. The clinical diagnosis of RVI was established by the bedside findings of elevated JVP, clear lung fields, and hypotension. Hemodynamic criteria included the finding of elevated right-sided filling pressures with normal or only minimally elevated left-sided pressures. This constellation of physical and hemodynamic signs overlaps with cardiac tamponade, however, closer scrutiny of the data revealed that the hemodynamic profile of RVI more closely resembled *constrictive*

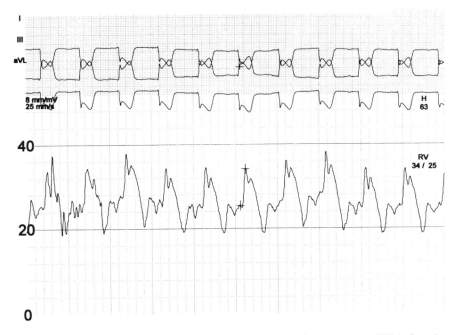

Figure 3. Right ventricular (RV) pressure tracing during acute RV infarction. The RV pressure is elevated (34/25 mm Hg) with the diastolic pressure equal to the RA pressure in Figure 2. The tracing during diastole is characterized by rapid filling during early diastole ("dip") followed by abrupt cessation during the remainder of diastole ("plateau"). This is also referred to as the "square root sign," also seen in constrictive pericardial disease. The pulmonary capillary wedge tracing (not shown) was notable for equalization of pressure between the RA and RV in diastole.

pericardial disease. These findings included a well-preserved and steep y descent in the RA pressure tracing (y descent is typically blunted in tamponade) and the characteristic RV dip and plateau or "square root sign" due to unimpeded early diastolic flow (Figures 2 and 3). The presence of RV dysfunction, chamber stiffness and noncompliance, and the restraining effects of the pericardium explain the restrictive pressure waveform in the setting of RVI.

Electrocardiogram

The standard 12-lead electrocardiogram is one of the most readily available tools for diagnosing myocardial ischemia. Inferior LV ischemia is identified by ST segment elevation in the standard inferior and inferior-posterior leads (II, III, aVF) (Figure 4). As first demonstrated by Erhardt et al., applying precordial lead CR_{4R} to the fifth right intercostal space can aid in the diagnosis of RVI.[36] Various other ECG criteria for diagnosing RVI have been proposed (Table 2).[36-48] The presence of > 1 mm ST segment elevation in right precordial lead V_{4R} is the most reliable and predictive of RVI (88% sensitivity, 78% specificity),[47] although others have proposed identification of ST elevation in lead III greater than lead II as an alternative. In fact, in one study of 24 patients with RVMI, there was no significant difference in the diagnostic accuracy of ST elevation in lead III exceeding that of lead II when compared with right chest leads.[46] It is noteworthy that the ST segment elevation in the setting of RVI appears to be a transient feature. In one series, resolution of this ECG finding within 10 hours from onset of symptoms was noted in 48% of patients.[40]

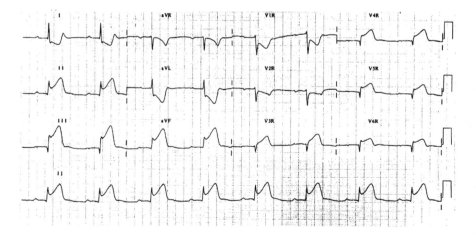

Figure 4. Electrocardiographic manifestations of right ventricular infarction. Twelve-lead electrocardiogram demonstrating significant ST segment elevation in the standard limb leads II, III, and aVF indicative of inferior myocardial infarction. The precordial leads are right-sided and demonstrate typical ST segment elevation in V_{4R} indicating RV ischemia (infarction). Courtesy of Dr. Eric Awtry.

Table 2.

Electrocardiographic Findings in Patients with Right Ventricular Infarction.*

Study	Date	No. of Patients	Finding Qualitative	Quantitative	Lead	Gold Standard	Sensitivity (%)	Specificity (%)	Positive Predictive Value (%)
Erhardt[37]	1974	21	ST segment elevation	1.0 mm	CR_{4R}[a]	Postmortem examination	83	89	91
Erhardt et al.[36]	1976	18	ST segment elevation	1.0 mm	CR_{4R}	Postmortem examination	70	100	100
Candell-Riera et al.[38]	1981	42	ST segment elevation	0.1 mV	V_{4R}	Hemodynamic measures or TPS	93	68	59
Croft et al.[39]	1982	33	ST segment elevation	0.1 mV	V_{4R}- V_{6R}	TPS or RVG	90	91	82
					V_{4R}		70	91	78
					V_2		10	87	25
					V_1		20	91	40
Braat et al.[40]	1983	67	ST segment elevation	1.0 mm	V_{3R}	TPS	69	97	95
					V_{4R}		93	95	93
					V_{5R}		90	92	90
					V_{6R}		83	92	89
Klein et al.[41]	1983	110	ST segment elevation	0.5 mm	V_{4R}	Postmortem examination or RVG + echocardiography, TPS, or hemodynamic measures	83	77	70
Braat et al.[42]	1984	42	ST segment elevation	1.0 mm	V_{4R}	Angiography[b]	100	87	92
Morgera et al.[43]	1984	28	ST segment elevation	0.5 mm	V_{4R}	Postmortem examination	76	86	94
			ST segment elevation	1.0 mm	V_{4R}		57	100	100
					V_{4R}		94	88	100
			Q waves		V_{4R}-V_{3R}		78	100	94

(continued)

Table 2. (continued)

Electrocardiographic Findings in Patients with Right Ventricular Infarction.*

Study	Date	No. of Patients	Finding Qualitative	Quantitative	Lead	Gold Standard	Sensitivity (%)	Specificity (%)	Positive Predictive Value (%)
Lopez-Sendon et al.[44]	1985	43	ST segment elevation	0.5 mm	V_{4R}	Postmortem examination	100	68	67
					V_{3R}		79	68	--
					V_1		43	46	--
					V_2		36	27	--
					V_{4R}		79	40	--
Lew et al.[45]	1986	68	Q waves ST segment depression (V_2) ST segment elevation (aVF)	50%	$V_2$and aVF	Angiography	79	91	82
Andersen et al.[46]	1989	24	ST segment elevation	1.0 mm	III>II[c]	Postmortem examination	63	88	91
Zehender et al.[47]	1993	200	ST segment elevation	1.0 mm	V_{4R}	Postmortem examination, TPS, angiography, or hemodynamic measures	88	78	79

TPS denotes technetium-99m pyrophosphate scintigraphy, and RVG radionuclide ventriculography.
[a] Lead is at fifth intercostal space, midclavicular line.
[b] Occlusion of right coronary artery proximal to the free wall branch.
[c] ST-segment elevation in lead III exceeds elevation in lead II.

Other findings on ECG include conduction abnormalities such as complete heart block and complete right bundle branch block.[48,49]

Other Imaging

Several noninvasive tests are useful in identifying patterns of RVI and RVMI. Chest roentgenography is notable for the absence of pulmonary congestion. Two-dimensional transthoracic echocardiography is useful in identifying RV chamber enlargement and wall motion abnormalities including hypokinesia, akinesia, or dyskinesia of the free wall.[50-52] Additionally, one can see paradoxical ventricular septal motion consistent with RV pressure and volume overload.[50-52] Complications of RVMI, including mural thrombi and tricuspid incompetence, can also be detected.[50] Two-dimensional echocardiography is also useful in detecting a pericardial effusion and tamponade which can clinically resemble RVMI. [35] First transit and gated equilibrium radionuclide angiographic studies typically demonstrate RV enlargement and regional wall motion abnormalities, often in combination with a depressed RV ejection fraction.[53,54] When performed early in patients with inferior MI, nuclear imaging can be useful in identifying hemodynamically significant RV infarction.[53]

Complications

There are a variety of complications of RVMI, the most severe of which are decreased cardiac output, hypotension, and shock. The incidence of high degree atrioventricular block (second- or third-degree AV block) with inferior MI is approximately 19%.[12] Mavric et al. studied patients with inferior infarction and complete heart block to determine whether the presence of RVMI impacted on survival. Of the 243 patients prospectively studied, patients with RVMI had a significantly higher mortality in the presence of complete heart block than those without RVMI (41% vs. 11%, $p < 0.05$).[49] Atrial fibrillation resulting from RA enlargement can compromise the atrial contribution to RV preload. Patients with RVMI may also be at an increased risk for ventricular tachycardia or ventricular fibrillation, particularly during pulmonary artery catheterization.[55] Intramural thrombus formation in a hypokinetic or akinetic right ventricle can lead to pulmonary embolus. Acute tricuspid regurgitation from papillary muscle infarction has been described with acute inferior wall infarction complicated by RVMI.[56] Right-to-left shunt through a patent foramen ovale leading to hypoxemia refractory to supplemental oxygen has also been described with RVMI.[57-59]

Treatment

Patients with RVMI should be admitted to a specialized cardiac unit with the capability for continuous electrocardiographic and hemodynamic

Table 3.

Treatment of Right Ventricular Infarction

Preload augmentation

Volume infusion
  Intravenous isotonic saline (goal right atrial pressure 10-14 mm Hg)
Maintenance of sinus rhythm
  Cardioversion for atrial fibrillation
Maintenance of AV synchrony
  Sequential dual chamber pacing

Inotropic support

Dobutamine (to increase biventricular contractility)
Afterload reduction (with significant left ventricular dysfunction)
Intra-aortic balloon pump counterpulsation
Vasodilator therapy (nitroprusside)

Reperfusion therapy

Thrombolytic therapy
Percutaneous transluminal coronary angioplasty (primary)
  Rescue percutaneous transluminal coronary angioplasty (for failed thrombolysis)

---

monitoring and frequent assessment. Successful treatment of RVMI differs from the conventional management of LV infarction (Table 3). Volume infusion is the mainstay of treating patients with RVMI and hypotension. Cohn and colleagues first observed this in their initial description in 1974.[8] In a series of patients with inferior MI and RVMI, Berisha and associates sought to determine the optimal RV filling pressure to maintain adequate cardiac performance in patients with inferior MI and RVMI.[60] They demonstrated that the right ventricle achieved its maximum cardiac and stroke work index when its filling pressure (mean RA pressure) was 10-14 mm Hg. In their series, the optimal PCW pressure was 16.8 mm Hg. Raising cardiac filling pressures stretches myocardial filaments to their optimal length for contraction, in accordance with Starling's Law. In the case of MI, it is the stretch of the remaining viable muscle fibers which presumably leads to improved cardiac performance.

Subsequently, Dell'Italia[33,61] and Lopez-Sendon[62] noted that, although volume expansion raised LV filling pressures, it did not invariably result in an improved cardiac index. In some cases, volume resuscitation can lead to increases in PCW pressure, but because of overdistension of the right ventricle and subsequent compression and impairment of LV filling, cardiac output does not significantly improve. [61] Additionally, although volume infusion increases LVEDP, the true distending pressure is dependent on the LV transmural pressure, as influenced by the intrapericardial pressure. Goldstein demonstrated this in the open and closed pericardial model of RV infarction in dogs.[25,56] In one series,[26] volume loading increased LV diastolic pressure but did not significantly improve cardiac index. Following pericardiotomy, diastolic filling pressures fell slightly, yet cardiac index improved.

In the setting of a low cardiac index, inotropic support with intravenous dobutamine can serve as an adjunct to volume loading once LV filling pressures have been optimized.[61] As previously mentioned, improved LV contractile performance increases the septal contribution to RV systolic performance as well, particularly when RV systolic function is depressed.[21,24]

Agents such as organic nitrates, morphine, and diuretics used commonly in acute LV infarction should be avoided in known or suspected RVI. These will only further compromise left-sided filling pressures, and can lead to profound systemic hypotension. Central hemodynamic monitoring can be helpful in assessing and guiding response to therapy. However, this should be undertaken with caution, as patients with RVMI may be at an increased risk for ventricular fibrillation during pulmonary artery catheterization.[55] In addition to avoiding excessive vasodilation on the venous side, maintaining atrioventricular (AV) synchrony and atrial contribution to RV filling is crucial in maximizing RV preload reserve. Augmented RA systolic function, as evidenced by the amplitude of the a wave, has been shown to serve as an important compensatory mechanism in RVMI and is associated with less hemodynamic compromise.[21] Heart block with atrial and ventricular dissociation should be corrected with temporary transvenous pacing to maintain the atrial contribution to ventricular end diastolic volume. Likewise, loss of atrial systolic function with the development of atrial fibrillation should be corrected with electrical cardioversion. Love et al. demonstrated that hypotension and shock could respond to restoration of sinus rhythm and/or AV synchrony by cardioversion or temporary pacing respectively in patients with RVMI.[63] Furthermore, Topol et al. demonstrated that sequential atrial and ventricular pacing, compared with ventricular pacing alone, is preferred in terms of maximizing cardiac output, further emphasizing the importance of atrial function in RVMI.[64]

Vasodilators, including sodium nitroprusside, are occasionally needed to decrease afterload when significant LV dysfunction and systemic arterial vasoconstriction are present. Intra-aortic balloon pump (IABP) counterpulsation should be considered when there is significant LV dysfunction associated with cardiogenic shock, ongoing ischemia, or persistent hemodynamic instability when all other measures fail. The IABP is synchronized to deflate just before the onset of systole to decrease afterload, and inflate during diastole thereby augmenting coronary perfusion.

Reperfusion

Restoration of coronary blood flow to ischemic myocardium, either with thrombolytic therapy or by percutaneous transluminal coronary angioplasty (PTCA), has led to dramatic improvements in outcomes of patients with LV MIs.[65-69] While choosing the most appropriate revascularization strategy involves a complicated assessment of patient suitability and resource availability, establishing early and complete patency of the infarct-related artery (IRA) has been repeatedly shown to decrease mortality from acute MI. This arguably represents one of the greatest advances in cardiovascular medicine in the last few decades.

Fibrinolytic Therapy

Although most large-scale randomized trials of reperfusion therapy for acute MI have demonstrated a survival benefit with effective coronary artery recanalization, the overall benefit of fibrinolytic therapy in patients with inferior wall infarction, and particularly those with RVMI, is more controversial and less clear.[70] First, reocclusion after thrombolytic therapy has been noted to be more common when the RCA is the IRA.[71] Secondly, coexisting bradycardia, heart block, hypotension, and shock with RVMI may impair delivery of the fibrinolytic agent to the site of coronary occlusion.[72] Additionally, mortality from acute inferior MI is considerably less than for anterior MI, and patients with inferior MI can further be divided into a spectrum of low or high risk subgroups based on ECG criteria.[12] Such a diverse group creates an inhomogenous study population of patients with inferior MI, and may in part explain why previous trials failed to show a treatment benefit with reperfusion therapy for inferior MI.[70] Finally, RV function has been noted to spontaneously improve over time following RVMI, even in the absence of reperfusion therapy.[54]

An early prospective study of patients undergoing intracoronary fibrinolytic therapy (n = 19 patients) demonstrated that those who had successful, early recanalization of the infarct-related artery (within 48 hours), had considerable improvements in RV function.[73] In contrast, patients in whom recanalization of the RCA was unsuccessful were found to have poor outcomes (death, cardiogenic shock) despite relatively intact LV systolic function, and did not recover RV function. In a similar study in patients with RCA occlusion receiving intracoronary streptokinase, early and late (3 months) RV ejection fraction was significantly better compared with those who did not receive reperfusion therapy.[74]

Retrospective analysis of 1110 patients enrolled in phase II of the Thrombolysis in Myocardial Infarction (TIMI) trial showed that fibrinolytic therapy reduced the frequency of RV dysfunction in patients with acute inferior LV infarction.[11] Right ventricular dysfunction, as detected by predischarge equilibrium radionuclide ventriculography, was more likely to be present in patients with persistent occlusion of IRA at the time protocol coronary angiography was performed (mean 18 to 48 hours).[11] Occlusion, as defined by TIMI 0 or 1 grade flow, was present in 48% of patients with RV wall motion abnormalities, compared with 14% of those without evident RV dysfunction.

Giannitsis et al.[75] prospectively studied 90 patients with acute inferior myocardial infarction to determine the efficacy of accelerated dose recombinant tissue-type plasminogen activator (rt-PA) in restoring patency of the IRA in patients with and without RVMI. Thirty-five (39%) patients fulfilled ECG criteria for RVI on admission, as defined by 0.1 mV ST elevation in right precordial lead V_{4R}. Patients received an accelerated dose regimen of rt-PA (100 mg) within 4 hours from the onset of chest pain, in addition to systemic heparinization and antiplatelet therapy for a minimum of 48 hours. Patients subsequently underwent coronary angiography at a mean interval of 12.8 days after admission. The main finding in this study was that normal coronary flow (TIMI grade 3) was present in 36 of 55 patients without RVMI (65%) but in only 10 of 35 patients (29%) with RVMI. Additionally, occlusion of the IRA (defined as TIMI grade 0 or 1 flow) was present in 69% of patients with RVMI and in 29% of patients without RVMI. Additionally, patients with RVMI had a higher incidence of in-hospital complications including hypotension, bradycardia, complete heart block, and ventricular fibrillation. The most striking finding in this study was the unacceptably low late patency rate (29% at 12 days) following accelerated dose rt-PA among patients with RVMI, suggesting that mechanical reperfusion may be a better initial strategy for restoring coronary arterial patency in acute RVMI.

Percutaneous Transluminal Coronary Angioplasty

Percutaneous transluminal coronary angioplasty (PTCA) has several advantages over fibrinolytic therapy, including better IRA patency rates, decreased recurrent ischemia, and lower incidence of major adverse events including intracerebral hemorrhage. Kinn and colleagues were the first to retrospectively analyze the effects of percutaneous reperfusion on hemodynamic status in patients with RVMI.[76] Patients in whom successful reperfusion of the infarct-related right coronary artery was achieved (TIMI 3 grade flow) had more rapid reduction in right atrial pressures. Persistently elevated right atrial pressure (>24 hours) in turn was associated with increased in-hospital mortality among patients with RVMI. Unfortunately, due to the small number of patients (n = 27), this study failed to demonstrate an overall mortality benefit with reperfusion.

In 1998, Bowers and colleagues sought to determine whether reperfusion by primary PTCA improved RV function and outcome.[77] Fifty-three patients presenting with acute inferior MI and RVI (defined by echocardiographic criteria of RV dysfunction, dilation, and segmental wall motion abnormalities) were taken for emergency PTCA. Complete reperfusion, which in this series was defined angiographically as restoration of flow to the major RV branches, was achieved in 41 patients (77%). Right ventricular performance was assessed serially at 1 hour, 1 day, and 1 month. At baseline, the echo studies were notable for severe RV dilation and encroachment on the LV cavity size. At end-systole, the RV free wall became dyskinetic and the septum exhibited paradoxical motion. Left ventricular function was intact. In the patients with successful reperfusion, recovery of RV function became evident as early as 1 hour, with improved RV free wall contraction and overall global RV systolic performance. By 1-month follow-up, RV size and systolic function had returned to normal in the group with successful reperfusion. The remaining patients with unsuccessful reperfusion had persistent hemodynamic compromise compared to the other group with regards to persistent hypotension and low cardiac output requiring prolonged inotropic support, and ultimate lack of recovery of RV function. The mortality rate was higher in the unsuccessful reperfusion group (58%) than the successful reperfusion group (2%). Interestingly, of the 12 patients who did not obtain successful reperfusion, the five who ultimately survived had no residual evidence of right heart failure. Hence, RV function recovered even in patients who survived despite being unsuccessfully reperfused.

Prognosis

It is generally believed that patients with acute inferior MI have a favorable long-term prognosis, even in the setting of RVMI. In the TIMI II trial, 1-year mortality was not statistically significant between the groups surviving acute inferior infarction regardless of whether RV dysfunction was present.[11] This may have been explained by the high rate of spontaneous resolution of RV wall motion abnormalities at 6 weeks in those patients who initially had RV dysfunction. Shah et al. similarly observed significant spontaneous improvement in global RV function over time in nearly 80% of patients with scintigraphically detected predominant RV dysfunction in the setting of acute MI.[54] However, elderly patients as a group are at increased risk of death when RVMI is present, largely due to a higher incidence of cardiogenic shock.[78]

Zeymer and colleagues stratified streptokinase-treated patients with inferior infarction based on the sum of ST segment elevation on the standard 12-lead electrocardiogram into large or small infarcts to determine whether the presence of RVMI had an impact on survival.[79] Their study showed that patients presenting with the sum of ST segment elevation from leads II, III, aVF, V_5, and $V_6 \leq 0.8$ mV and no precordial ST segment depression ("small infarcts") had a low overall mortality (< 1%) regardless of whether RVMI was present. Higher 30-day cardiac mortality with RVMI (5.9% vs. 2.5%) was related to larger total ST elevation and larger infarct size. They concluded that patients with small infarcts and RVMI would likely not benefit from fibrinolytic therapy. Furthermore, the presence of RVMI was not found to be an independent predictor of 30-day mortality in this study.

Zehender and colleagues studied 200 patients with acute inferior MI to assess both in-hospital and long-term outcomes with respect to the presence or absence of RVI, as defined by ST segment elevation in right precordial lead V_4.[47] Additionally, they sought to determine the diagnostic accuracy of ST segment elevation in V_{4R} for diagnosing RVMI. Of the 200 patients with inferior MI, 107 patients (54%) had at least 1 mm ST elevation in V_{4R}. When compared with autopsy, angiography, technetium-99, or hemodynamics, the sensitivity, specificity, and diagnostic accuracy were 88%, 78%, and 83%, respectively. The second analysis was to determine the prognostic effect of this ST elevation in V_{4R}. Overall in-hospital mortality was significantly higher when ST elevation in V_{4R} was present (31%) compared to when it was absent (6%). Major complications (ventricular fibrillation, sustained ventricular tachycardia, shock, myocardial rupture/tamponade, high degree AV block, or need for pacing) were also very high and significantly more common in the presence of ST elevation in V_{4R} (64% versus 28%). Multivariate analysis demonstrated that only ST elevation in V_{4R} and the presence of cardiogenic shock were predictive of major in-hospital complications; age (> 70) or whether thrombolytic therapy was given were not. At long-term follow-up (mean 37 months), only age and myocardial reinfarction were predictive of increased mortality after hospital discharge. Thus, ST segment elevation in V_{4R} accurately diagnosed RV involvement in the presence of inferior MI, and was a strong independent predictor of in-hospital mortality and major complications. However, ST elevation in V_{4R} was not a prognostic predictor after long-term follow-up in those who survived and were discharged from the hospital.

Conclusion

In conclusion, RVMI is an important clinical entity to consider when a patient presents with acute MI and cardiogenic shock. It is most often present in association with concomitant infarction of the inferior wall of the left ventricle. Rapid bedside assessment with focused attention to the cardio-pulmonary examination, and accurate ECG interpretation with right-sided precordial leads, can often support the diagnosis before invasive hemodynamic monitoring is available. Initial therapy should focus on averting hemodynamic collapse by vigorous volume expansion and inotropic support when signs of peripheral hypoperfusion are present (cool, clammy extremities, oliguria, narrow pulse pressure, mental obtundation). We, the authors, strongly believe that reperfusion therapy should be considered in all patients, either PTCA or fibrinolysis, as guided by local availability. Importantly, RV infarction still represents one of the potentially reversible causes of cardiogenic shock if recognized early and treated aggressively.

References

1. Sanders AO. Coronary thrombosis with complete heart-block and relative ventricular tachycardia. A case report. *Am Heart J* 1930-31; 6:820-823.

2. Starr I, Jeffers WA, Meade RH. The absence of conspicuous increments of venous pressure after severe damage to the right ventricle of the dog, with a discussion of the relation between clinical congestive failure and heart disease. *Am Heart J* 1943; 26:291-301.

3. Bakos ACP. The question of the function of the right ventricular myocardium: An experimental study. *Circulation* 1950; 1:724-732.

4. Kagan A. Dynamic responses of the right ventricle following extensive damage by cauterization. *Circulation* 1952; 5:816-823.

5. Fontan F, Baudet E. Surgical repair of tricuspid atresia. *Thorax* 1971; 26:240-248.

6. Sade RM, Castenada AR. The dispensible right ventricle. *Surgery* 1975; 77:624-631.

7. Cohn JN. Right ventricular infarction revisited. *Am J Cardiol* 1979; 43:666-668.

8. Cohn JN, Nabil G, Martin B, et al. Right ventricular infarction: Clinical and hemodynamic features. *Am J Cardiol* 1974; 33:209-214.

9. Isner JM, Roberts WC. Right ventricular infarction complicating left ventricular infarction secondary to coronary artery disease: Frequency, location, associated findings and significance from analysis of 236 necropsy patients with acute or healed myocardial infarction. *Am J Cardiol* 1978; 42:885-894.

10. Andersen HR, Falk E, Nielsen D. Right ventricular infarction: Frequency, size, and topography in coronary heart disease. *J Am Coll Cardiol* 1987; 10:1223-1232.

11. Berger PB, Ruocco NA, Ryan TJ, et al. Frequency and significance of right ventricular dysfunction during inferior wall left ventricular myocardial infarction treated with thrombolytic therapy. *Am J Cardiol* 1993; 71:1148-1152.

12. Berger PB, Ryan TJ. Inferior myocardial infarction. High-risk subgroups. *Circulation* 1990; 81:401-411.

13. Wackers FJ, Lie KI, Sokole EB, et al. Prevalence of right ventricular involvement in inferior wall infarction associated with myocardial imaging with thallium-201 and technetium-99m pyrophosphate. *Am J Cardiol* 1978; 42:358-362.

14. Cabin HS, Clubb S, Wackers FJ, et al. Right ventricular myocardial infarction with anterior wall left ventricular infarction: An autopsy study. *Am Heart J* 1987; 113:16-23.

15. Roberts N, Harrison DG, Reimer KA, et al. Right ventricular infarction with shock but without significant left ventricular infarction: A new clinical syndrome. *Am Heart J* 1985; 110:1047-1052.

16. Kahn JK, Bernstein M, Bengston JR. Isolated right ventricular myocardial infarction. *Ann Intern Med* 1993; 118:708-711.

17. Kinch JW, Ryan TJ. Right ventricular infarction. *N Engl J Med* 1994; 330:1211-1217.

18. Isner JM. Right ventricular myocardial infarction. *JAMA* 1988; 259:712-718.

19. Hess DS, Bache RJ. Transmural right ventricular myocardial blood flow during systole in the awake dog. *Circ Res* 1979; 45:88-94.

20. Shiraki H, Yoshikawa T, Anzai T, et al. Association between preinfarction angina and a lower risk of right ventricular infarction. *N Engl J Med* 1998; 338:941-947.

21. Goldstein JA, Barzilai B, Rosamond TL, et al. Determinants of hemodynamic compromise with severe right ventricular infarction. *Circulation* 1990; 82:359-368.

22. Santamore WP, Dell'Italia LJ. Ventricular interdependence: Significant left ventricular contributions to right ventricular systolic function. *Prog Cardiovasc Dis* 1998; 40(4):289-308.

23. Dell'Italia LJ, Santamore WP. Can indicies of left ventricular function be applied to the right ventricle? *Prog Cardiovasc Dis* 1998; 40(4):309-324.

24. Brookes C, Ryan H, White P, et al. Acute right ventricular dilation in response to ischemia significantly impairs left ventricular systolic performance. *Circulation* 1999; 100:761-767.

25. Goldstein JA, Vlahakes GJ, Verrier ED, et al. Volume loading improves low cardiac output in experimental right ventricular infarction. *J Am Coll Cardiol* 1983; 2:270-278.

26. Goldstein JA, Vlahakes GJ, Verrier ED, et al. The role of right ventricular systolic dysfunction and elevated intrapericardial pressure in the genesis of low output in experimental right ventricular infarction. *Circulation* 1982; 65:513-522.

27. Dell'Italia LJ. Reperfusion from right ventricular infarction. *N Engl J Med* 1998; 338:978-980.

28. Armour JA, Pace JB, Randall WC. Interrelationship of architecture and function of the right ventricle. *Am J Physiol* 1970; 218:174-179.

29. Maughan WL, Shoukas AA, Sagawa K, et al. Instantaneous pressure-volume relationship of the canine right ventricle. *Circ Res* 1979; 44:309-315.

30. Dell'Italia LJ, Walsh RA. Application of a time varying elastance model to right ventricular performance in man. *Cardiovasc Res* 1988; 22:864-874.

31. Dell'Italia LJ, Starling MR, O'Rourke RA. Physical examination for the exclusion of hemodynamically important right ventricular infarction. *Ann Intern Med* 1983; 99:608-611.

32. Lloyd EA, Gersh BJ, Kennelly BM. Hemodynamic spectrum of "Dominant" right ventricular infarction in 19 patients. *Am J Cardiol* 1981; 48:1016-1022.

33. Dell'Italia LJ, Starling MR, Crawford MH, et al. Right ventricular infarction: Identification by hemodynamic measurements before and after volume loading and correlation with noninvasive techniques. *J Am Coll Cardiol* 1984; 4:931-939.

34. Lopez-Sendon J, Coma-Canella I, Gamallo C. Sensitivity and specificity of hemodynamic criteria in the diagnosis of acute right ventricular infarction. *Circulation* 1981; 64:515-525.

35. Lorell B, Leinbach RC, Pohost GM, et al. Right ventricular infarction. Clinical diagnosis and differentiation from cardiac tamponade and pericardial constriction. *Am J Cardiol* 1979; 43:465-471.

36. Erhardt LR, Sjogren A, Wahlberg I. Single right-sided precordial lead in the diagnosis of right ventricular involvement in inferior myocardial infarction. *Am Heart J* 1976; 91:571-576.

37. Erhardt LR. Clinical and pathological observations in different types of acute myocardial infarction: A study of 84 patients deceased after treatment in a coronary care unit. *Acta Med Scand Suppl* 1974; 560:1-78.

38. Candell-Riera J, Figueras J, Valle V, et al. Right ventricular infarction: Relationships between ST segment elevation in V4R and hemodynamic, scintigraphic, and echocardiographic findings in patients with acute inferior wall myocardial infarction. *Am Heart J* 1981; 101:281-287.

39. Croft CH, Nicod P, Corbett JR, et al. Detection of acute right ventricular infarction by right precordial electrocardiography. *Am J Cardiol* 1982; 50:421-427.

40. Braat SH, Brugada P, de Zwaan C, et al. Value of lead V4R for recognition of the infarct coronary artery in acute inferior myocardial infarction. *Br Heart J* 1983; 49:368-372.

41. Klein HO, Tordjman T, Ninio R, et al. The early recognition of right ventricular infarction: Diagnostic accuracy of the electrocardiographic V4R lead. *Circulation* 1983; 67:558-565.

42. Braat SH, Brugada P, den Dulk K, et al. Value of lead V4R for recognition of the infarct coronary artery in acute inferior myocardial infarction. *Am J Cardiol* 1984; 53:1538-1541.

43. Morgera T, Alberti E, Silverstri F, et al. Right precordial ST and QRS changes in the diagnosis of right ventricular infarction. *Am Heart J* 1984; 108:13-18.

44. Lopez-Sendon J, Coma-Canella I, Alcasena S, et al. Electrocardiographic findings in acute right ventricular infarction: Sensitivity and specificity of electrocardiographic alterations in right precordial leads V4R, V3R, V1, V2, and V3. *J Am Coll Cardiol* 1985; 6:1273-1279.

45. Lew AS, Laramee P, Shah PK, et al. Ratio of ST-segment depression in lead V2 to ST-segment elevation in lead aVF in evolving inferior acute myocardial infarction: An aid to the early recognition of right ventricular ischemia. *Am J Cardiol* 1986; 57:1047-1051.

46. Andersen HR, Nielsen D, Falk E. Right ventricular infarction: Diagnostic value of ST elevation in lead III exceeding that of lead II during inferior/posterior infarction and comparison with right-chest leads V3R to V7R. *Am Heart J* 1989; 117:82-86.

47. Zehender M, Kasper W, Kauder E, et al. Right ventricular infarction as an independent predictor of prognosis after acute inferior myocardial infarction. *N Engl J Med* 1993; 328:981-988.

48. Robalino BD, Whitlow PL, Underwood DA, et al. Electrocardiographic manifestations of right ventricular infarction. *Am Heart J* 1989; 118:138-144.

49. Mavric Z, Zaputovic L, Matana A, et al. Prognostic significance of complete atrioventricular block in patients with acute inferior myocardial infarction with and without right ventricular involvement. *Am Heart J* 1990: 119; 823-828.

50. D'Arcy B, Nanda NC. Two-dimensional echocardiographic features of right ventricular infarction. *Circulation* 1982; 65:167-173.

51. Jugdutt BI, Sussex BA, Sivaram CA, et al. Right ventricular infarction: Two-dimensional echocardiographic evaluation. *Am Heart J* 1984; 107:505-518.

52. Bellamy GR, Rasmussen HH, Nasser FN, et al. Value of two-dimensional echocardiography, electrocardiography, and clinical signs in detecting right ventricular infarction. *Am Heart J* 1986; 112:304-309.

53. Starling MR, Dell'Italia LJ, Chaudhuri TK, et al. First transit and equilibrium radionuclide angiography in patients with inferior transmural myocardial infarction: Criteria for the diagnosis of associated hemodynamically significant right ventricular infarction. *J Am Coll Cardiol* 1984; 4:923-930.

54. Shah PK, Maddahi J, Berman DS, et al. Scintigraphically detected predominant right ventricular dysfunction in acute myocardial infarction: Clinical and hemodynamic correlates and implications for therapy and prognosis. *J Am Coll Cardiol* 1985; 6:1264-1272.

55. Lopez-Sendon J, Lopez de Sa E, Gonzalez Maqueda I, et al. Right ventricular infarction as a risk factor for ventricular fibrillation during pulmonary artery catheterization using Swan-Ganz catheters. *Am Heart J* 1990; 119:207-209.

56. Korr KS, Levinson H, Bough EW, et al. Tricuspid valve replacement for cardiogenic shock after acute right ventricular infarction. *JAMA* 1980; 244:1958-1960.

57. Morris AL, Donen N. Hypoxia and intracardiac right-to-left shunt complicating inferior myocardial infarction with right ventricular extension. *Arch Intern Med* 1978; 138:1405-1406.

58. Manno BV, Bemis CE, Carver J, et al. Right ventricular infarction complicated by right to left shunt. *J Am Coll Cardiol* 1983; 1:554-557.

59. Bansal RC, Marsa RJ, Holland D, et al. Severe hypoxemia due to shunting through a patent foramen ovale: A correctable complication of right ventricular infarction. *J Am Coll Cardiol* 1985; 5:188-192.

60. Berisha S, Kastrati A, Goda A, et al. Optimal value of filling pressure in the right side of the heart in acute right ventricular infarction. *Br Heart J* 1990; 63:98-102.

61. Dell'Italia LJ, Starling MR, Blumhardt R, et al. Comparative effects of volume loading, dobutamine, and nitroprusside in patients with predominant right ventricular infarction. *Circulation* 1985; 72:1327-1335.

62. Lopez-Sendon J, Coma-Canella I, Adanez JV. Volume loading in patients with ischemic right ventricular dysfunction. *Eur Heart J* 1981; 2:329-339.

63. Love JC, Hafajee CI, Gore JM, et al. Reversibility of hypotension and shock by atrial or atrioventricular sequential pacing in patients with right ventricular infarction. *Am Heart J* 1984; 108:5-13.

64. Topol EJ, Goldschlager N, Ports TA, et al. Hemodynamic benefit of atrial pacing in right ventricular myocardial infarction. *Ann Int Med* 1982; 96:594-597.

65. Gruppo Italiano per lo Studio della Streptochinasi Nell'Infarto Miocardico (GISSI). Effectiveness of intravenous thrombolytic treatment in acute myocardial infarction. *Lancet* 1986; 1:397-401.

66. ISIS-2 (Second International Study of Infarct Survival) Collaborative Group. Randomized trial of intravenous streptokinase, oral aspirin, both, or neither among 17,187 cases of suspected acute myocardial infarction. ISIS-2. *Lancet* 1988; 2:349-360.

67. GUSTO Investigators. An international randomized trial comparing four thrombolytic strategies for acute myocardial infarction. *N Engl J Med* 1993; 329:673-682.

68. Grines CL, Browne KF, Marco J, et al. A comparison of immediate angioplasty with thrombolytic therapy for acute myocardial infarction. *N Engl J Med* 1993; 328:673-679.

69. Fibrinolytic Therapy Trialists (FTT) Collaborative Group. Indications for Fibrinolytic therapy in suspected acute myocardial infarction: Collaborative overview of early mortality and major morbidity results from all randomized trials of more than 1000 patients. *Lancet* 1994; 343:311-322.

70. Bates ER. Revisiting reperfusion therapy in inferior myocardial infarction. *J Am Coll Cardiol* 1997; 30:334-342.

71. Bates ER, Califf RM, Stack RS, et al. Thrombolysis and angioplasty in myocardial infarction (TAMI-1) trial: Influence of infarct location on arterial patency, left ventricular function, and mortality. *J Am Coll Cardiol* 1989; 13:12-18.

72. Prewitt RM, Gu S, Garger PJ, et al. Marked systemic hypotension depresses coronary thrombolysis induced by intracoronary administration of recombinant tissue-type plasminogen activator. *J Am Coll Cardiol* 1992; 20:1626-1633.

73. Schuler G, Hofmann M, Schwarz F, et al. Effect of successful thrombolytic therapy on right ventricular function in acute inferior wall myocardial infarction. *Am J Cardiol* 1984; 54:951-957.

74. Braat SH, Ramentol M, Halders S, et al. Reperfusion with streptokinase of an occluded right coronary artery: Effects of early and late right and left ventricular ejection fraction. *Am Heart J* 1987; 113:257-260.

75. Giannitsis E, Potratz J, Wiegand U, et al. Impact of early accelerated dose tissue plasminogen activator on in-hospital patency of the infarcted vessel in patients with acute right ventricular infarction. *Heart* 1997; 77(6):512-516.

76. Kinn JW, Aljuni SC, Samyn JG, et al. Rapid hemodynamic improvement after reperfusion during right ventricular infarction. *J Am Coll Cardiol* 1995; 26:1230-1234.

77. Bowers TR, O'Neill WW, Grines C, et al. Effect of reperfusion on biventricular function and survival after right ventricular infarction. *N Engl J Med* 1998; 338:933-940.

78. Bueno H, Lopez-Palop R, Bermejo J, et al. In-hospital outcome of elderly patients with acute inferior myocardial infarction and right ventricular involvement. *Circulation* 1997; 96(2):436-441.

79. Zeymer U, Neuhaus KL, Wegscheider K, et al. Effects of thrombolytic therapy in acute inferior myocardial infarction with and without right ventricular involvement. *J Am Coll Cardiol* 1998; 32:876-881.

Chapter 11

Mechanical Causes of Cardiogenic Shock

Edward B. Savage, MD

Introduction

The heart is a muscle-powered pump with a simple function: to convert chemical energy to mechanical work so as to circulate blood. The heart usually performs this function efficiently and reliably, but its function can be disrupted by alterations in the mechanical structure of the heart. Essential to the task of the heart is adequate muscle function to provide the conversion of chemical to mechanical energy, a system of integrated chambers that perform a capacitance function, and valves that provide direction to the mechanical energy imparted to the blood by the myocardium. This chapter will focus on syndromes of acute mechanical dysfunction that result in cardiogenic shock, with brief consideration of certain chronic syndromes that can lead to a low output state.

Mechanical causes of cardiogenic shock can be defined as conditions that result from structural changes in the heart or external mechanical stresses placed on the heart. These can result from complications of infarction, infection, trauma, cancer and other disease processes. Acute mechanical dysfunction can be broken down into three major classes: (1) ventricular dysfunction either due to muscular dysfunction or loss of structural integrity, (2) valvular dysfunction due to valve destruction or dysfunction or destruction of the support apparatus, and (3) extracardiac causes due to external compression.

Ventricular Dysfunction

Acute Myocardial Ischemia

Most acute causes of ventricular muscle dysfunction are complications of ischemic disease. Acute myocardial ischemia is discussed in detail

From: Hollenberg SM, Bates ER. *Cardiogenic Shock*. Armonk, NY: Futura Publishing Co., Inc.; ©2002.

in other chapters, yet some comment is merited here. Acute ischemia in the absence of infarction leads to severe dysfunction that may be reversible with revascularization. When a region becomes ischemic the area ceases to contract, and may instead passively expand under the stress of systolic function. Other myocardial regions may be subject to ischemia from inadequate cardiac perfusion secondary to hypotension. As the heart dilates and regional wall function worsens, the support apparatus for the mitral valve can become distorted or dysfunctional, leading to valvular insufficiency, discussed further below. This scenario of reversible ischemia-induced myocardial dysfunction is most striking in the operating room when a patient with severe coronary diseases decompensates, developing severe hypotension and then cardiogenic shock prior to surgery, and then can be weaned from cardiopulmonary bypass and regains normal cardiac function after revascularization.

Myocardial Disruption Syndromes

The two acute myocardial disruption syndromes are ventricular free wall rupture and ventricular septal rupture. Myocardial disruption syndromes are sequelae of myocardial infarction (MI). Pathologically, the defects in the myocardium develop in a large transmural infarction with a large area of necrosis.[1] The endocardium is disrupted, with formation of a hematoma in the myocardium. Blood dissects through the myocardium either through the free wall or into the right ventricle, completing the defect. Although these syndromes are usually apparent and often fatal in the acute phase, they can become chronic. An incomplete or contained free wall rupture may develop into a ventricular pseudoaneurysm, or a small ventricular septal rupture with limited symptomatology and compromise may become a chronic acquired ventricular septal defect.

Acute and Subacute Free Wall Rupture

Ventricular free wall rupture is uncommon and often fatal, although there are reports of successful operation, even if the patient presents with cardiogenic shock. Acute rupture refers to sudden frank large rupture with immediate tamponade and rapid death. Subacute rupture refers to a smaller tear, with a slow or intermittent leak that causes progressive tamponade. Most ruptures occur within the first 2 weeks, with peak incidence at 5 days.[2] The use of thrombolytics decreases the risk of rupture, but may hasten its occurrence.[3] Rupture more commonly occurs with a lateral infarction, especially with associated inferior or posterior infarction, in the presence of persistent ST elevation, with pericarditis, repetitive emesis, restlessness or agitation, hypertension, and in patients above 65 years of age.[4,5] The clinical scenario is that of a patient recovering from a recent MI who suffers sudden cardiovascular collapse. Cardiovascular function is compromised secondary to pericardial tamponade (discussed further below). If the patient is compromised but stable, echocardiography will help identify rupture. The only therapy for rupture, however, is immediate repair. Any delay will reduce the chance of success.

With the onset of cardiovascular collapse, whatever the etiology, an intra-aortic balloon pump should be inserted, with the institution of inotropic support as necessary to maintain systemic pressure and perfusion. If rupture is suspected, it may be prudent to consider immediate transfer to the operating room, where multiple mechanical issues can be diagnosed by transesophageal echocardiography and addressed surgically. Another approach to consider, particularly if coronary angiography is desired or if the patient has had previous cardiac surgery, is placement of a transportable system to provide percutaneous cardiopulmonary support. This will provide circulatory support to stabilize the patient so as to allow further diagnostic workup (e.g., cardiac catheterization) if necessary.

Acute Ventricular Septal Rupture

Perhaps more familiarly known as postinfarction ventricular septal defect, the formation of a connection between the left and right ventricles in the setting of an acute MI is more appropriately termed acute ventricular septal rupture. This is because the pathology, implications, and management are very different in the acute stage than with congenital ventricular septal defects.

Ventricular septal rupture can occur in the anterior or posterior septum, depending on the coronary artery involved in the infarction. Anteroapical or anteroseptal rupture, secondary to infarction in the left anterior descending distribution, comprises 60% to 80% of ruptures in most series. These are usually direct, through and through perforations with a fairly well circumscribed defect.[6] Inferoposterior rupture, secondary to infarction in the distribution of a dominant right coronary or dominant left circumflex artery, results from the completion of a serpigineous dissection of blood through the myocardium. The entry point is often remote from the septum, in the posterior wall.

Acute septal rupture is associated with first MI, the absence of the development of collateral circulation, and complete coronary occlusion, which predisposes to a larger and transmural infarction with significant necrosis.[7,8] When anterior, there are often significant stenoses in the right coronary system, limiting collateral supply to the anterior septum.[9] Posterior ventricular septal rupture is often associated with significant mitral insufficiency as the postero-medial papillary muscle can be involved in the infarction. Posterior ventricular septal rupture can also be associated with right ventricular infarction, which may have more prognostic significance than the defect in the septum. Rupture can occur at any time in the first 2 weeks, and is most common 1–3 days after MI. Once rupture occurs, 25% of untreated patients will die within 24 hours, 50% within the first week, 70% within two weeks, and 80% within 4 weeks.[10] In the SHOCK (SHould we emergently revascularize Occluded Coronaries in cardiogenic shocK) trial, of 939 patients with cardiogenic shock analyzed, 55 had an associated septal rupture.[11] In comparison to those patients with left ventricular (LV) shock, those with septal rupture had a higher mortality (87% vs. 61%, p < 0.001). Of 31 patients treated surgically, 6 (19%) survived; of 24 treated medically, only 1 survived (4%).

Similar to ventricular free wall rupture, rupture of the ventricular septum presents with acute cardiovascular collapse. However, the mechanism is quite different. Large portions of the LV output will preferentially traverse the defect in the septum to the low resistance pulmonary circulation, creating an acute increase in pulmonary blood flow and an acute decrease in systemic blood flow. This is manifested as pulmonary edema and systemic hypotension and hypoperfusion. If left untreated, most patients with persistent low cardiac output will develop peripheral organ failure.

The clinical scenario when septal rupture occurs is in the setting of a recent MI. Chest pain is associated with the onset of a new pan-systolic murmur at the left lower sternal border. Septal rupture must be differentiated from acute mitral incompetence due to papillary muscle rupture (see below), which can have an identical clinical presentation. Transthoracic or transesophageal echocardiography can rapidly differentiate between the two pathologic processes. Prior to the widespread use of echocardiography, the syndromes were differentiated with right heart catheterization. The oxygen saturation of blood from the right ventricle or pulmonary artery compared to the right atrium will increase more than 9% from the left-to-right shunt associated with septal rupture.[12]

For acute septal rupture, immediate therapeutic interventions include the institution of inotropic support and initiation of intra-aortic balloon pump support and possibly percutaneous cardiopulmonary support. Immediate coronary angiography is essential prior to surgery to identify the need for and map targets for coronary bypass grafting. If coronary catheterization is not possible, blind bypass surgery to major arterial targets is possible but not ideal.

The presence of an acute septal rupture, with rare exception, is an absolute indication for emergency surgery. The rare exception is the rupture that creates a very small defect with a limited shunt causing no systemic hemodynamic disturbance. In this scenario, if the repair can be delayed the operation is easier and more secure once the infarct has had time to heal. The criteria for delaying operation include adequate systemic cardiac output, the absence of fluid retention, and the maintenance of renal function. Unless these criteria are met, emergent operation is mandatory. In the presence of systemic compromise, any delay will lengthen the time the peripheral organs are subject to hypoperfusion, reducing chances for survival.[13] In certain advanced situations, surgery will not influence ultimate outcome; these include prolonged hypotension and hypoperfusion, neurologic impairment, severe renal dysfunction, or complete right ventricular infarction.

At the time of surgery, all stenotic major coronary arteries should be bypassed. The septal defect is approached through the infarction and closed with a patch of Dacron or pericardium (Figure 1). Early hospital mortality rates range from 10% to 30%. Posterior ruptures carry a higher mortality rate (34%) than anterior ruptures (15%) in most series.[14] Risk

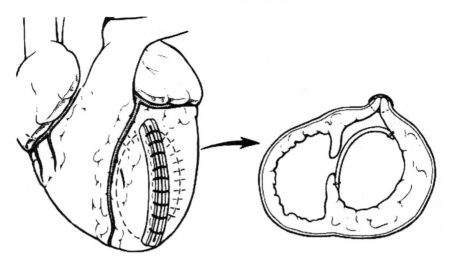

Figure 1. Completed repair of ventricular septal rupture, technique of infarct exclusion . (From Madsen JC, Daggett WM: Postinfarction ventricular septal defect and free wall rupture. In Edmunds LH (ed): Cardiac Surgery in the Adult. NewYork, McGraw-Hill, 1997, p. 643.)

factors for operative mortality include the presence of cardiogenic shock, more proximal location in the ventricle, associated mitral regurgitation, associated right ventricular infarction, early rupture, and age.[15] The causes of death include persistent low cardiac output, cerebrovascular accident, ventricular dysrhythmias, and renal failure. Concurrent revascularization will not impact 30-day mortality, but significantly improves long-term survival. A residual or recurrent septal defect will be present in 10% to 25% of patients.[16] Depending on the degree of shunt and symptoms, this may need to be addressed.

Left Ventricular Pseudoaneurysm

Nonfatal, untreated free wall ruptures will progress to form a pseudoaneurysm. This is characterized by a narrow defect in the ventricular wall leading to an aneurysm cavity. By definition, the sac containing the aneurysm, in contrast to a true ventricular aneurysm, will contain no myocardial cells and will usually have a narrow neck (Figure 2). Pseudoaneurysms usually occur posteriorly. Most patients will present with heart failure secondary to cardiac compression and steal of systolic ejection into the pseudoaneurysm. The presence of a pseudoaneurysm is usually an indication for surgery, as most continue to enlarge and eventually rupture. Small, incidentally discovered pseudoaneurysms (< 3 cm) can be closely observed if asymptomatic.

Chronic Postinfarction Ventricular Septal Defect

Patients will occasionally present with a chronic mature postinfarction ventricular septal defect. This occurs either due to a small known

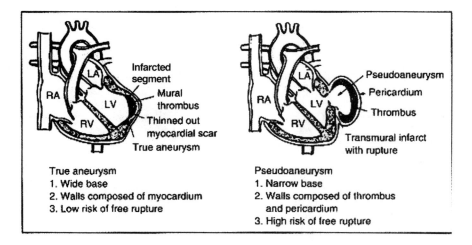

Figure 2. Comparison of true and pseudo- left ventricular aneurysm. (Adapted from Shah PK: Complications of acute myocardial infarction. In Parmley W, Chatterjee K (eds): Cardiology. Philadelphia, J. B. Lippincott, 1987.)

rupture at the time of infarction without significant hemodynamic compromise, or with a rupture that remained undetected at the time of infarction. About one-half will have an associated LV aneurysm. These patients present with congestive heart failure symptoms including shortness of breath, fatigue, edema, and angina. A systolic murmur suggests the diagnosis. Unless the shunt is quite small, the defect should be repaired in most symptomatic patients, usually along with coronary artery bypass and aneurysm resection.

Ventricular Aneurysm

Although not usually a cause of classic cardiogenic shock, ventricular aneurysm as a sequel to MI, a mechanical cause of chronic cardiac dysfunction, merits brief mention. Ventricular aneurysms are inconsistently defined as differing changes in regional and global ventricular geometry. The healed results of a MI include: (1) a scar, which is not discrete, composed predominantly of muscle with minimal wall thinning and characterized by akinesis; (2) a classic aneurysm, a well-delineated transmural fibrous scar, thinned with very little muscle, often with a neck, characterized by dyskinesis; or (3) an alternatively defined aneurysm composed of a large area of myocardial thinning contributing to cardiac enlargement and reduced ejection fraction (< 35%), characterized either by akinesis or dyskinesis.[17]

Pathologically, the aneurysm is composed of a thin white fibrous scar, which may be calcified. The endocardium is smooth and non-trabeculated. Eighty-five percent are located in the anteroapex and septum, and 5% to 10% are posterobasal, usually with associated mitral incompetence.[18] The

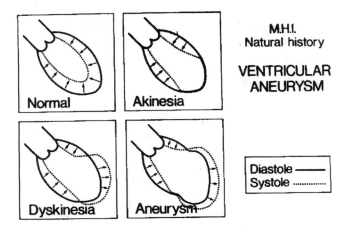

Figure 3. Various wall motion abnormalities that can cause ventricular dysfunction. (From Grondin P, Kretz JG, Bical O, et al. Natural history of saccular aneurysms of the left ventricle. *J Thorac Cardiovasc Surg* 1979;77:57.)

incidence of ventricular aneurysm was 10% to 30% in the past, but is much lower now due to the use of ACE inhibitors and thrombolytic therapy. Risk factors for the development of a ventricular aneurysm include hypertension and the use of corticosteroids.

An aneurysm can be focal and dyskinetic causing minimal to moderate ventricular enlargement, or large and akinetic causing severe global enlargement (Figure 3). In the first scenario, symptoms result from enlargement and competitive filling of the dyskinetic aneurysm requiring more work to maintain adequate cardiac output. In the second scenario, gradual ventricular enlargement changes chemico-mechanical energy relationships. The function-limiting fuel for myocardial function is oxygen, which is dependent on myocardial blood flow. Oxygen demand is proportional to wall stress, which is proportional to chamber radius and pressure and inversely proportional to wall thickness according to the Laplace law:

$$O_2\ demand \approx \sigma \approx \frac{rP}{2h}$$

(where σ is wall stress, r is radius, p is pressure, and h is wall thickness)

Thus as radius increases, so does wall stress; as the ventricular wall thins, wall stress increases. In the ventricle that has enlarged in response to an aneurysm, oxygen requirements begin to outstrip oxygen delivery. The goal of surgery is to reverse these changes (Figure 4).

Ventricular aneurysms can be diagnosed with echocardiography or ventriculography. The first aneurysm type with focal enlargement and a neck is easily identified. However, the second type is often not recognized as an aneurysm, but rather as an "enlarged ventricle, severely reduced ejection fraction, with large anterior scar" belying the potential for operative therapy. Surgery should be considered in the symptomatic patient.

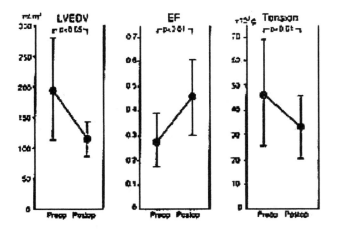

Figure 4. Effect of linear aneurysmectomy. (From Kawachi K, Kitamura S, Kawata R, et al. Hemodynamic assessment during exercise after left ventricular aneurysmectomy. *J Thorac Cardiovasc Surg* 1994; 107:178.)

Despite the fact that 50% of aneurysms will have thrombus, thromboembolism is uncommon and the presence of thrombus is not an indication for surgery. Severe angina is the most common symptom; most of the patients will have associated three-vessel coronary artery disease. Patients with a dilated enlarged heart secondary to aneurysms may more commonly have congestive heart failure as a presenting symptom. If the patient is referred for coronary artery bypass graft (CABG) surgery, small aneurysms should not be resected, but large aneurysms should be addressed.

Operative approaches include the classic linear repair (Figure 5) and more recently adopted patch techniques (Figure 6). The goal of aneurysm repair is to reduce cavity size and, in the case of the focal aneurysm,

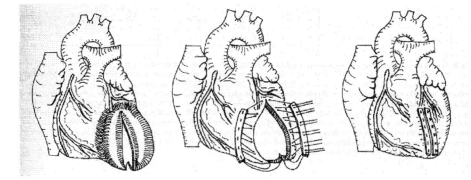

Figure 5. Linear repair of left ventricular aneurysm. (From Mickleborough LL, Maruyama H, Lim P, et al. Results of left ventricular aneurysmectomy with tailored scar excision and primary closure technique. *J Thorac Cardiovasc Surg* 1994;107:690.)

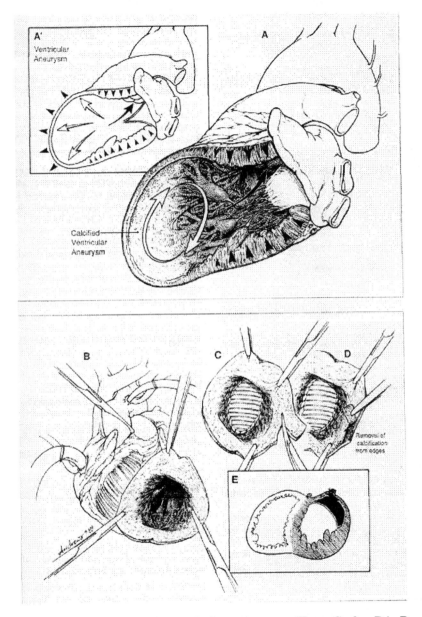

Figure 6. Patch repair of left ventricular aneurysm. (From Cooley DA. Repair of the calcified ventricular aneurysm. *Ann Thorac Surg* 1990;49:489.)

eliminate the volume sink. In the case of the nonfocal aneurysm, the additional goal is to return the ventricular geometry from the less efficient spherical shape to the more efficient elliptical or bullet shape. This can be done with a linear repair or patch repair depending on ventricular shape.

Cardiac Trauma

Blunt and penetrating trauma can cause multiple injuries to the heart that in turn can cause mechanical dysfunction. The heart is generally well protected, resting behind the sternum and left lower rib cage. Nevertheless, it is vulnerable to injury. Deceleration injuries with impact to the sternal area and penetrating weapons can result in cardiac contusion, injury to coronary arteries, rupture of valves, and dissections. All of the injuries can lead to mechanical dysfunction based on mechanisms described above and below.

Valvular Dysfunction

Slowly progressive, chronic valvular dysfunction is often well tolerated for prolonged periods of time. However acute alterations in valvular function are poorly tolerated and some can result in frank cardiogenic shock. Valvular dysfunction may result from disruption or immobilization of valve leaflets or disruption of the valve supporting structures. Causes include endocarditis, thrombosis or dysfunction of prosthetic valves, trauma, and other syndromes described below.

Aortic Valve

Acute Aortic Regurgitation

Acute aortic regurgitation is usually a result of endocarditis, trauma or aortic dissection. Aortic regurgitation increases preload, wall tension, and myocardial oxygen consumption.[19] Reduced diastolic pressure and prolonged systole compromise coronary flow reserve.[20] This results in oxygen demand/supply mismatch. With chronic aortic insufficiency, the heart is able to adapt by dilating. In contrast, acute aortic insufficiency is poorly tolerated and can result in cardiogenic shock. Since the regurgitant volume fills a normal sized ventricle that cannot acutely dilate, net forward flow is drastically reduced. The only way to maintain cardiac output is to increase heart rate to compensate for reduced stroke volume. Thus, these patients will present with weakness, dyspnea, hypotension, tachycardia, peripheral vasoconstriction, and possibly cyanosis and pulmonary edema. Minimal or absent are classic peripheral signs of aortic insufficiency. Pulse pressure is only slightly widened. Early death is frequent in these patients, and so prompt operative intervention is required.

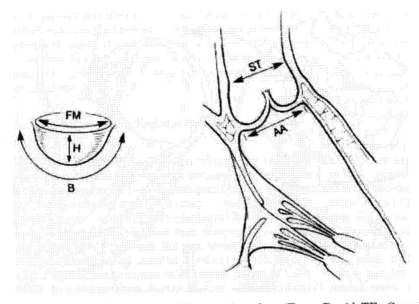

Figure 7. Structural anatomy of the aortic valve. (From David TE. Complex Operations of the Aortic Root. In Edmunds LH (ed): Cardiac Surgery in the Adult. New York, McGraw-Hill, 1997, p. 948.)

Depending on the etiology of the aortic insufficiency, different operative approaches are applicable. The normal aortic valve is a three dimensional structure. The aortic annulus is poorly defined; instead, the leaflets are suspended in the aorta with semilunar attachments to the aortic wall. (Figure 7). In the presence of endocarditis, a portion of the valve has usually been destroyed by the infective process, requiring replacement. With aortic dissection, the valvular leaflets are intact, and the insufficiency is due to disruption of the suspensory apparatus of the valve as the dissection causes one or two commissures to prolapse into the lumen allowing the leaflet to prolapse through the valve annulus. This can often be repaired by resuspending the valve commissure.

Mitral Valve

Acute Mitral Regurgitation

Acute mitral regurgitation may result from endocarditis, chordal rupture, papillary muscle rupture, trauma, or ischemic dysfunction. Similar to acute aortic regurgitation, acute mitral regurgitation is poorly tolerated, and can result in pulmonary edema or cardiogenic shock. Normally, the mitral valve provides stiff resistance during ejection, maintaining impedence. In the presence of mitral regurgitation, impedence to flow during ejection is drastically reduced due to the low pressure of the left atrium. As a result, ventricular emptying is increased, but retrograde flow through the mitral orifice is increased, and antegrade flow through the aortic valve is reduced. Acutely, the heart can only compensate to maintain output by increasing heart rate, whereas chronically the heart dilates to increase stroke volume. In the acute situation, the left atrium is usually of normal size and compliance, so the elevated back-pressure is conveyed to the lungs and causes pulmonary edema, elevated pulmonary vascular resistance, and right heart failure. Cardiac size is usually normal on chest X-ray and echocardiogram, however ejection fraction is usually increased in response to decreased impedence to emptying. Principles of treatment include afterload reduction and intra-aortic balloon pump placement to shift the balance of aortic ejection to forward flow. Early surgical intervention is usually indicated.

Ischemia Induced Mitral Regurgitation

Ischemia-induced mitral regurgitation associated with myocardial infarction can be severe leading to cardiogenic shock. When severe, peri-infarction acute mitral regurgitation causing cardiogenic shock has a significant impact on prognosis, and significantly increases the mortality of MI.[21] If the patient can be supported, however, the mitral regurgitation will often resolve as the infarct heals.

Mitral regurgitation is fairly common within the first 24 to 48 hours after both anterior and posterior MI. With posterior infarction, mitral regurgitation tends to be of greater severity. Most often this will resolve as the infarct matures and remodels, however 15% will have varying degrees of residual regurgitation.[22] In uncommon scenarios, the regurgitation is quite severe and in combination with ventricular dysfunction can lead to cardiogenic shock.

The less common but more easily understood cause of mitral regurgitation is partial or complete papillary muscle rupture. The mechanism of failure of mitral competency can be compared to a parachute. The chordae attached to the papillary muscle tether and support the leaflet and control leaflet motion and position. Once ruptured, the support apparatus cannot support and retain the leaflet(s), allowing them to "billow in the wind." This can be understood by reviewing the anatomy of the mitral valve (Figure 8). The anterolateral papillary muscle receives blood from diagonal and obtuse marginal branch coronary arteries. The posteromedial papillary muscle receives blood from the posterior descending and postero-lateral circulation, whether derived from the left circumflex or right coronary artery. Seventy-five percent of ruptures involve the postero-medial papillary muscle, 25% the antero-lateral papillary muscle.[23] Papillary muscle rupture is responsible for 5% of fatal infarctions. Depending on the degree of regurgitation, partial papillary muscle rupture may be well-tolerated, however complete rupture will reliably cause severe acute re-gurgitation and cardiogenic shock.

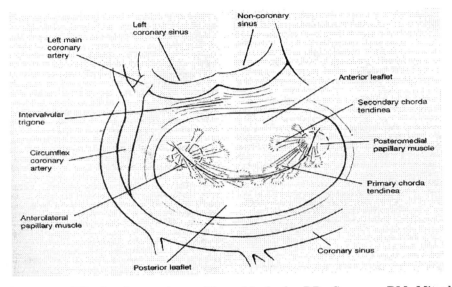

Figure 8. Mitral valve anatomy. (From Muehrcke DD, Cosgrove DM. Mitral Valvuloplasty. In Edmunds LH (ed): Cardiac Surgery in the Adult. NewYork, McGraw-Hill, 1997, p. 995.)

More common than papillary muscle rupture is the occurrence of regurgitation secondary to primary muscle dysfunction. A commonly held misconception is that the leak is due to dysfunction of the papillary muscle itself. Experimentally, isolated papillary muscle infarction does not cause regurgitation. Instead, infarction of the ventricular muscle to which the papillary muscle is attached influences the occurrence and character of the regurgitation. Acutely, wall infarction leads to stiffening and paradoxical motion, which causes tethering and retraction of the leaflet into the ventricle, limiting leaflet motion and coaptation. As the infarct heals, multiple effects can influence the function of the valve. For example, as the infarct stiffens and heals, retraction may lessen, reducing regurgitation. In contrast, if the ventricle dilates, it may cause further retraction of the leaflets or annular dilation, worsening the leak.

Clinically, peri-infarction mitral regurgitation can go undetected. The presence of a new murmur is suggestive, although a murmur may be absent with massive regurgitation. Papillary muscle rupture usually occurs within a few hours to 14 days after infarction.[23] The symptoms of rupture can range from mild congestive failure to pulmonary edema or acute profound shock. In the absence of muscle rupture, regurgitation is seldom severe enough to produce profound shock and cardiovascular collapse.

The natural history is often related to the severity of presentation. Patients with total papillary muscle rupture without intervention have a poor chance for survival, (25% at 24 hours). Partial papillary muscle rupture has lower mortality with a 70% survival at 24 hours, and 50%

survival at 1 month without intervention.[23] Regurgitation in the absence of papillary muscle rupture carries a much better short-term prognosis. Acute medical interventions include percutaneous transluminal coronary angioplasty (PTCA) of the infarct artery and intra-aortic balloon pump placement for support. The requirement for surgery is guided by the severity of symptoms and the etiology of regurgitation.

In general, urgent surgery for ischemic mitral regurgitation carries a significant operative mortality risk. In the SHOCK trial registry,[24] 98 of 1190 patients with cardiogenic shock had severe mitral regurgitation. When compared to patients in cardiogenic shock with LV failure alone, mortality was not increased in the group with severe mitral regurgitation (55% vs. 61%, p = 0.277). In this registry, both treatment approaches carried a high mortality; 71% of patients treated medically died, and 40% of those treated surgically died. It was noted by the authors, however, that surgery was offered only to patients felt more likely to benefit, with the sicker cohort not offered surgery.

Surgery is usually required in the presence of papillary muscle rupture, much less commonly in the absence of rupture. In general, if the patient can be supported while the infarct heals, the regurgitation may resolve, allowing simple coronary bypass without adding a mitral valve operation to the procedure. Furthermore, the mitral valve in this scenario is more difficult to repair and more often requires replacement because the valve is morphologically normal and the mitral annulus is not dilated.

Acute Chordal Rupture

By a mechanism akin to that of papillary muscle rupture, rupture of major valve-supporting chordae may result in severe regurgitation. Causes include spontaneous rupture and excessive mechanical stress as may occur with sudden hypertension or trauma. In the absence of previous regurgitation, this is often poorly tolerated. These valves are usually diseased and by their nature are more amenable to repair.

Prosthetic Valve Failure

Prosthetic valves fail with either stenosis or, more commonly, with regurgitation. All prosthetic valves are at risk of infection, which varies with different types of valves. Infection will usually cause regurgitation either by destroying valve components, allowing a leak through the valve, or by causing disruption of suture lines securing the valve, allowing a leak around the valve. Cusps of bioprosthetic valves can tear. These leaks can be acute and severe, at time causing shock and requiring urgent operation. All valves can thrombose acutely, but this occurs more commonly with mechanical valves. This will usually cause stenosis but can also cause regurgitation. Chronic progressive stenosis caused by excessive tissue proliferation, which encroaches on the valve structure and limits movement of the functional parts of the valve, can present as low output extending to cardiogenic shock, also requiring urgent valve replacement.

Extracardiac Causes

Tamponade

Cardiac tamponade resulting in cardiogenic shock can be acute or chronic. Cardiac tamponade is protean in nature. Classically, acute tamponade is associated with a rapid accumulation of fluid in the minimally expansible constraining parietal pericardium. The mechanism is the restriction of cardiac filling, as the limiting space of the pericardium is filled with extracardiac fluid raising intrapericardial pressure and limiting chamber expansion during diastole. However, focal accumulations of fluid or thrombus can have a similar effect. For example, after cardiac surgery a large thrombus behind and compressing the left atrium or next to and compressing the right atrium can limit atrial inflow and ventricular output.

Tension Pneumothorax or Hemothorax

Similar to tamponade, when air or fluid accumulates rapidly and is trapped in the nonexpansile chest, intrathoracic pressure increases, limiting venous return to the heart and causing cardiogenic shock. This can be rapidly reversed by releasing the air or fluid.

References

1. Hutchins GM. Rupture of the interventricular septum complicating myocardial infarction: Pathological analysis of 10 patients with clinically diagnosed perforations. *Am Heart J* 1979; 97:165-173.

2. Batts KP, Ackermann DM, Edwards WD. Postinfarction rupture of the left ventricular free wall: Clinicopathologic correlates in 100 consecutive autopsy cases. *Hum Pathol* 1990; 21:530-535.

3. Honan MB, Harrell FE Jr., Reimer KA, et al. Cardiac rupture, mortality and the timing of thrombolytic therapy: A meta-analysis. *J Am Coll Cardiol* 1990; 16:359-367.

4. Oliva PB, Hammill SC, Edwards WD. Cardiac rupture, a clinically predictable complication of acute myocardial infarction: Report of 70 cases with clinicopathologic correlations. *J Am Coll Cardiol* 1993; 22:720-726.

5. Pollak H, Diez W, Spiel R, et al. Early diagnosis of subacute free wall rupture complicating acute myocardial infarction. *Eur Heart J* 1993; 14:640-648.

6. Edwards BS, Edwards WD, Edwards JE. Ventricular septal rupture complicating acute myocardial infarction: Identification of simple and complex types in 53 autopsied hearts. *Am J Cardiol* 1984; 54:1201-1205.

7. Skehan JD, Carey C, Norrell MS, et al. Patterns of coronary artery disease in post-infarction ventricular septal rupture. *Br Heart J* 1989; 62:268-272.

8. Miller S, Dinsmore R, Grenne R, et al. Coronary, ventricular, and pulmonary abnormalities associated with rupture of the interventricular septum complicating myocardial infarction. *Am J Radiol* 1978; 131:571.

9. Berger T, Blackstone E, Kirklin J. Postinfarction ventricular septal defect. In: Kirklin J, Barratt-Boyes B, eds. Cardiac Surgery. New York: Churchill Livingstone, 1993:403-413.

10. Sanders R, Kern W, Blount S. Perforation of the interventricular septum complicating myocardial infarction. *Am Heart J* 1956; 51:736.

11. Menon V, Webb JG, Hillis LD, et al. Outcome and profile of ventricular septal rupture with cardiogenic shock after myocardial infarction: A report from the SHOCK Trial Registry. SHould we emergently revascularize Occluded Coronaries in cardiogenic shocK? *J Am Coll Cardiol* 2000; 36:1110-1116.

12. Hillis LD, Firth BG, Winniford MD. Variability of right-sided cardiac oxygen saturations in adults with and without left-to-right intracardiac shunting. *Am J Cardiol* 1986; 58:129-132.

13. Heitmiller R, Jacobs ML, Daggett WM. Surgical management of postinfarction ventricular septal rupture. *Ann Thorac Surg* 1986; 41:683-691.

14. Komeda M, Fremes SE, David TE. Surgical repair of postinfarction ventricular septal defect. *Circulation* 1990; 82:IV243-247.

15. Madsen J, Daggett W. Postinfarction ventricular septal defect and free wall rupture. In: Edmunds L, ed. Cardiac Surgery in the Adult. New York: McGraw-Hill, 1997:647.

16. Skillington PD, Davies RH, Luff AJ, et al. Surgical treatment for infarct-related ventricular septal defects. Improved early results combined with analysis of late functional status. *J Thorac Cardiovasc Surg* 1990; 99:798-808.

17. Johnson R, Draggett WJ. Heart failure resulting from coronary artery disease. In: Johnson R, Haber E, Austen W, eds. The Practice of Cardiology. Boston: Little, Brown, 1980:455-491.

18. Left Ventricular Aneurysm. In: Kirklin J, Barratt-Boyes B, eds. Cardiac Surgery. New York: Churchill Livingstone, 1993:383-402.

19. Urschel CW, Covell JW, Graham TP, et al. Effects of acute valvular regurgitation on the oxygen consumption of the canine heart. *Circ Res* 1968; 23:33-43.

20. Dehmer GJ, Firth BG, Hillis LD, et al. Alterations in left ventricular volumes and ejection fraction at rest and during exercise in patients with aortic regulation. *Am J Cardiol* 1981; 48:17-27.

21. Tcheng JE, Jackman JD, Jr., Nelson CL, et al. Outcome of patients sustaining acute ischemic mitral regurgitation during myocardial infarction. *Ann Intern Med* 1992; 117:18-24.

22. Hickey MS, Smith LR, Muhlbaier LH, et al. Current prognosis of ischemic mitral regurgitation. Implications for future management. *Circulation* 1988; 78:I51-59.

23. Mitral incompetence from ischemic heart disease. In: Kirklin J, Barratt-Boyes B, eds. Cardiac Surgery. New York: Churchill Livingston, 1993:415-424.

24. Thompson CR, Buller CE, Sleeper LA, et al. Cardiogenic shock due to acute severe mitral regurgitation complicating acute myocardial infarction: A report from the SHOCK Trial Registry. SHould we use emergently revascularize Occluded Coronaries in cardiogenic shocK? *J Am Coll Cardiol* 2000; 36:1104-1109.

Chapter 12

Rhythm Disturbances in Cardiogenic Shock

Sergio L. Pinski, MD and Michael Shapiro, MD

Introduction

Guidelines for prophylactic intervention, optimal treatment, and follow-up management of arrhythmias in patients with cardiogenic shock are not firmly established. For obvious reasons, these matters are difficult to study according to the modern standard of randomized, double-blind, placebo-controlled, intention-to-treat, well-powered studies. Therapeutic algorithms are often based on pathophysiological considerations, observational evidence, and extrapolation from more stable clinical scenarios. In this chapter, we review clinical presentation, distinctive pathophysiology, and treatment of rhythm disturbances causing or associated with cardiogenic shock in different clinical settings. Because extensive acute myocardial infarction (MI) is the most common pathologic state associated with cardiogenic shock, we will place emphasis on its electrophysiologic correlates.

It is clinically useful to attempt the somewhat arbitrary distinction between primary arrhythmias causing hemodynamic collapse, and secondary arrhythmias occurring in the setting of cardiogenic shock. In the former, successful arrhythmia control should result in rapid restoration of normal or near-normal hemodynamic status. In the later, arrhythmia control, although a necessary therapeutic step, may not result in significant hemodynamic improvement.

Determinants of the Hemodynamic Response During Tachyarrhythmias

The hemodynamic effects of a tachyarrhythmia depend on multiple factors: ventricular rate, tachycardia duration, the atrio-ventricular (AV)

From: Hollenberg SM, Bates ER. *Cardiogenic Shock*. Armonk, NY: Futura Publishing Co., Inc.; ©2002.

Table 1.
Determinants of the Hemodynamic Impact of Arrhythmias.

Ventricular rate
Atrioventricular relationship
Ventricular activation pattern
Systolic and diastolic ventricular function
Concomitant drugs
Induced myocardial ischemia
Peripheral responses
    Reflex vasoconstriction
    Paradoxical vasodilatation

relation, activation pattern (e.g., normal vs. aberrant QRS), the severity of any underlying heart disease, concurrent hemodynamically active medications, and the adaptations of peripheral vascular resistance (Table 1). The ventricular rate is the main determinant of the hemodynamic response during tachycardia. At fast rates, the diastolic filling time drops significantly, resulting in a decreased end-diastolic volume and stroke volume.[1] Furthermore, inotropic reserve (i.e., the increase in left ventricular [LV] contractility secondary to an increase in the rate) is significantly impaired in patients with LV systolic dysfunction.[2]

Both incomplete filling and incoordinate contraction contribute to impaired hemodynamics during sustained ventricular tachycardia (VT).[3] There is rapid deterioration in the contractile function of the left ventricle, as evidenced by a fall in peak systolic pressure and +dP/dt, despite an increase in end-diastolic pressure.[4] The site of origin of VT may also influence hemodynamics. For example, rapid pacing from the right ventricular outflow tract results in more favorable LV hemodynamics, compared to those from the right ventricular apex.[5] Pulse deficit, where the electrical rate is faster than pulse rate (determined by palpation, arterial catheterization, or Doppler flow), is common during rapid tachyarrhythmias. This denotes a failure to open the aortic valve due to insufficient filling time and mechanical alternans, but can paradoxically result in better stroke volume and blood pressure.

The degree of hemodynamic recovery during spontaneous or simulated VT is lower in the presence of AV dissociation.[6] Ventricular tachycardia beats preceded by a dissociated (but optimally timed) P wave generate a larger stroke volume.[7] During tachycardias with 1:1 AV relationship, the timing of the P wave influences the hemodynamic response. In typical AV nodal reentry tachycardia, for example, atrial and ventricular systole occur simultaneously, impeding ventricular filling.[8] A long RP' interval results in better maintenance of blood pressure, despite less sympathetic activation.[9] Reflex vasodilatation secondary to activation of cardiopulmonary baroreceptors can contribute to the hypotension seen with simultaneous atrial and ventricular contraction.[9]

A critical determinant of the hemodynamic response to an arrhythmia lies in the reflex responses triggered.[10] An abrupt increase in ventricular rate results in declines in cardiac output and in blood pressure. Typically, this is followed within 30 seconds by a rise in blood pressure, although usually not to baseline levels. The initial drop in blood pressure is sensed by aortic and carotid baroreceptors and triggers reflex sympathetic activation.[11] The resulting α-adrenergic vasoconstriction and β-adrenergic augmentation of contraction and relaxation tends to restore the blood pressure and maintain vital organ perfusion.[12] Baroreflex gain predicts the degree of recovery of blood pressure during simulated VT (i.e., rapid pacing) in the individual patient.[13] However, other less adaptive responses can contribute to hemodynamic compromise. An increase in atrial pressure can stimulate central cardiopulmonary baroreceptors with vagal afferents and result in profound reflex vasodilatation.[14] The combination of arrhythmia-induced depressed cardiac output and reflex vasodilatation can be synergistic in producing hypotension. Tachyarrhythmias also induce rate-related increases in myocardial oxygen consumption. Simultaneously, coronary blood flow decreases due to a drop in the coronary perfusion pressure and shortening of the diastolic interval during which most of coronary flow occurs. Myocardial ischemia can occur,[15] even in patients without obstructive coronary disease. Any ischemic insult further impairs myocardial contractility, leading, if unchecked, to the deadly spiral of cardiogenic shock. Angina, ECG changes, and other usual markers of myocardial ischemia may be absent.

Arrhythmias that Can Cause Hemodynamic Collapse Even in the Normal Heart

Several primary rhythm disturbances can cause decompensation in the presence of a structurally normal or minimally diseased heart. When these same arrhythmias occur in patients with significant systolic or diastolic myocardial dysfunction or significant (especially obstructive) valvular lesions, they are even more poorly tolerated. Also, a persistent tachycardia of any mechanism can induce myocardial dysfunction: the well-recognized tachycardia-induced cardiomyopathy.[16] The induced myocardial dysfunction is generally reversible with appropriate and timely rate control. However, the cardiomyopathy can predispose to other rhythm disturbances, and, more importantly, makes the causative arrhythmia much less well tolerated.

Incessant Atrial Tachycardias

Sinus tachycardia is an expected compensatory response in the hemodynamically compromised patient and should not be directly treated. It is exceptional for sinus tachycardia to cause hemodynamic decompensation *per se*, although when persistent it can result in cardiomyopathy. In the acutely decompensated tachycardic patient, the question of sinus tachycardia versus a treatable primary atrial tachycardia often arises. With rapid rates, superimposition of the T and P waves makes morphological analysis difficult. When the QRS is wide and a previous ECG is not available, even the diagnosis of VT may be entertained. Every attempt at a definitive diagnosis should be undertaken before empiric administration of antiarrhythmic drugs or cardioversion is undertaken. Useful maneuvers include review of previous ECG tracings, recording of a highly-amplified precordial bipolar lead, and responses to carotid sinus massage and IV adenosine. Sinus tachycardia will transiently slow and then reaccelerate after adenosine. When given during atrial tachycardia, adenosine typically causes transient AV block without change in atrial cycle length, allowing better analysis of P wave morphology. More rarely, atrial tachycardia is terminated by adenosine.[17] It should be remembered that the P wave during certain atrial tachycardias (including those arising from common foci such as the high *crista terminalis* and the right superior pulmonary vein) can be indistinguishable from the sinus P wave. When in doubt, electrophysiological consultation and intracardiac mapping aimed at curative ablation should be considered. Contemporary interventional electrophysiologic techniques make ablative procedures possible even in cardiogenic shock patients. Electrophysiology laboratory experience in dealing with critically ill patients, such as those requiring mechanical ventilation and intra-aortic balloon counterpulsation, is mandatory if such procedures are to be considered.

Paroxysmal Supraventricular Tachycardias

The common forms of paroxysmal supraventricular tachycardia (PSVT), namely AV nodal reentry and orthodromic AV reentry, generally occur in the absence of significant structural heart disease and rarely cause acute hemodynamic collapse. Severe decompensation only occurs when the rates are excessively fast, when there is significant structural heart disease, or in the occasional patient in whom arrhythmia onset triggers a vasodepressor response instead of the more normal compensatory vasoconstriction.

The treatment of the PSVTs associated with cardiogenic shock is challenging. If the diagnosis is correct, termination, achieved by any means, should result in almost immediate improvement. On the other hand, drugs with negative inotropic effects such as verapamil, diltiazem, beta-blockers, or class I agents can be catastrophic if they fail to restore sinus rhythm. Vagal maneuvers should be tried first; they are more often effective in children and in patients with AV reentry.[18] Adenosine is highly effective (> 90 %) in acutely terminating PSVT and is the drug of choice in the unstable patient because of its very short half-life.[19,20] Incremental doses should be given, starting at 6 mg up to a maximum dose of 18 mg in adults. Administration via a central line is more effective, and an initial dose of 3 mg is recommended.[21] The main concerning side effect of adenosine is the potential for induction of atrial fibrillation.[22] This is particularly detrimental in the patient with severe diastolic disease or with an unsuspected Wolff-Parkinson-White (WPW) syndrome. Digoxin is less effective at acutely terminating PSVT. Other treatments used in the past such as IV edrophonium or phenylephrine are no longer recommended.

Overdrive pacing termination should be considered if there is a permanent or temporary pacemaker in place. Transesophageal atrial pacing is very effective in terminating PSVTs at the bedside.[23] It is minimally invasive, can be performed with little or no sedation, and is hemodynamically well tolerated. It is especially useful in infants, children, or the frail elderly. Emergent direct-current (DC) cardioversion of PSVT should rarely be necessary, but is always an option. In patients with shock and PSVT who require cardioversion, antiarrhythmic drug therapy should be initiated concomitantly to prevent recurrences.

PSVT often recurs shortly after adenosine administration, and longer acting drugs become necessary. Intravenous diltiazem is useful in this situation, although it may not be tolerated in patients with severe LV dysfunction. Intravenous amiodarone is also effective but slower acting for the common PSVTs.[24] An effect can often be seen within an hour if an initial loading dose of 5 to 10 mg/kg is given. Exceptionally, PSVT will be refractory even to intravenous amiodarone and urgent catheter ablation will become necessary.

Atrial Fibrillation and Flutter

It is rare for atrial fibrillation and flutter to present with hemodynamic deterioration in patients with normal or minimally diseased hearts (e.g., mild hypertensive LV hypertrophy with preserved systolic function).[25] On the other hand, both are common causes of acute decompensation in patients with severe LV systolic or diastolic dysfunction, stenotic valvular lesions (especially mitral stenosis), or after palliative operations for congenital heart disease such as the Fontan procedure. Atrial fibrillation is a common cause of hemodynamic decompensation in patients with hypertrophic cardiomyopathy.[26] All other conditions being equal, an excessively fast ventricular rate is the main determinant of hemodynamic deterioration during atrial tachyarrhythmias. Concealed conduction to the AV node makes this unlikely in atrial fibrillation, in the absence of an accessory pathway or so-called "enhanced AV nodal conduction" (spontaneous or catecholamine-induced). One-to-one conduction is relatively more common during atrial flutter. Usually, this occurs as a form of pharmacological proarrhythmia after the administration of class I antiarrhythmic drugs (quinidine, flecainide, propafenone) for atrial fibrillation or flutter without adequate AV nodal blockade (Figure 1).[27] The drugs slow intra-atrial conduction and organize the rhythm into a slower atrial flutter (rates < 225 beats/min), which can then conduct one-to-one through the AV node. The ECG diagnosis of atrial flutter with one-to-one conduction can be difficult. The fast rates frequently result in functional intraventricular aberrancy. Also, the use-dependent conduction slowing caused by class I drugs (i.e., more sodium channel block at faster rates) can cause the QRS to be very bizarre and suggestive of VT.

The treatment of atrial fibrillation in the cardiogenic shock patient is critical. The first component of therapy is usually controlling the ventricular response. In the presence of severe systolic or diastolic dysfunction,

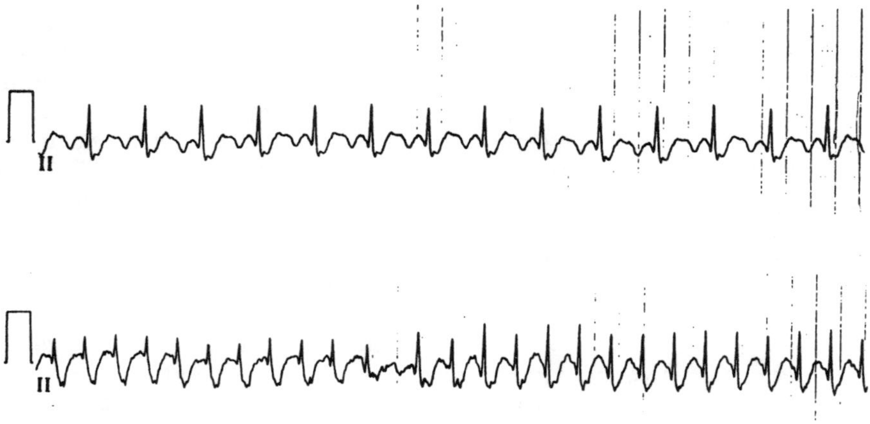

Figure 1. Atrial flutter with 1:1 conduction. A patient presented with atrial flutter (atrial cycle length 240 ms) with 2:1 conduction, resulting in a ventricular rate of 125 beats/min (upper tracing). He was given oral propafenone. Two hours later, he developed progressive hypotension. The atrial flutter cycle length was now 280 ms. This allowed 1:1 ventricular conduction with a ventricular rate of 215 beats/min (lower tracing). Emergent cardioversion was needed.

the contribution of the atrial systole is crucial to maintain adequate cardiac output. The less stable the patient, the more critical restoration of sinus rhythm becomes. It should be remembered that reestablishing a normal rhythm is often the best way to achieve rate control.

Restoration of sinus rhythm should be strongly considered in hemodynamically unstable patients with atrial fibrillation or flutter. Two modalities are available in the intensive care unit: direct current external cardioversion or pharmacological conversion. Additionally, pace-termination can be attempted in atrial flutter. This is easiest in post-operative patients with epicardial atrial wires in place[28] or in patients with a permanent atrial or dual-chamber pacemaker. In medical patients, the success rate of overdrive atrial pacing is lower.[29] Therefore, insertion of a transvenous or transesophageal pacing wire just to terminate atrial flutter is not recommended as an initial maneuver.

The relative merits of electrical versus pharmacological conversion of atrial tachyarrhythmias in patients with cardiogenic shock are not clear.[30] To our knowledge, head-to-head comparisons of these therapies have not been performed. Furthermore, because hemodynamic instability is often an exclusion criterion in randomized pharmaceutical trials, the true efficacy of antiarrhythmic drugs in this setting remains unknown. There is no doubt that electrical cardioversion remains the most effective way of restoring sinus rhythm in patients with atrial flutter or fibrillation and should be attempted first in the acutely decompensated patient.[31] However, the high incidence of early recurrence makes it less desirable as a sole therapeutic modality. Furthermore, the need for short-term anesthesia or deep sedation (with the added risk of hypotension) complicates its use in the unstable patient.

Pharmacological conversion of atrial tachyarrhythmias is more likely to be successful when the arrhythmia is of recent onset (less than 48 hours). Attempts at pharmacological conversion of atrial tachyarrhythmias in patients in shock should use intravenous agents. Inconsistent absorption rules out use of oral agents that are useful in more stable settings. In the United States, only procainamide, ibutilide, and amiodarone are widely available in intravenous form. More options, including disopyramide, flecainide, propafenone, sotalol, and dofetilide[32] are available in other countries. Intravenous procainamide often causes hypotension and is therefore dangerous in the already hypotensive patient. Although ibutilide has emerged as the intravenous drug of choice for the acute termination of atrial tachyarrhythmias, there is little experience with its use in hemodynamically unstable patients. Preliminary evidence suggests that it may be less effective in patients with a history of congestive heart failure.[33] Likewise, the risk of torsade de pointes (its most common side effect) appears higher in patients with severe LV dysfunction.[34] At the present time, ibutilide cannot be widely recommended to convert atrial tachyarrhythmias in the hypotensive patient.[35] It may have a role in facilitating electrical conversion of otherwise refractory atrial fibrillation. As it is a "single-use" agent with a short duration of action, it has no role in the maintenance of sinus rhythm after conversion. An intravenous class III agent that could be given as a continuous infusion would be valuable in this setting.

Although not approved in the United States for this indication, intravenous amiodarone is frequently used worldwide for the conversion of atrial tachyarrhythmias in the critically ill patient. Placebo-controlled trials have demonstrated that a significant effect is first seen after the first few hours of infusion and does not reach a plateau until at least 48 hours. Therefore, the main role of intravenous amiodarone in patients with atrial fibrillation and cardiogenic shock is as an adjuvant to DC cardioversion. The drug should be initiated as soon as possible after the need for cardioversion is identified in an attempt to decrease the incidence of recurrence.

Frequently, sinus rhythm cannot be restored or holds for only short periods of time, and rate control becomes the therapeutic goal. Rate control is difficult because the most effective drugs (diltiazem, verapamil, beta-blockers) are relatively contraindicated in the hypotensive patient. However, if a very rapid ventricular rate is the main determinant of a low cardiac output, rate control with one or more of these agents can result in an increase in stroke volume, cardiac output, and blood pressure. Due to its ultra-short half-life, esmolol may be particularly useful in the unstable patient.[36] Esmolol often results in conversion in hyperadrenergic settings, such as the postoperative period.[37,38] Although still indicated in patients with pump failure and atrial tachyarrhythmias, intravenous digoxin rarely achieves rate control when used alone. Limited evidence suggests that pharmacological doses of magnesium sulfate can reduce the ventricular response during atrial fibrillation without inducing hypotension.[39] Concomitant use with digoxin can achieve additive effects.[40] Intravenous amiodarone is also useful in controlling the ventricular response in criti-

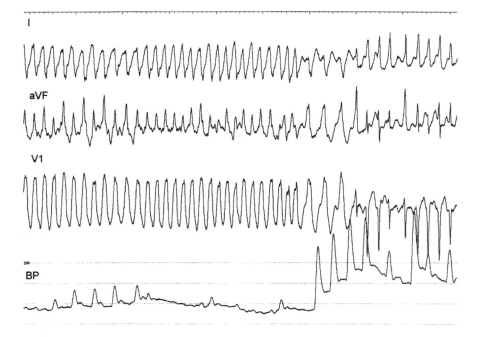

Figure 2. Atrial fibrillation with rapid conduction in a patient with WPW syndrome. Note that most beats during periods of very rapid conduction do not generate a blood pressure waveform. Blood pressure recovers somewhat in beats preceded by a longer filling time. The patient was emergently cardioverted. The left lateral accessory pathway was successfully ablated.

cally ill patients with atrial fibrillation.[41] This effect, although not immediate, is evident sooner (1-2 hours) than the effect on conversion rates. Often, repeated loading doses are needed to achieve the desired response. Left ventricular dysfunction is a risk factor for thromboembolic events in patients with atrial fibrillation. Critically ill patients with atrial fibrillation should be anticoagulated with heparin if there is no contraindication.

Atrial Tachyarrhythmias in the Wolff-Parkinson-White Syndrome

Accessory AV pathways, the anatomical substrate for the WPW syndrome, can have a very short anterograde refractory period. Bypassing the rate-limiting safety properties of the AV node can allow extremely rapid AV conduction during atrial tachyarrhythmias. Atrial fibrillation with very rapid ventricular response in the WPW syndrome often causes cardiovascular collapse. Degeneration to ventricular fibrillation (VF) can also occur. The ECG shows a very rapid and grossly irregular wide-complex tachycardia (Figure 2). The predominant QRS complex is very wide and bizarre, ruling out aberrant conduction; it represents complete ventricular pre-excitation. With a left free wall accessory pathway (the most common location), the QRS typically shows positive concordance in the precordial leads. Interspersed QRS complexes of other morphologies represent different degrees of fusion between activation via the normal conduction system and the accessory pathway. Pre-excited atrial fibrillation is usually much more irregular than most ventricular tachycardias, facilitating the differential diagnosis. Other atrial tachyarrhythmias, such as atrial flutter, can also conduct with a one-to-one ratio to the ventricles via an accessory pathway. In these cases, the resulting tachyarrhythmia is generally regular. Most WPW patients with rapid atrial tachyarrhythmias have a previous history of recurrent paroxysmal supraventricular tachycardia. However, it is occasionally their first manifestation, especially in elderly patients.

Treatment of these patients must be expeditious. External DC cardioversion should be used when there is severe hemodynamic compromise. A brief trial of pharmacological treatment is reasonable in more stable patients. Digitalis, verapamil, diltiazem, and adenosine can cause a paradoxical increase in ventricular response rates and are contraindicated (Figure 3). Intravenous procainamide is the traditional agent of choice.[42] It can prolong the refractory period and slow conduction in the accessory pathway[43] and atrial tissue, resulting in a slower ventricular response or even conversion. There is much less experience with intravenous ibutilide,[44] although its favorable electrophysiological and hemodynamic profile[45] should make it very useful for this indication. When drugs are used, one should be prepared for emergency external countershock, in case collapse or ventricular fibrillation occur. Catheter ablation of the accessory pathway is curative and represents the first choice for chronic management of these patients.

Wide-Complex Tachycardia

Wide complex tachycardias represent a diagnostic challenge (Table 2). Several studies have chronicled the frequent misdiagnosis of VT as supraventricular tachycardia with aberrancy in patients who initially present with well-tolerated wide-complex tachycardia. In the 1980s, intravenous verapamil was frequently administered in this situation, and often resulted in hemodynamic deterioration and need for emergent cardioversion.[46,47] With the availability of intravenous adenosine, verapamil is rarely given for wide-complex tachycardia. Although adenosine is unlikely to produce hemodynamic embarrassment, it should not be used routinely for undiagnosed wide-complex tachycardia, as it can delay more appropriate treatment. Emphasis should be placed instead in establishing a positive diagnosis on the basis of clinical and 12-lead ECG data. Sustained monomorphic VT is the most common cause of regular wide QRS tachycardia in the conscious adult patient, especially when there is a history of remote myocardial infarction.[48] Recognition of this simple principle and careful examination of the 12-lead electrocardiogram will prevent the misapplication of pharmacotherapy. Several ECG diagnostic algorithms with acceptable discriminatory power have been published,[49,50] and the

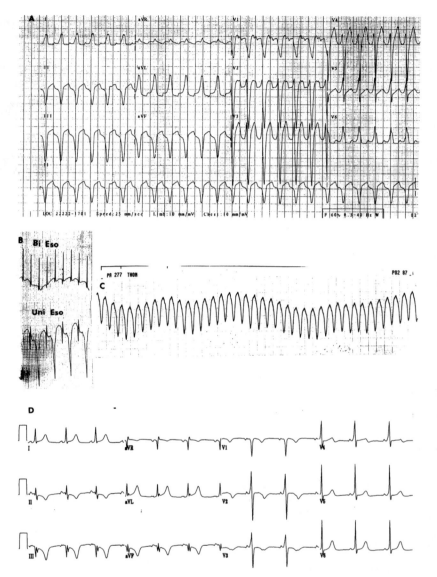

Figure 3. Hazards of calcium channel blockers in patients with pre-excited tachy-cardias. A teenager presented with a wide-complex tachycardia with a left bundle branch pattern at a rate of 140 beats/min (**A**). There was no response to carotid sinus massage or adenosine. An esophageal recording demonstrated atrial flutter with 2:1 conduction (**B**). The mistaken diagnosis of atrial flutter with left bundle branch aberrancy was made. The patient was given IV diltiazem (10 mg). Shortly thereafter, he developed 1:1 conduction with a ventricular rate of 280 beats/min, requiring emergent cardioversion (**C**). The 12-lead ECG after conversion shows WPW syndrome with a right lateral accessory pathway (**D**). In retrospect, the diagnosis of aberrancy could have been excluded by careful analysis of the QRS complex during tachycardia (i.e., wide initial R wave in leads V_1 and V_2). Bi eso: bipolar esophageal recording; Uni eso: unipolar esophageal recording.

Table 2.

Classification of the Most Common Forms
of Regular Wide-Complex Tachycardia.

Ventricular tachycardia
Supraventricular tachycardia with aberrancy due to intraventricular conduction delay*
    Sinus tachycardia
    Atrial tachycardia
    Atrial flutter with fixed AV block
    AV nodal reentry tachycardia
    AV reentry tachycardia (orthodromic)
    Junctional tachycardia
Preexcited tachycardia (associated with or mediated by an accessory pathway)
    Atrial tachycardia
    Atrial flutter
    AV reentry tachycardia (antidromic)
Paced tachycardias¶
    Tracking of supraventricular tachyarrhythmias
    Endless-loop tachycardia
    Sensor-mediated tachycardias

---

* The intraventricular conduction delay could be due to fixed or rate-related bundle branch block, or to diffuse conduction delay due to pharmacological agents (e.g., class I antiarrhythmic drugs) or metabolic factors (e.g., hyperkalemia, acidosis).

¶ With bipolar pacing and low amplitude pacing pulses, the pacing artifact can be almost imperceptible in standard ECGs.

intensivist should become familiar with at least one of them. The algorithms, however, have less value in patients with preexistent bundle branch block.[51,52] An esophageal recording, by demonstrating AV dissociation, can help diagnose VT in unclear cases.[53] Adenosine should be given when supraventricular tachycardia with aberrancy is strongly suspected. The treatment of confirmed or strongly suspected VT is given below. Empirical treatment of wide-complex tachycardia of unknown origin involves broad-spectrum antiarrhythmic agents. Agents such as procainamide, amiodarone (and perhaps ibutilide) are efficacious against VT, PSVT, and accessory pathway conduction. On the other hand, agents that predominantly block the AV node (notably verapamil or diltiazem) are hazardous in patients with VT or preexcited tachycardia and are absolutely contraindicated for the empirical treatment of wide-complex tachycardia.

Ventricular Tachycardia

Although it constitutes up to 10% of patients with VT referred for electrophysiological evaluation, idiopathic VT rarely causes collapse. On the other hand, VT is a frequent cause of hemodynamic deterioration in patients with structural heart disease. Hemodynamically unstable VT requires immediate termination with synchronized cardioversion. Often times, the patient is "hemodynamically stable" (i.e., there is no clinical evidence of tissue hypoperfusion or shock) on initial presentation. In these

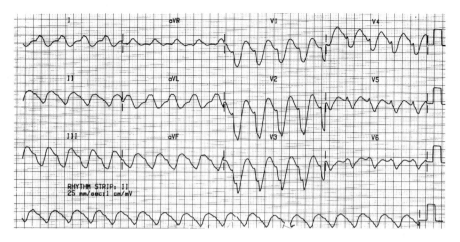

Figure 4. Wide-complex tachycardia in a patient with cardiovascular collapse and flecainide intoxication. Note the very wide QRS and the sinusoidal appearance of the waveforms. In this case, it represented sinus tachycardia with very slowed intraventricular conduction. The patient recovered with alkalinization and supportive treatment.

cases, there is sufficient time to allow pharmacological intervention. It should be remembered however, that subtle decompensation can progress rapidly to full-blown hemodynamic collapse in the patient with left ventricular dysfunction.[54] Treating personnel should be prepared for emergent cardioversion if the need arises.

Sustained monomorphic VT generally occurs in the patient with remote myocardial infarction or cardiomyopathy, but is less often associated with AMI. Although lidocaine can be administered rapidly with minimal effect on blood pressure, it is relatively ineffective for termination.[55,56] In randomized controlled trials, both procainamide[57] and sotalol[58] have been more effective than lidocaine in terminating VT. Magnesium is ineffective.[59] The effectiveness of intravenous amiodarone for hemodynamically unstable VT is well proven,[60] and by extrapolation it is assumed safe and effective for patients with stable VT. Current guidelines recommend intravenous amiodarone (especially when there is concomitant left ventricular dysfunction), intravenous procainamide, and intravenous sotalol (not available in the United States) for the treatment of patients with sustained monomorphic VT that is not pulseless.[61]

Overdosing with a variety of drugs with sodium channel blocking activity, including class I antiarrhythmic drugs and tricyclic antidepressants, can induce VT. Hemodynamic collapse is common, even in patients without structural heart disease. In typical cases, these tachycardias are relatively slow and have a characteristic sinusoidal pattern, but at times it is difficult to differentiate drug-induced VT from sinus tachycardia with impaired intraventricular conduction (Figure 4). When sudden conversion to a wider-complex rhythm occurs with hypotension, drug-induced VT is likely and cardioversion is indicated. However, these VTs are often incessant and recur immediately after cardioversion. Hypertonic saline and systemic alkalinization often reverse the adverse electrophysiological effects of poisoning with sodium channel blocking agents.[62] Hypertonic sodium bicarbonate is particularly valuable because it both provides hypertonic saline and systemic alkalinization. When this antidote is used, the goal is an arterial pH of 7.50 to 7.55. Respiratory alkalosis can be used as a temporary measure until the appropriate degree of metabolic alkalosis can be attained with sodium bicarbonate. Current guidelines recommend establishing the target arterial pH with repetitive boluses of 1 to 2 mEq/kg of sodium bicarbonate and then maintaining the alkalinization via a titrated infusion of a solution consisting of 3 ampules of sodium bicarbonate (150 mEq) and KCl (30 mEq) in 850 mL of D_5W.[63]

Ventricular Electrical Storm

Ventricular electrical storm is a serious but treatable clinical syndrome of recurrent severe ventricular tachyarrhythmias.[64] Although the definitions are still evolving, hemodynamically unstable VT or VF recurring within 24 hours characterizes the condition. It most often occurs in patients with coronary artery disease, previous MI and LV dysfunction. Frequent precipitants of electrical storm include recent worsening of heart failure, hypokalemia, changes in antiarrhythmic drug therapy, and myocardial ischemia. There is evidence that increased sympathetic tone, triggered by physical or psychological stress, often contributes to the severity of this syndrome. Although torsade de pointes can present as electrical storm, its etiology, management, and prognosis is very different. Intravenous magnesium sulfate and temporary overdrive pacing are specifically useful in this context.[65] The management of electrical storm in implantable cardioverter-defibrillator recipients is discussed elsewhere.[66]

Specific triggers should be searched for and corrected if possible. Antiarrhythmic drugs represent the first line of therapy and should be initiated after the first recurrence or even after the initial episode if the risk of recurrence is felt to be very high. Intravenous amiodarone is the drug of choice in most forms of ventricular electrical storm (except in torsades de pointes). Sympathetic blockade, if tolerated, is also useful.

The multiple electrophysiological effects of intravenous amiodarone effects make it a "broad-spectrum" agent. The immediate effects after initial administration consist of slowing of AV nodal conduction, blockade, and sympathetic antagonism. Prolongation of action potential duration and refractoriness in atrial and ventricular myocardium appear later. The hemodynamic profile of intravenous amiodarone can complicate its administration in the hypotensive patient. The drug has significant vasodilatory properties. Worsening of hypotension is common and requires slowing of the infusion rate. Also, the vehicle for dissolving this highly lipophilic agent, a polysorbate compound, likely has its own vasodilating properties. The hemodynamic and antiarrhythmic effects of an aqueous preparation of amiodarone are the focus of ongoing research. Intravenous amiodarone has little or no negative inotropic effects. In patients with severe LV dysfunction in sinus rhythm, it often results in increased cardiac output secondary to afterload reduction.

Intravenous amiodarone is administered as 150 mg over 10 minutes; followed by 1 mg/min infusion for 6 hours and then 0.5 mg/min. Supplementary infusions of 150 mg can be repeated as required for recurrent or resistant arrhythmias to a maximum manufacturer-recommended total daily dose of 2 g. Higher doses, including initial infusions of 5 to 10 mg/kg over 30 to 60 minutes are in common use outside the United States.[67] The major side effects from intravenous amiodarone are hypotension and bradycardia, which can be prevented by slowing the rate of infusion or treated with fluids, pressors, chronotropic agents, or temporary pacing. Prolonged peripheral infusions often cause phlebitis. A central line should be considered when the drug is to be infused for more than a few hours.

Myocardial injury, as indicated by elevations in cardiac isoenzymes and troponin levels, is often detectable after multiple external or internal countershocks.[68,69] In humans, shocks produce a strength-dependent transient drop in cardiac index.[70] Diastolic dysfunction is more prominent than systolic dysfunction after multiple shocks.[71] In animal models, multiple shocks over short periods of time produce cumulative tissue damage.[72] A similar phenomenon (although not well documented) is likely in humans. It appears that biphasic shocks (now available in external defibrillators) induce less myocardial dysfunction than conventional monophasic shocks.[73]

Pace termination of frequently recurring monomorphic VT is very useful in the intensive care unit[74] and is preferred to repeat external DC cardioversions.[75] A temporary ventricular pacing wire should be inserted early on in this situation. Antitachycardia pacing is most effective for VT with rates below 200 beats/min, with a success rate of > 80% and a low risk (< 5%) of tachycardia acceleration.[76] Preparations should be made for prompt external defibrillation in case acceleration occurs. Self-adhesive, preapplied defibrillation pads are recommended. Under ECG monitoring, ventricular pacing is initiated at a rate 10 to 20 beats/min faster than the VT. Pacing is then abruptly stopped after confirming capture for 2 to 10 seconds. If VT persists, pacing is repeated, increasing the pacing rate by 10 beats/min after each failed attempt. However, pacing rates $\geq$ 250 beats/min should be avoided because they are very likely to cause acceleration. Antitachycardia pacing can serve as a bridge to definitive antiarrhythmic therapy (catheter ablation, device implantation, or optimized antiarrhythmic drugs). A permanent antitachycardia pacemaker can be connected externally to the temporary ventricular wire after manually delivered therapy is proved effective in terminating VT. The device is then programmed to deliver effective antitachycardia pacing sequences automatically or upon placing a magnet on top of it by nursing personnel after recognition of VT.[77]

In some patients, VT is incessant (i.e., it recurs almost immediately after pace or shock termination). Here, it is essential to maintain the circulation with pharmacological or nonpharmacological means until the arrhythmia can be "cooled down" or definite percutaneous or surgical treatment performed. Mechanical ventilation and sedation are helpful. Inotropes, on the other hand, can make the VT faster and less well tolerated. Appropriately timed atrial pacing during VT to restore synchrony can increase blood pressure and cardiac index significantly.[78] The technique should be attempted in patients with pre-existent atrial and ventricular temporary pacing wires. Intra-aortic balloon counterpulsation can also help control refractory ventricular arrhythmia, allowing time for the institution of more definitive treatment.[79]

Incessant monomorphic VT is often a successful target for catheter ablation, if the circulation can be sustained during the relatively long mapping procedure.[80] If not available locally, early patient transfer to an electrophysiology center experienced with this technique is recommended. In occasional patients, bundle branch reentry is the mechanism responsible for incessant VT. The arrhythmia can be suspected from surface ECG. Ablation of the right bundle branch is simple and curative.[81] "Heroic" measures, including surgical VT ablation,[82] percutaneous transcoronary chemical ablation,[83] insertion of an LV assist device,[84] or cardiac transplantation should be considered only if catheter ablation fails or is contraindicated.

Bradycardias

The hemodynamic consequences of sinus bradycardia are related primarily to the slow ventricular rate. Ventricular filling is well preserved in most instances, and an adequate or enhanced stroke volume is present at rest. Bradyarrhythmias rarely cause hemodynamic collapse in patients with structurally normal hearts unless the ventricular rate is below 30 beats/min. Even patients with significant heart disease often tolerate rates of 40 beats/min or less at rest. The treatment of bradyarrhythmias causing hemodynamic compromise is straightforward. Temporary transvenous ventricular pacing should be initiated as soon as possible. External transcutaneous pacing or isoproterenol can be used as a "bridge" until transvenous pacing is established. A discussion of the techniques, results and complications of temporary pacing is beyond the scope of this chapter. The reader is referred to recent comprehensive reviews.[85,86]

A relatively common cause of bradyarrhythmia and hypotension (even in patients with structurally normal hearts) is acute intoxication with beta-blockers or calcium channel blockers. All beta-blockers can cause profound bradycardia and high-degree AV block in overdose. Among calcium channel blockers, verapamil and diltiazem cause bradycardia and heart block more frequently and severely than the dihydropyridine agents, which require massive overdoses as sometimes seen in suicide attempts. Not only bradycardia, but also myocardial depression and peripheral vasodilatation contribute to the profound hypotension seen with calcium channel blocker or beta-blocker overdose. Consideration should be given to specific antidotes. Glucagon is often effective for beta-blocker intoxication. Bradyarrhythmias due to calcium-channel blocker intoxication may respond to intravenous calcium chloride or gluconate and sympathomimetics. However, a temporary pacing wire will often be necessary, especially when the ingestion involves sustained-release preparations.

Patients with a malfunctioning pacemaker can present with a compromising bradyarrhythmia if the escape rhythm is too slow. The causes of pacing malfunction can be divided into output failure and capture failure. Output failure is suspected in the presence of intrinsic rhythm with a heart rate that is lower than the programmed lower rate limit and with no spikes visible. Causes of output failure are multiple. They include battery depletion, circuit failure, lead fracture, incompatible lead or header, and oversensing of external (electromagnetic) or internal (e.g., myopotential) interference. Differentiation between absence of pulse generation and pulse transmission is relatively easy using telemetry of the internal markers from the device. When there is failure to transmit the pulse, markers will indicate a scheduled paced event. Oversensing can be confirmed in the emergency setting with the use of a magnet. If oversensing was causing output inhibition, magnet application results in asynchronous pacing. Although component failure is in general rare with modern devices, it is more likely to occur in hospitalized patients subjected to a variety of therapeutic procedures including external cardioversion or defibrillation, electrocautery, and radiation therapy. It is important to rule out pseudo-nonoutput caused by nonvisible bipolar spikes, hysteresis, oversensing, artifact, or automatic mode switching.

Pacemaker spikes not followed by a depolarization suggest loss of capture. The causes of noncapture vary with the time elapsed since implantation. When an intermittent or persistent high stimulation threshold is detected within the first 48 hours, lead dislodgment or malposition is likely. Within the first 6 weeks after a pacemaker implant, a rise in the pacing threshold is not uncommon and results from inflammation surrounding the endocardium-lead interface. The problem can be corrected by increasing the output until the pacing threshold becomes normal. In stable patients, capture failures detected after this initial period suggest lead fracture or battery depletion. However, in the acutely ill patient, factors external to the pacemaker system can also cause an increase in the pacing threshold leading to noncapture. These include class I antiarrhythmic drugs, myocardial infarction or ischemia, DC cardioversion, and metabolic problems, such as acidosis or hyperkalemia. Correction of these factors is often all that is needed to restore capture (Figure 5).

Arrhythmias Associated with Cardiogenic Shock in Acute Myocardial Infarction

Though the incidence of complications in acute MI has changed dramatically as the eras have progressed from observation to reperfusion, rhythm disturbances are still very common in the patient with extensive infarction. The discussion of the causes of demise in fatal cardiogenic shock is difficult and tautological, as unless electromechanical dissociation develops, no patient dies without an arrhythmia. However, it is clinically useful to classify arrhythmias (especially ventricular ones) in acute MI as primary or secondary. Primary arrhythmias occur early on, are often a direct consequence of myocardial ischemia, and when treated successfully, carry less adverse prognostic implication. Secondary arrhythmias occur in the setting of severe pump failure, are associated with a spiral of

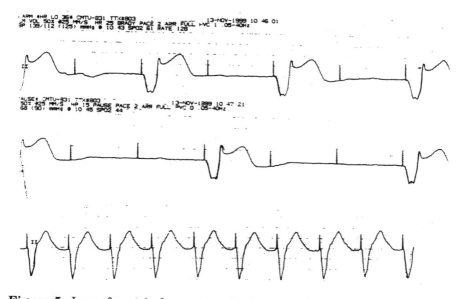

Figure 5. Loss of ventricular capture due to metabolic disturbances. A patient with an implantable cardioverter defibrillator programmed for back-up VVI pacing at 40 beats/min developed severe pneumonia and became bradycardic. Severe hypoxemia and acidosis were present. There was sudden loss of ventricular capture in a 2:1 pattern (upper tracing) and then in a 3:1 pattern (middle tracing). Note that capture beats are very wide. Ventricular capture was restored after mechanical ventilation and correction of the metabolic disturbances. The pacing rate was also increased to 70 beats/min. The paced QRS complex narrowed significantly (bottom tracing).

detrimental hemodynamic and metabolic derangements, and have a poor short- and long-term prognosis, even when successfully treated. Multiple care issues need to be simultaneously addressed while diagnosing and treating arrhythmias in the patient with acute MI and cardiogenic shock. Prompt opening of the acutely occluded coronary artery, tailored treatment of hemodynamic derangements, and comprehensive supportive care are all crucial for a positive outcome.

Sinus Tachycardia

Due to reflex adrenergic activation, most patients with cardiogenic shock secondary to acute MI present with significant sinus tachycardia. A rapid sinus rate remains one of the strongest predictors of mortality in acute MI. In principle, no specific treatments are indicated for this sinus tachycardia in cardiogenic shock, though use of digoxin is nearly universal. Unlike hemodynamically stable acute MI patients, of course, beta-blockade is specifically contraindicated in patients with cardiogenic shock.

Atrial Tachyarrhythmias

Atrial tachyarrhythmias are an important cause of hemodynamic deterioration in patients with acute MI. The incidence of atrial fibrillation in unselected patients with acute MI ranges from 10% to 16%. Thrombolysis reduces the incidence of new-onset atrial fibrillation.[87] Atrial fibrillation is more prevalent (22%) among elderly acute MI patients, and is present on arrival (and presumably chronic) in approximately half of those cases.[88] Atrial flutter or atrial tachycardia is much less frequent.

The pathogenesis of atrial fibrillation associated with acute MI is protean. Atrial fibrillation developing in the first few hours is relatively uncommon and often results from acute atrial ischemia or infarction.[89] Thus, it tends to occur more often in patients with inferior wall acute MI, especially when the circumflex artery is the culprit vessel.[90] Other studies have found a relation with compromise of the sinus node artery, irrespective of its origin from the right or circumflex coronary artery.[91] Early atrial fibrillation is often associated with sinus bradycardia, AV block, or both, reflecting concurrent ischemia of the sinoatrial and AV nodes. A rapid ventricular response is therefore rare. Hemodynamic decompensation does not occur[92] unless there are concomitant mechanical complications such as acute mitral regurgitation or right ventricular infarction.[93]

Atrial fibrillation occurring later in the course of acute MI is generally associated with extensive infarction and heart failure. An increase in pulmonary capillary wedge pressure is a frequent harbinger of late atrial fibrillation in acute MI.[94] A hyperadrenergic state often results in rapid ventricular response. Atrial fibrillation is more common in patients with infarct-associated pericarditis.[95] However, this may be a result of larger infarct size rather than a direct effect of atrial epicardial inflammation.[96,97]

Patients developing atrial fibrillation during acute MI are older, have more extensive infarction, and have a higher incidence of congestive heart failure, hypotension, ventricular arrhythmias, and AV block. Despite these associations, atrial fibrillation (especially when of new-onset and associated with anterior wall acute MI) independently portends a worse prognosis.[87,88,98] Thus, it is possible that its prevention and management may improve outcome.

There are few controlled studies of the treatment of atrial fibrillation in acute MI. Prompt cardioversion is recommended when there is severe hemodynamic compromise. However, the incidence of early recurrence is high, and concomitant pharmacological therapy aimed at rate control and maintenance of sinus rhythm is often needed. In patients with concomitant bradyarrhythmias, the use of negative chronotropic or dromotropic agents is problematic in the absence of a pacemaker. In a small randomized study, intravenous amiodarone was more effective in controlling the ventricular response and restoring sinus rhythm than intravenous digoxin.[99] Atrial fibrillation is a powerful risk factor for the development of ischemic stroke in patients with acute myocardial infarction.[100] One half of embolic events occur on the first day and more than 90% occur by the fourth day.[101] Short-term prophylactic anticoagulation with heparin is recommended.

AV Block

Complete heart block in the setting of inferior wall acute MI occurs at the level of the AV node and can be classified as early and late. Early AV block is often due to increased parasympathetic discharge and develops abruptly within 6 hours of infarct onset.[102] Not infrequently, it is precipitated by pharmacological or mechanical reperfusion.[103] Because of the often-slow ventricular escape rate plus the associated vasodilatation, hypotension is common. However, the prompt response to atropine makes the need of temporary pacing rare.[104] Patients who develop AV block after 6 hours of infarction usually do so gradually, and the return to normal sinus rhythm is equally slow. The ventricular escape rhythm has a relatively high rate, and the response to atropine is poor. The most likely mechanism is reversible AV nodal (i.e., "proximal") ischemia. Necrosis (irreversible damage) of the AV node is rare owing to its extensive collateral circulation,[105] as well as a low metabolic rate. Adenosine, an endogenous ischemic metabolite with negative chronotropic and dromotropic effects, may be a mediator of bradyarrhythmias associated with inferior acute MI. Aminophylline is a competitive A_1 receptor antagonist and can acutely reverse atropine-resistant AV block in these patients.[106] A loading dose of 5 mg/kg should be considered, and a continuous infusion initiated afterwards if there is a favorable response. However, temporary transvenous pacing is often necessary.

Complete AV block is common in patients with inferior AMI and right ventricular compromise.[107] It may be partly or entirely responsible for hypotension or shock in this setting. Ventricular pacing often does not improve hemodynamics because the atrial contribution to right ventricular filling is crucial in these patients. Restoration of AV synchrony via AV sequential pacing may dramatically increase blood pressure, cardiac output, and stroke volume.[108] In patients with bradyarrhythmias and right ventricular infarction, pacing at relatively fast rates (100 to 130 beats/min) results in significant hemodynamic improvement in comparison to the usual rate of 70 beats/min.[109]

The higher in-hospital mortality of patients with inferior acute MI and late AV block (compared to patients without arrhythmic complications) does not result from the bradyarrhythmia itself, but generally from a larger myocardial infarction. Permanent pacing is very rarely needed after inferior acute MI. Atrioventricular block may take as long as 3 weeks to subside, especially if reperfusion was not achieved acutely. Implantation of a permanent pacemaker should not be considered before day 16, except in the rare patient in whom intra- or infrahisian block is confirmed. Patients with inferior wall acute MI who require temporary pacing and survive to hospital discharge have a good subsequent prognosis.

In contrast, AV block in patients with anterior wall acute MI is "distal." It is the result of dysfunction of the trifascicular intraventricular conduction system, usually from proximal occlusion of the left anterior descending coronary artery. Patients with anterior wall acute MI and second or third degree AV block have a high incidence of heart failure, asystole, and ventricular tachyarrhythmias, with a mortality rate of 40% to 50%. Autopsy studies show extensive septal necrosis encompassing the His bundle and the bundle branches. However, AV block in patients with anterior acute MI may also result from ischemia rather than necrosis of the proximal infranodal tissue.[110] Reversion of intraventricular conduction defects in patients undergoing thrombolysis is not infrequent[111] and is associated with an improved prognosis.[112] Onset of complete AV block in patients with anterior acute MI is often abrupt, with poor ventricular escape and no response to atropine. Progression to AV block can generally be predicted by the presence of new, often combined, intraventricular conduction defects.[113] Prophylactic pacing is generally indicated for new bifascicular or trifascicular block or alternating bundle branch block complicating anterior wall acute MI. Blocks of indeterminate onset should be considered new. A useful clinical prediction rule to assess the potential for progression to complete AV block in patients with acute MI assigns a score of 1 to each of the following ECG findings: first-degree AV block, second-degree (types I and II) AV block, right bundle branch block, left bundle branch block, left anterior fascicular block, and left posterior fascicular block.[114] Patients with a total score of 3 or more have a high (> 36 %) risk of progression to complete AV block and should receive a prophylactic temporary wire. Patients with intermediate scores of 1 and 2 have rates of occurrence of 7.8% and 25%, respectively, and should be considered for prophylactic transcutaneous pacing.[115] It should be noted that these algorithms represent the "natural" history of acute MI. Mechanical or pharmacological reperfusion decreases the incidence, severity, and duration of AV block and should raise the threshold for insertion of a transvenous pacing wire. Patients with left bundle branch block can develop complete AV block during right-heart catheterization if the catheter induces right bundle branch block. A prophylactic pacing wire is not warranted, but a pulmonary artery catheter with pacing capabilities should be considered,[116] and transcutaneous pacing should be immediately available.

Atropine is contraindicated in the hypotensive patient with anterior wall acute MI and AV block. Isoproterenol can accelerate the ventricular escape, but it should be used only as a temporizing measure because it increases myocardial oxygen consumption, promotes tachyarrhythmias, and induces vasodilatation that can worsen coronary perfusion. A temporary pacing wire should be inserted emergently while the patient is supported with isoproterenol or transcutaneous pacing. AV block regresses in the majority of surviving patients, although residual intraventricular conduction defects are common. Implantation of a permanent pacemaker in these patients is recommended.[117]

Ventricular Ectopy

Complex ventricular ectopy, including runs of nonsustained VT, is almost universal in the patient with extensive acute MI and pump failure.

When persistent or very frequent, suppression of ectopy can improve cardiac output. More often, the question of prophylaxis against more sustained tachyarrhythmias arises. Systematic prospective studies have shown that in coronary care unit patients, complex ventricular ectopy has poor positive and negative predictive values for subsequent VF, suggesting that selective prophylaxis in patients exhibiting these rhythms is not warranted. Meta-analyses of prophylactic lidocaine have shown that although it reduces the incidence of VF, it may adversely affect mortality rates.[118,119] Its routine use is not recommended and has decreased considerably worldwide.[120] It should be noted that the meta-analyses of routine prophylaxis with lidocaine have not reported separate results in patients with pump failure, in whom the risk-benefit ratio could be different. Prophylactic high-dose intravenous amiodarone started in the first few hours of an uncomplicated acute MI results in a significant increase in mortality, while a lower-dose regimen is associated with mortality similar to that of placebo.[121] Beta-blockers are effective in preventing ventricular arrhythmias in acute MI,[122] but their hemodynamic profile preclude widespread use in cardiogenic shock.

Sustained Monomorphic Ventricular Tachycardia

Sustained monomorphic VT is rare (< 2 %) during the first 48 hours of acute MI. It is often associated with extensive myocardial damage and severe congestive heart failure or cardiogenic shock. It is frequently recurrent and is an independent predictor of in-hospital mortality.[123] In the GUSTO study of patients undergoing fibrinolysis, 20% of patients with sustained VT and 34% of patients with both sustained VT and VF had cardiogenic shock.[124] Late sustained monomorphic VT (i.e., > 48 hours after acute MI) is also uncommon and associated with large infarcts and pump failure.[125] Despite the use of fibrinolysis, the mortality of patients with sustained VT during AMI remains high (30%-50%). The treatment of monomorphic VT causing immediate hypotension is DC synchronized cardioversion with 100 J. Although lidocaine and procainamide are still recommended for more stable patients, there is little evidence of their efficacy and safety in this setting. Intravenous amiodarone is probably a better choice.

Ventricular Fibrillation

Primary VF has been defined as an arrhythmia that occurs during the first 48 hours of an acute MI in a patient who is otherwise stable and without signs of pump failure. In the pre-thrombolytic era its incidence was around 2%.[126] It is not clear if its incidence is higher in patients undergoing thrombolysis, probably reflecting triggering by reperfusion. Its prognostic impact is often misunderstood. It is widely acknowledged that prompt defibrillation in the Coronary Care Unit is compatible with full recovery. However, in many patients primary VF can be the first manifestation of subtle decompensation. For example, some studies have found that patients with primary VF have larger infarcts and a higher incidence of subsequent AV block and atrial fibrillation. Furthermore, treatment, including multiple external shocks (in the 10%-15% of patients with recurring arrhythmia) and antiarrhythmic drugs can have deleterious effects of their own. Most large studies have concluded that primary VF exerts an independent, significant effect on in-hospital mortality.[127] Prognosis after discharge is not affected. Fibrinolytic treatment affords protection against secondary VF most probably by a limitation of infarct size.[128] The arrhythmia is associated with an adverse short-term outcome.

Post-myocardial infarction polymorphic VT is in general not related to an abnormally long QT interval, sinus bradycardia, preceding sinus pauses, or electrolyte abnormalities. It has a variable response to class I antiarrhythmics but may be suppressed by intravenous amiodarone therapy. It is often associated with signs or symptoms of recurrent myocardial ischemia. Furthermore, coronary revascularization appears to be effective in preventing the recurrence of polymorphic VT when associated with recurrent postinfarction angina.[129]

There are no firm data to help define an optimal management strategy for prevention of recurrences in patients who have sustained an initial episode of VF in the setting of acute MI. It seems prudent to correct any electrolyte and acid-base disturbances and (if not contraindicated) administer beta-blocking agents. If infusion of an antiarrhythmic drug is initiated, it should probably be maintained for only 6 to 24 hours and then discontinued so that the patient's ongoing need for antiarrhythmic treatment can be reassessed. Rarely, patients with AMI develop recurrent drug-refractory, sustained polymorphic VT or VF. Sympathetic blockade (achieved with intravenous β-blockade or left stellate ganglion blockade) supplemented with intravenous amiodarone is much more effective than conventional antiarrhythmic drugs in patients with electrical storm and a recent myocardial infarction.[130]

References

1. Benchimol A, Desser KB, Raizada V, et al. Simultaneous left ventricular echocardiography and aortic blood velocity during rapid right ventricular pacing in man. *Am J Med Sci* 1977; 273:55-62.

2. Yamakado T, Yamada N, Tarumi T, et al. Left ventricular inotropic and lusitropic responses to pacing-induced tachycardia in patients with varying degrees of ventricular dysfunction. *Am Heart J* 1998; 135:584-591.

3. Lima JA, Weiss JL, Guzman PA, et al. Incomplete filling and incoordinate contraction as mechanisms of hypotension during ventricular tachycardia in man. *Circulation* 1983; 68:928-398.

4. Saksena S, Ciccone JM, Craelius W, et al. Studies on left ventricular function during sustained ventricular tachycardia. *J Am Coll Cardiol* 1984; 4:501-508.

5. Kolettis TM, Kyriakides ZS, Popov T, et al. Importance of the site of ventricular tachycardia origin on left ventricular hemodynamics in humans. *Pacing Clin Electrophysiol* 1999; 22:871-879.

6. Peuhkurinen KJ, Uusimaa PA, Ruskoaho H, et al. Hemodynamic recovery, atrial natriuretic peptide, and catecholamines during simulated ventricular tachycardia: Effects of ventriculoatrial conduction. *Pacing Clin Electrophysiol* 1995; 18:75-82.

7. Maloney J, Khoury D, Simmons T, et al. Effect of atrioventricular synchrony on stroke volume during ventricular tachycardia in man. *Am Heart J* 1992; 123:1561-1568.

8. Sganzerla P, Fabbiocchi F, Grazi S, et al. Electrophysiologic and haemodynamic correlates in supraventricular tachycardia. *Eur Heart J* 1989; 10:32-39.

9. Hamdan MH, Zagrodzky JD, Page RL, et al. Effect of P-wave timing during supraventricular tachycardia on the hemodynamic and sympathetic neural response. *Circulation* 2001; 103:96-101.

10. Smith ML, Joglar JA, Wasmund SL, et al. Reflex control of sympathetic activity during simulated ventricular tachycardia in humans. *Circulation* 1999; 100:628-634.

11. Smith ML, Ellenbogen KA, Beightol LA, et al. Sympathetic neural responses to induced ventricular tachycardia. *J Am Coll Cardiol* 1991; 18:1015-1024.

12. Feldman T, Carroll JD, Munkenbeck F, et al. Hemodynamic recovery during simulated ventricular tachycardia: Role of adrenergic receptor activation. *Am Heart J* 1988; 115:576-587.

13. Hamdan MH, Joglar JA, Page RL, et al. Baroreflex gain predicts blood pressure recovery during simulated ventricular tachycardia in humans. *Circulation* 1999; 100:381-386.

14. Leitch JW, Klein GJ, Yee R, et al. Syncope associated with supraventricular tachycardia: An expression of tachycardia rate or vasomotor response? *Circulation* 1992; 85:1064-1071.

15. Peuhkurinen KJ, Huikuri HV, Linnaluoto M, et al. Changes in myocardial metabolism and transcardiac electrolytes during simulated ventricular tachycardia: Effects of beta-adrenergic blockade. *Am Heart J* 1994; 128:96-105.

16. Shinbane JS, Wood MA, Jensen DN, et al. Tachycardia-induced cardiomyopathy: A review of animal models and clinical studies. *J Am Coll Cardiol* 1997; 29:709-715.

17. Chen SA, Chiang CE, Yang CJ, et al. Sustained atrial tachycardia in adult patients: Electrophysiological characteristics, pharmacological response, possible mechanisms, and effects of radiofrequency ablation. *Circulation* 1994; 90:1262-1268.

18. Mehta D, Wafa S, Ward DE, et al. Relative efficacy of various physical manoeuvres in the termination of junctional tachycardia. *Lancet* 1988; 1:1181-1185.

19. Pinski SL, Maloney JD. Adenosine: A new drug for acute termination of supraventricular tachycardia. *Clev Clin J Med* 1990; 57:383-388.

20. Melio FR, Mallon WK, Newton E. Successful conversion of unstable supraventricular tachycardia to sinus rhythm with adenosine. *Ann Emerg Med* 1993; 22:709-713.

21. McIntosh-Yellin NL, Drew BJ, Scheinman MM. Safety and efficacy of central intravenous bolus administration of adenosine for termination of supraventricular tachycardia. *J Am Coll Cardiol* 1993; 22:741-745.

22. Strickberger SA, Man KC, Daoud EG, et al. Adenosine-induced atrial arrhythmia: A prospective analysis. *Ann Intern Med* 1997; 127:417-22. (Erratum in: *Ann Intern Med* 1998 Mar 15; 128:511).

23. Deal BJ. Esophageal pacing. In: Ellenbogen KA, Kay GN, Wilkoff BW, eds. Clinical Cardiac Pacing. Philadelphia, W.B. Saunders: 1995, pp. 701-705.

24. Cybulski J, Kulakowski P, Makowska E, et al. Intravenous amiodarone is safe and seems to be effective in termination of paroxysmal supraventricular tachyarrhythmias. *Clin Cardiol* 1996; 19:563-566.

25. Lok LS, Lau CP. Presentation and management of patients admitted with atrial fibrillation: A review of 291 cases in a regional hospital. *Int J Cardiol* 1995; 48:271-278.

26. Robinson K, Frenneaux MP, Stockinns B, et al. Atrial fibrillation in hypertrophic cardiomyopathy: A longitudinal study. *J Am Coll Cardiol* 1990; 15:1279-1285.

27. Pinski SL, Helguera ME. Antiarrhythmic drug initiation in patients with atrial fibrillation. *Prog Cardiovasc Dis* 1999; 42:75-90.

28. Waldo AL, Henthorn RW, Plumb VJ. Temporary epicardial wire electrodes in the diagnosis and treatment of arrhythmias after open heart surgery. *Am J Surg* 1984; 148:275-283.

29. Peters RW, Shorofsky SR, Pelini M, et al. Overdrive atrial pacing for conversion of atrial flutter: Comparison of postoperative with nonpostoperative patients. *Am Heart J* 1999; 137:100-103.

30. Van Gelder IC, Tuinenburg AE, Schoonderwoerd BS, et al. Pharmacologic versus direct-current electrical cardioversion of atrial flutter and fibrillation. *Am J Cardiol* 1999; 84(9A):147R-151R.

31. Trohman RG, Parrillo JE. Direct current cardioversion: Indications, techniques and recent advances. *Crit Care Med* 2000; 28(Suppl):N170-173.

32. Norgaard BL, Wachtell K, Christensen PD, et al. Efficacy and safety of intravenously administered dofetilide in acute termination of atrial fibrillation and flutter: A multicenter, randomized, double-blind, placebo-controlled trial. *Am Heart J* 1999; 137:1062-1069.

33. Zaqqa M, Afshar H, Rasekh A, et al. Predictors of conversion to sinus rhythm using ibutilide for atrial fibrillation or flutter. *Am J Cardiol* 2000; 85:112-114.

34. Oral H, Souza JJ, Michaud GF, et al. Facilitating transthoracic cardioversion of atrial fibrillation with ibutilide pretreatment. *N Engl J Med* 1999; 340:1849-1854.

35. Varriale P, Sedighi A. Acute management of atrial fibrillation and atrial flutter in the critical care unit: Should it be ibutilide? *Clin Cardiol* 2000; 23:265-268.

36. Barbier GH, Shettigar UR, Appunn DO. Clinical rationale for the use of an ultra-short acting beta-blocker: Esmolol. *Int J Clin Pharmacol Ther* 1995; 33:212-218.

37. Balser JR, Martinez EA, Winters BD, et al. Beta-adrenergic blockade accelerates conversion of postoperative supraventricular tachyarrhythmias. *Anesthesiology* 1998; 89:1052-1059.

38. Mooss AN, Wurdeman RL, Mohiuddin SM, et al. Esmolol versus diltiazem in the treatment of postoperative atrial fibrillation/atrial flutter after open heart surgery. *Am Heart J* 2000; 140:176-180.

39. Moran JL, Gallagher J, Peake SL, et al. Parenteral magnesium sulfate versus amiodarone in the therapy of atrial tachyarrhythmias: A prospective, randomized study. *Crit Care Med* 1995; 23:1816-1824.

40. Hays JV, Gilman JK, Rubal BJ. Effect of magnesium sulfate on ventricular rate control in atrial fibrillation. *Ann Emerg Med* 1994; 24:61-64.

41. Clemo HF, Wood MA, Gilligan DM, et al. Intravenous amiodarone for acute heart rate control in the critically ill patient with atrial tachyarrhythmias. *Am J Cardiol* 1998; 81:594-598.

42. Shettigar UR. Management of rapid ventricular rate in acute atrial fibrillation. *Int J Clin Pharmacol Ther* 1994; 32:240-245.

43. Leitch JW, Klein GJ, Yee R, et al. Differential effect of intravenous procainamide on anterograde and retrograde accessory pathway refractoriness. *J Am Coll Cardiol* 1992; 19:118-124.

44. Varriale P, Sedighi A, Mirzaietehrane M. Ibutilide for termination of atrial fibrillation in the Wolff-Parkinson-White syndrome. *Pacing Clin Electrophysiol* 1999; 22:1267-1269.

45. Murray KT. Ibutilide. *Circulation* 1998; 97:493-497.

46. Stewart RB, Bardy GH, Greene HL. Wide complex tachycardia: Misdiagnosis and outcome after emergent therapy. *Ann Intern Med* 1986; 104:766-771.

47. Rankin AC, Rae AP, Cobbe SM. Misuse of intravenous verapamil in patients with ventricular tachycardia. *Lancet* 1987; 2:472-474.

48. Steinman RT, Herrera C, Schuger CD, et al. Wide QRS tachycardia in the conscious adult. Ventricular tachycardia is the most frequent cause. *JAMA* 1989; 261:1013-1016.

49. Akhtar M, Shenasa M, Jazayeri M, et al. Wide QRS complex tachycardia: Reappraisal of a common clinical problem. *Ann Intern Med* 1988; 109:905-912.

50. Brugada P, Brugada J, Mont L, et al. A new approach to the differential diagnosis of a regular tachycardia with a wide QRS complex. *Circulation* 1991; 83:1649-1659.

51. Littman L, McCall MM. Ventricular tachycardia can masquerade as supraventricular tachycardia in patients with preexistent bundle branch block. *Ann Emerg Med* 1995; 26:98-101.

52. Alberca T, Almendral J, Sanz P, et al. Evaluation of the specificity of morphological electrocardiographic criteria for the differential diagnosis of wide QRS complex tachycardia in patients with intraventricular conduction defects. *Circulation* 1997; 96:3527-3533.

53. Shaw M, Niemann JT, Haskell RJ, et al. Esophageal electrocardiography in acute cardiac care: Efficacy and diagnostic value of a new technique. *Am J Med* 1987; 82:689-696.

54. Domanovits H, Paulis M, Nikfardjam M, et al. Sustained ventricular tachycardia in the emergency department. *Resuscitation* 1999; 42:19-25.

55. Armengol RE, Graff J, Baerman JM, et al. Lack of effectiveness of lidocaine for sustained, wide QRS complex tachycardia. *Ann Emerg Med* 1989; 18:254-257.

56. Nasir N, Jr., Taylor A, Doyle TK, et al. Evaluation of intravenous lidocaine for the termination of sustained monomorphic ventricular tachycardia in patients with coronary artery disease with or without healed myocardial infarction. *Am J Cardiol* 1994; 74:1183-1186.

57. Gorgels AP, van den Dool A, Hofs A, et al. Comparison of procainamide and lidocaine in terminating sustained monomorphic ventricular tachycardia. *Am J Cardiol* 1996; 78:43-46.

58. Ho DS, Zecchin RP, Richards DA, et al. Double-blind trial of lignocaine versus sotalol for acute termination of spontaneous sustained ventricular tachycardia. *Lancet* 1994; 344:18-23.

59. Farouque HM, Sanders P, Young GD. Intravenous magnesium sulfate for acute termination of sustained monomorphic ventricular tachycardia associated with coronary artery disease. *Am J Cardiol* 2000; 86:1270-1272.

60. Kowey PR, Marinchak RA, Rials SJ, et al. Intravenous amiodarone. *J Am Coll Cardiol* 1997; 29:1190-1198.

61. International Consensus on Science. Guidelines 2000 for cardiopulmonary resuscitation and emergency cardiovascular care. Pharmacology I: Agents for arrhythmias. *Circulation* 2000; 102(Suppl I):I-112-128.

62. Brown TCK. Tricyclic antidepressant overdosage: Experimental studies on the management of circulatory complications. *Clin Toxicol* 1976; 9:255-272.

63. International Consensus in Science. Guidelines 2000 for cardiopulmonary resuscitation and emergency cardiovascular care. Toxicology in ECC. *Circulation* 2000; 102(Suppl I); I-223-228.

64. Dorian P. An overview of the management of electrical storm. *Can J Cardiol* 1997; 13(Suppl A):13A-17A.

65. Viskin S. Long QT syndromes and torsade de pointes. *Lancet* 1999; 354:1625-1633.

66. Pinski SL. Emergencies related to implantable cardioverter-defibrillators. *Crit Care Med* 2000; 28 (Suppl.):N175-N180.

67. Cotter G, Blatt A, Kaluski E, et al. Conversion of recent onset paroxysmal atrial fibrillation to normal sinus rhythm: The effect of no treatment and high-dose amiodarone: A randomized, placebo-controlled study. *Eur Heart J* 1999; 20:1833-1842.

68. Hurst TM, Hinrichs M, Braidenbach C, et al. Detection of myocardial injury during transvenous implantation of automatic cardioverter-defibrillators. *J Am Coll Cardiol* 1999; 34:402-408.

69. Joglar JA, Kessler DJ, Welch PJ, et al. Effects of repeated electrical defibrillations on cardiac troponin I levels. *Am J Cardiol* 1999; 83:270-272.

70. Tokano T, Bach D, Chang J, et al. Effect of ventricular shock strength on cardiac hemodynamics. *J Cardiovasc Electrophysiol* 1998; 9:791-797.

71. Runsio M, Bergfeldt L, Brodin LA, et al. Left ventricular function after repeated episodes of ventricular fibrillation and defibrillation assessed by transoesophageal echocardiography. *Eur Heart J* 1997; 18:124-131.

72. Patton JN, Allen JD, Pantridge JF. The effects of shock energy, propranolol, and verapamil on cardiac damage caused by transthoracic countershock. *Circulation* 1984; 69:357-368.

73. Tang W, Weil MH, Sun S, et al. The effects of biphasic and conventional monophasic defibrillation on postresuscitation myocardial function. *J Am Coll Cardiol* 1999; 34:815-822.

74. Oldroyd KG, Rankin AC, Rae AP, et al. Pacing termination of spontaneous ventricular tachycardia in the coronary care unit. *Int J Cardiol* 1992; 36:223-226.

75. Stoddard MF, Labovitz AJ, Stevens LL, et al. Effects of electrophysiologic studies resulting in electrical countershock or burst pacing on left ventricular systolic and diastolic function. *Am Heart J* 1988; 116:364-370.

76. Maloney JD, Vanerio G, Pinski SL, et al. Chronic pacing for the management of tachyarrhythmias: Basic and clinical aspects. In: Mandel WJ (ed). Cardiac Arrhythmias: Their Mechanisms, Diagnosis, and Management, 3rd edition. Philadelphia: J. B. Lippincott, 1995: 1095-1116.

77. Ahern TS, Nydegger C, Greenspon AJ, et al. Programmable external automatic antitachycardia pacing as a bridge to definitive therapy in patients with recurrent sustained ventricular tachycardia. Pacing Clin Electrophysiol 1992; 15:1258-1265.

78. Hamer AW, Zaher CA, Rubin SA, et al. Hemodynamic benefits of synchronized 1:1 atrial pacing during sustained ventricular tachycardia with severely depressed ventricular function in coronary heart disease. Am J Cardiol 1985; 55:990-994.

79. Fotopoulos GD, Mason MJ, Walker S, et al. Stabilisation of medically refractory ventricular arrhythmia by intra-aortic balloon counterpulsation. Heart 1999; 82:96-100.

80. Cao K, Gonska BD. Catheter ablation of incessant ventricular tachycardia: Acute and long-term results. Eur Heart J 1996; 17:756-763.

81. Mehdirad AA, Keim S, Rist K, et al. Long-term clinical outcome of right bundle branch radiofrequency catheter ablation for treatment of bundle branch reentrant ventricular tachycardia. Pacing Clin Electrophysiol 1995; 18:2135-2143.

82. Hobson CE, DiMarco JP, Haines DE, et al. The influence of preoperative shock on outcome in sequential endocardial resection for ventricular tachycardia. J Thorac Cardiovasc Surg 1991; 102:348-353.

83. Okishige K, Andrews TC, Friedman PL Suppression of incessant polymorphic ventricular tachycardia by selective intracoronary ethanol infusion. Pacing Clin Electrophysiol 1991; 14:188-195.

84. Kullick DM, Bolman RM 3rd, Salerno CT, et al. Management of recurrent ventricular tachycardia with ventricular assist device placement. Ann Thorac Surg 1998; 66:571-573.

85. Gammage MD. Temporary cardiac pacing. Heart 2000; 83:715-720.

86. Pinski SL. Temporary cardiac pacing. In: Parrillo JE, Dellinger RP, eds. Critical Care Medicine: Principles of Diagnosis and Management. Mosby-Yearbook, 2001 pp. 64-81.

87. Wong CK, White HD, Wilcox RG, et al. New atrial fibrillation after acute myocardial infarction independently predicts death: the GUSTO-III experience. Am Heart J 2000; 140:878-885.

88. Rathore SS, Berger AK, Weinfurt KP, et al. Acute myocardial infarction complicated by atrial fibrillation in the elderly: Prevalence and outcomes. Circulation 2000; 101:969-974.

89. Nielsen FE, Andersen HH, Gram-Hansen P, et al. The relationship between ECG signs of atrial infarction and the development of supraventricular arrhythmias in patients with acute myocardial infarction. Am Heart J 1992; 123:69-72.

90. Hod H, Lew AS, Keltai M, et al. Early atrial fibrillation during evolving myocardial infarction: A consequence of impaired left atrial perfusion. Circulation 1987; 75:146-150.

91. Kyriakidis M, Barbetseas J, Antonopoulos A, et al. Early atrial arrhythmias in acute myocardial infarction. Role of the sinus node artery. Chest 1992; 101:944-947.

92. Serrano CV Jr, Ramires JA, Mansur AP, et al. Importance of the time of onset of supraventricular tachyarrhythmias on prognosis of patients with acute myocardial infarction. *Clin Cardiol* 1995; 18:84-90.

93. Sugiura T, Iwasaka T, Takahashi N, et al. Atrial fibrillation in inferior wall Q-wave acute myocardial infarction. *Am J Cardiol* 1991; 67:1135-1136.

94. Sugiura T, Iwasaka T, Ogawa A, et al. Atrial fibrillation in acute myocardial infarction. *Am J Cardiol* 1985; 56:27-29.

95. Widimsky P, Gregor P. Recent atrial fibrillation in acute myocardial infarction: A sign of pericarditis. *Cor Vasa* 1993; 35:230-232.

96. Nagahama Y, Sugiura T, Takehana K, et al. The role of infarction-associated pericarditis on the occurrence of atrial fibrillation. *Eur Heart J* 1998; 19:287-292.

97. Sugiura T, Iwasaka T, Takahashi N, et al. Factors associated with atrial fibrillation in Q wave anterior myocardial infarction. *Am Heart J* 1991; 121:1409-1412.

98. Crenshaw BS, Ward SR, Granger CB, et al. Atrial fibrillation in the setting of acute myocardial infarction: The GUSTO-I experience. Global Utilization of Streptokinase and TPA for Occluded Coronary Arteries. *J Am Coll Cardiol* 1997; 30:406-413.

99. Cowan JC, Gardiner P, Reid DS, et al. A comparison of amiodarone and digoxin in the treatment of atrial fibrillation complicating suspected acute myocardial infarction. *J Cardiovasc Pharmacol* 1986; 8:252-256.

100. Mahaffey KW, Granger CB, Sloan MA, et al. Risk factors for in-hospital nonhemorrhagic stroke in patients with acute myocardial infarction treated with thrombolysis: Results from GUSTO-I. *Circulation* 1998; 97:757-764.

101. Behar S, Zahavi Z, Goldbourt U, et al. Long-term prognosis of patients with paroxysmal atrial fibrillation complicating acute myocardial infarction: SPRINT Study Group. *Eur Heart J* 1992; 13:45-50.

102. Feigl D, Ashkenazy J, Kishon Y. Early and late atrioventricular block in acute myocardial infarction. *J Am Coll Cardiol* 1984; 4:35-38.

103. Clemmensen P, Bates ER, Califf RM, et al. Complete atrioventricular block complication inferior wall acute myocardial infarction treated with reperfusion therapy. *Am J Cardiol* 1991; 67:225-230.

104. Swart G, Brady WJ, Jr., DeBehnke DJ, et al. Acute myocardial infarction complicated by hemodynamically unstable bradyarrhythmia: Prehospital and ED treatment. *Am J Emerg Med* 1999; 17:647-652.

105. Kennel AJ, Titus JL. The vasculature of the human atrioventricular conduction system. *Mayo Clin Proc* 1972; 47:562-566.

106. Goodfellow J, Walker PR. Reversal of atropine-resistant atrioventricular block with intravenous aminophylline in the early phase of inferior wall acute myocardial infarction following treatment with streptokinase. *Eur Heart J* 1995; 16:862-865.

107. Zehender M, Kasper W, Kauder E, et al. Right ventricular infarction as an independent predictor of prognosis after acute inferior myocardial infarction. *N Engl J Med* 1993; 328:981-988.

108. Matangi MF. Temporary physiologic pacing in inferior wall acute myocardial infarction with right ventricular damage. *Am J Cardiol* 1987; 59:1207-1208.

109. Vrouchos GT, Kiulpalis A, Trullakis GA, et al. High-rate cardiac pacing increases blood pressure and decreases right atrial pressure in patients with hemodynamic significant acute right ventricular myocardial infarction and bradyarrhythmia. *Clin Cardiol* 1997; 20:41-46.

110. Wilber D, Walton J, O'Neill W, et al. Effects of reperfusion on complete heart block complicating anterior myocardial infarction. *J Am Coll Cardiol* 1984; 4:1315-1321.

111. Sgarbossa EB, Pinski SL, Gates KB, et al. Predictors of in-hospital bundle branch block reversion after presenting with acute myocardial infarction and bundle branch block. *Am J Cardiol* 1998; 82:373-374

112. Sgarbossa EB, Pinski SL, Topol EJ, et al. Acute myocardial infarction and complete bundle branch block at hospital admission: Clinical characteristics and outcome in the thrombolytic era. *J Am Coll Cardiol* 1998; 31:105-110.

113. Hindman MC, Wagner GS, JaRo M, et al. The clinical significance of bundle branch block complicating acute myocardial infarction. 2. Indications for temporary and permanent pacemaker insertion. *Circulation* 1978; 58:689.

114. Lamas GA, Muller JE, Turi ZG, et al. A simplified method to predict occurrence of complete heart block during acute myocardial infarction. *Am J Cardiol* 1986; 57:1213-1219.

115. Ryan TJ, Antman EM, Brooks NH, et al. ACC/AHA guidelines for the management of patients with acute myocardial infarction: 1999 update: A report of the American College of Cardiology/American Heart Association Task Force on Practice Guidelines (Committee on Management of Acute Myocardial Infarction). *J Am Coll Cardiol* 1999; 34:890-911.

116. Sprung CL, Elser B, Schein RM, et al. Risk of right bundle-branch block and complete heart block during pulmonary artery catheterization. *Crit Care Med* 1989; 17:1-3.

117. Gregoratos G, Cheitlin MD, Conill A, et al. ACC/AHA guidelines for implantation of cardiac pacemakers and antiarrhythmia devices: A report of the American College of Cardiology/American Heart Association Task Force on Practice Guidelines (Committee on Pacemaker Implantation). *J Am Coll Cardiol* 1998; 31:1175-1209.

118. MacMahon S, Collins R, Peto R, et al. Effects of prophylactic lidocaine in suspected acute myocardial infarction. An overview of results from the randomized, controlled trials. *JAMA* 1988; 260:1910-1916.

119. Sadowski ZP, Alexander JH, Skrabucha B, et al. Multicenter randomized trial and a systematic overview of lidocaine in acute myocardial infarction. *Am Heart J* 1999; 137:792-798.

120. Alexander JH, Granger CB, Sadowski Z, et al Prophylactic lidocaine use in acute myocardial infarction: Incidence and outcomes from two international trials. *Am Heart J* 1999; 137:799-805.

121. Elizari MV, Martinez JM, Belziti C, et al. Morbidity and mortality following early administration of amiodarone in acute myocardial infarction. *Eur Heart J* 2000; 21:198-205.

122. Ryden L, Ariniego R, Arnman K, et al. A double-blind trial of metoprolol in acute myocardial infarction. Effects on ventricular tachyarrhythmias. *N Engl J Med* 1983; 308:614-618.

123. Mont L, Cinca J, Blanch P, et al. Predisposing factors and prognostic value of sustained monomorphic ventricular tachycardia in the early phase of acute myocardial infarction. *J Am Coll Cardiol* 1996; 28:1670-1676.

124. Newby KH, Thompson T, Stebbins A, et al. Sustained ventricular arrhythmias in patients receiving thrombolytic therapy: Incidence and outcomes. *Circulation* 1998; 98:2567-2573.

125. Emori T, Ohe T, Haze K, et al. Clinical and electrophysiological characteristics of sustained ventricular tachycardia occurring 3 to 21 days after acute myocardial infarction. *Jpn Circ J* 1995; 59:257-263.

126. Behar S, Goldbourt U, Reicher-Reiss H, et al. Prognosis of acute myocardial infarction complicated by primary ventricular fibrillation. *Am J Cardiol* 1990; 66:1208-1211.

127. Volpi A, Cavalli A, Santoro L, et al. Incidence and prognosis of early primary ventricular fibrillation in acute myocardial infarction--results of the Gruppo Italiano per lo Studio della Sopravvivenza nell'Infarto Miocardico (GISSI-2) database. *Am J Cardiol* 1998; 82:265-271.

128. Volpi A, Cavalli A, Santoro E, et al. Incidence and prognosis of secondary ventricular fibrillation in acute myocardial infarction. Evidence for a protective effect of thrombolytic therapy. *Circulation* 1990; 82:1279-1288.

129. Wolfe CL, Nibley C, Bhandari A, et al. Polymorphous ventricular tachycardia associated with acute myocardial infarction. *Circulation* 1991; 84:1543-1551.

130. Nademanee K, Taylor R, Bailey WE, et al. Treating electrical storm:Sympathetic blockade versus advanced cardiac life support-guided therapy. *Circulation* 2000(15); 102:742-747.

Chapter 13

Mechanical Circulatory Assist Devices

Joseph G. Salloum, MD and
Richard W. Smalling, MD, PhD

Introduction and General Principles

Cardiogenic shock is a life-threatening clinical situation. Mechanical circulatory assistance is a very important therapeutic approach once the arsenal of pharmacologic therapy is exhausted.

Conceptually, mechanical circulatory assistance revolves around two main objectives: maintenance of organ perfusion at a level compatible with end-organ salvage, and protection of injured myocardium to an extent that permits recovery. The importance of maintenance of adequate blood flow is self-evident. Assist devices use pneumatic or electrical energy to propel blood at a flow rate and pressure that ensure adequate blood supply to vital organs. The successful operation of an assist device is manifested by an improvement in organ system function.

Recovery of myocardial function is achieved mainly through unloading. This concept is especially relevant in the context of cardiogenic shock resulting from massive acute myocardial infarction (MI). Nevertheless, a small population of chronic, end-stage heart failure patients have recovered myocardial function after extended mechanical support and chronic unloading.

Unloading refers to diminishing myocardial wall stress through a reduction in systolic and diastolic pressures and volumes. Because elevated wall stress increases cardiac oxygen requirements and contributes to the reduction of oxygen supply, injury to myocardial cells, especially

From: Hollenberg SM, Bates ER. *Cardiogenic Shock.* Armonk, NY: Futura Publishing Co., Inc.; ©2002.

in the subendocardial region, is perpetuated and myocardial recovery is nearly impossible. In addition to myocardial damage, elevated cardiac pressures produce elevated pressures in the pulmonary circulation, leading to direct lung injury and impaired gas exchange.

In the setting of acute MI, mechanical unloading prior to reperfusion in the experimental setting has been shown to reduce infarct size, especially when coupled with full reperfusion of the jeopardized myocardium.[1,2] This, however, is not a unanimous finding,[3] although it does seem to be the consensus. The long-term effects of early unloading on the ventricle in terms of remodeling are unclear at this time.

The vast majority of mechanical assist devices are capable of unloading the ventricle. Naturally, the extent of this unloading varies. A notable exception is percutaneous arterio-venous cardiopulmonary bypass. Unlike open bypass, percutaneous bypass has even been associated with elevated intra-cardiac pressures. The details of this hemodynamic profile will be discussed below.

The assist devices currently available can be viewed in two main categories. One includes devices that can be applied without the need for complicated surgery. They can be inserted percutaneously, in the cardiac catheterization laboratory or even at the bedside. Their advantages are evident. They are especially, although not exclusively, helpful in the cardiogenic shock patient who presents abruptly, as in cases of massive acute MI. The anticipated duration of support, during which recovery of function is expected, is usually no more than a few days. Otherwise, another support device or cardiac transplantation is contemplated. The downside of these devices is the relatively limited degree of circulatory support they provide, and their limitation to patient mobility.

The second group comprises those devices that are implanted by means of complicated thoracic surgery. The characteristics of patients in need of such support contribute further to the high-risk character of this surgery. They are usually chronic heart failure patients who have progressed in their clinical course to a point where mechanical support is imperative. These devices assume complete responsibility for circulatory support and permit greater patient mobility. The expected duration of support is in terms of months or even years. They are, however, costly and complex, and function at the risk of a range of complications that can potentially yield disastrous consequences. Furthermore, they are viewed as a bridge to the final form of therapy, cardiac transplantation. Some devices that we have included with this second group are designed for hemodynamic support of no more than 1 to 2 weeks. These, however, share with this group the need for surgical implantation and the complete support of systemic circulation.

A complete discussion of all available assist devices is beyond the scope of this chapter. The general principles covered are probably of much greater benefit than an exhaustive enumeration of all available and experimental assist devices. These principles would probably allow the reader to approach any mechanical support device one may encounter in clinical practice with a more comprehensive insight and a better grasp of the subject matter.

The Intra-aortic Balloon Pump (IABP)

With nearly 100,000 IABP catheters inserted in 1993 in the United States alone, intra-aortic balloon counterpulsation is by far the most commonly used mechanical assist device. The first successful clinical application of balloon counterpulsation was reported by Kantrowitz et al in 1968.[4] Percutaneous insertion of IABP was described by Bregman and Casarella in 1980.[5] The IABP has proven itself beneficial in multiple clinical settings including cardiogenic shock, myocardial ischemia or infarction, high-risk percutaneous revascularization, perioperatively in high-risk cardiac surgery patients, and in heart transplantation. The use of IABP in cardiogenic shock is reviewed in Chapter 5.

The IABP has been useful in high-risk patients undergoing cardiac surgery. These include patients undergoing emergency cardiac operations in the setting of mechanical complications of acute MI,[6] patients with low cardiac output preoperatively,[7] and patients undergoing redo operations with poor systolic function or with left main stenosis.[8] The IABP has been found useful both in the stabilization of the hemodynamic status of these patients before surgery and in improving their chances of survival during and after surgery. Insertion of the IABP a few hours before a planned high-risk cardiac operation decreases the incidence of postoperative low output syndrome.

The IABP has also been found to be of benefit in those patients awaiting heart transplantation. The discrepancy between the growing number of candidates for heart transplantation and the limited availability of donor organs translates into a longer waiting period. Some patients inevitably reach a point where they cannot maintain central perfusion without mechanical assistance. As early as 1986, the IABP had been found a suitable assist device for these patients. Its risk-benefit profile has clearly favored its use as a "bridge" from the time the hemodynamic status of transplant candidates deteriorates to the point where the donor organ takes over, for as long as 37 days.[9] Other assist devices have evolved for this specific role. The IABP, however, still maintains obvious advantages in that it can be inserted at the bedside, it has a relatively simple mechanical design, and the potential risk of life threatening complications is low.

With the advent of circulatory assist devices that are capable of ensuring organ perfusion without the contribution of the left ventricle, it is necessary to recognize those patients for whom IABP therapy alone is not sufficient. These patients require IABP but are found to remain in a precarious hemodynamic condition despite aortic counterpulsation. Normal and coworkers[10] compiled the experience of several tertiary care institutions and were able to draw a profile for post-cardiotomy low-output patients who uniformly survived with IABP alone, those who were much more likely to survive with counterpulsation alone, and those who invariably perished despite IABP therapy. The first group consists of patients who maintain a cardiac index better than 2.1 L/min/m^2 on IABP, together with a systemic vascular resistance less than 2,100 dynes·sec·cm^{-5}. This group of patients is expected to survive their shock situation with the assistance of the balloon pump. The next group of patients showed a survival of 80% on the IABP. It consists of patients with cardiac index less than 2.1 L/min/m^2 but greater than 1.2 L/min/m^2, with a systemic resistance less than 2,100 dynes·sec·cm^{-5}. The third group of patients invariably dies as a direct consequence of hemodynamic shock, despite the assistance of the IABP. These patients have a cardiac index less than 2.1 L/min/m^2 and a systemic vascular resistance greater than 2,100 dynes·sec·cm^{-5} or a cardiac index less than 1.2 L/min/m^2, regardless of systemic resistance. These data illustrate the limitations of IABP therapy. Accordingly, patients with unfavorable hemodynamics on the IABP would be recognized and offered alternative means of circulatory assistance before they reach dire consequences. These data should be used to prevent the situation whereby such patients are not offered assist devices initially, on the account that IABP is expected to reverse their shock, and then, when it is too late to change the clinical course, assist devices are used as a desperate measure.

Percutaneous Cardiopulmonary Bypass

History and Description

Cardiopulmonary bypass is historically the first circulatory assist device. Its use was proposed by John Gibbon as early as 1937[11] and its first successful experimental utilization reported two years later by Gibbon himself.[12] The first human application occurred at the hand of the same surgeon on May 15, 1953 when it was used in the closure of an atrial septal defect.

A percutaneous cardiopulmonary bypass (PCB) system became available for clinical use in 1986.[13] In essence, PCB consists of inflow and outflow cannulae, a blood pump, a heat exchanger, an oxygenator, and connecting tubing. The venous (inflow) cannula is inserted via the femoral vein over a dilator with the tip reaching the right atrium, and the arterial (outflow) cannula is inserted via the femoral artery. The blood pump provides positive pressure for non-pulsatile arterial flow as well as negative pressure for venous inflow. A flow probe follows in series with the pump for monitoring purposes, in addition to a heat exchanger and an oxygenator.[14]

Insertion of the PCB begins with accessing the femoral vein and subsequent placement of right-sided monitoring catheters before the insertion of the venous cannula. The common femoral artery is accessed next and an iliac and femoral angiogram is performed (usually using a pigtail catheter) using about 20 mL of contrast. This is done to ascertain patency of the vessels, identify the common femoral rather than the profunda or superficial femoral artery, and to assess for tortuosity, which may affect cannula insertion and flow rates. The artery and vein are then sequentially dilated and the respective cannula inserted over a guidewire, followed by the intravenous administration of 5,000 U heparin. Care must be taken to avoid air embolization during manipulation of the cannulae and the different dilators. The arterial and venous cannulae are then connected to the appropriate tubing and the system primed with saline to eliminate any air. Heparin is then re-administered at a dose of 300 U/ kg body weight for full anticoagulation, with an activated clotting time maintained at levels greater than 400 seconds, and bypass is initiated. The relatively small cannulae used by PCB allow flows between 3 and 4 L/min, which should offer adequate organ perfusion in most patients (Figure 1).[13]

PCB insertion and function is not achieved without the risk of complications. Local complications are related to the site of vascular access: vascular perforation, femoral nerve injury, bleeding, atrio-ventricular (AV) fistula formation, and arterial or venous thrombosis. Systemic complications include air embolism, infection, acute renal failure, gastrointestinal ischemia and bleeding, in addition to transient cerebral ischemia. Prolonged PCB support using the relatively smaller cannulae has a notable deleterious effect on red blood cells. In fact, significant hemolysis limits the use of PCB beyond 6 hours.

A more important systemic complication to CPB is known as "whole body inflammatory response" or "post perfusion syndrome."[15] It is believed that neutrophils are activated upon exposure to the bypass circuit, resulting in the release of proteases, the formation of free radicals, and the secretion of inflammatory cytokines, resulting in the development of a state of systemic inflammatory reaction, including complement activation. The ensuing consequences are manifest mainly at the level of the microcir-

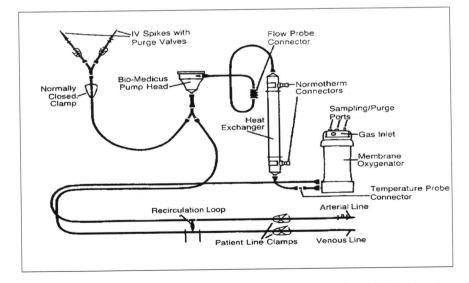

Figure 1. Diagram illustrating the components of percutaneous cardiopulmonary bypass. The IV spikes connect to normal saline for priming the circuit. When the pump is inserted but not operating, the patient lines are clamped and the recirculation loop "short-circuits" the connections in order to prevent stasis in the different components. (Reproduced with permission.[14])

culation, triggering an insufficiency in organ function. The lung appears to be most vulnerable to this chain of events, resulting in prolonged ventilator dependence and elevated pulmonary vascular resistance.[16]

Hemodynamic Principles

It is most important to keep in mind that PCB bypass is unable to unload the left ventricle. PCB does not drain the left ventricle directly (like the Hemopump [Medtronic, Inc. Minneapolis, MN] does, for instance), nor does it allow the ventricle to empty itself more easily (like the IABP does). With complete circulatory support, the aortic valve does not open at all. The ventricular pressure and volume can even increase, since blood cannot evacuate the left ventricle. If the aortic valve does open, it would do so against an *increased* afterload caused by the relatively high pressure in the arterial tree resulting from its filling from the femoral artery cannula.[17,18]

Some investigators, however, have indicated that PCB can effectively unload the left ventricle if pulsatile flow is used in synchronous pulsation.[19] An ingenious way to unload the ventricle is by inducing pulmonary valve regurgitation using a special catheter. In the presence of concomitant mitral regurgitation, quite common in those patients in cardiogenic shock, the left ventricle would be adequately vented in a retrograde fashion. Not only the left ventricle, but also the pulmonary circulation would have lower pressures. Both myocardium and lung tissue would thus be protected.[20] Although still at an experimental stage, this clever way of venting the left ventricle during PCB may find clinical application in the future.

On the other hand, PCB is capable of offering complete circulatory support and adequate blood oxygenation. The driving pump of PCB is usually a centrifugal pump, the hemodynamic characteristics of which are discussed in detail in the appropriate section below.

Indications and Clinical Experience with PCB

The adaptation of cardiopulmonary bypass into a system that allows full percutaneous insertion permits the catheterization laboratory to benefit from its many advantages (Table 1). PCB can support the circulation to allow patient survival until a more definitive form of therapy, be it surgery or permanent ventricular assist device (VAD), is implemented. It may be viewed as a safety net should angioplasty fail or should any other catastrophe happen during the course of a procedure. It is also very helpful to those patients whose presentation is profound circulatory decompensation. The systemic effects of bypass membranes and cannulae are reviewed briefly in the section on long-term assist devices entitled Operative and Perioperative Considerations, below.

Many series describing experience with the PCB have been published. In one such series, PCB was used for coronary angioplasty in a group of

Table 1.

Main Indications for Percutaneous Coronary Bypass.[14,21]

- Cardiogenic shock (with or without anatomically correctable causes like postinfarction ventricular septal defect)
- High-risk angioplasty/valvuloplasty
- Failed angioplasty with hemodynamic compromise
- Temporary ventricular assist or bridging to other ventricular assist systems
- Trauma with hemodynamic collapse
- Minimally invasive cardiac surgery
- Organ donor preservation

11 high-risk patients. Nine of these patients survived for 1 year after the procedure.[22] Another series[23] summarized data with 187 patients from 17 institutions. PCB was instituted for multiple indications: 67% for cardiac arrest, 24% for cardiogenic shock, 5% for pulmonary insufficiency, and other causes. Of the total number of patients, 34% needed other modes of circulatory assist, while weaning from bypass was successful in 31% of cases. The overall survival at 30 days was 21%.

As the scope of percutaneous interventions in the catheterization laboratory widens, so should familiarity with ventricular support systems. As more and more daring interventions are envisaged in high-risk patient populations, PCB clearly offers an edge to the interventional cardiologist for partial or total hemodynamic support both during the procedure itself, or as a bailout should a crisis occur.

The Hemopump

History and Description

The Hemopump (HP [Medtronic Inc., Minneapolis, MN]) is a rotary left ventricular (LV) assist device. It was conceived by Dr. Richard Wampler in 1975 and the design accomplished in 1982. In 1988, the study of the HP in human subjects was approved in the setting of an Investigational Device exemption by the Food and Drug Administration. Three HP devices were evaluated: HP31, HP21, and HP14, differing in insertion site and cannula size.

The HP cannula was inserted in the cavity of the left ventricle with the outflow port crossing the aortic valve. At the distal tip of the cannula, a disposable rotor was attached to a drive cable and inserted in a nondisposable stator. Power was generated by a paracorporeal electromagnetic motor and was transmitted to the rotor via the drive cable. Dextran solution was infused into a plastic sheath surrounding the drive cable as a lubricant.[24,25] A bedside console contained the lubricant roller pump, the motor control electronics, alarm systems, and rechargeable batteries for back-up power. It provided seven levels of support, (27,600 rpm to

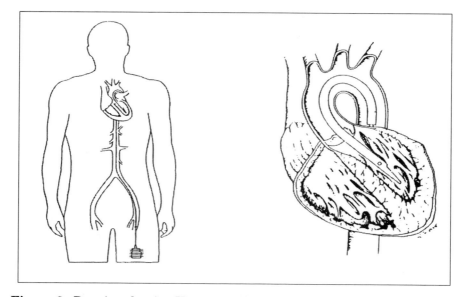

Figure 2. Drawing showing Hemopump placement via the femoral artery. The outflow of the pump cannula is located in the proximal descending aorta. (Reproduced with permission.[29])

45,000 rpm) and heparin was usually used to avoid thrombotic complications (Figure 2).

Despite its usefulness, ease of operation and relative low cost, the HP is not available at the present time. Nonetheless, understanding the principles behind the function of the HP will help with the understanding of other, very promising, axial flow devices. The technology and knowledge that have been accumulated from the HP experience in the United States and Europe may hopefully play a role in the evolution of future strategies for hemodynamic support.

Hemodynamic Principles

The HP is a rotary, non-pulsatile, blood pump that offers a constant blood pressure in the aorta. Nonetheless, blood flow through the HP is far from a simple continuous stream that drains the left ventricle into the aorta. Elegant animal experiments have allowed us an increasing understanding of blood circulation in the presence of the HP in the normal and in the failing heart. The determining variables of HP flow are preload, arterial vascular resistance, and rotary pump speed.

Preload

The HP inlet cannula is positioned in the LV cavity. If preload decreases, the output of the HP is adversely affected. Furthermore, a smaller

LV cavity, as would be expected with a reduced preload, would increase the resistance to blood aspiration by the inlet cannula, thus contributing further to the decrease in HP output.[26] The systolic function of the right ventricle, in addition to intravascular volume and pulmonary vascular resistance, are the main determinants of LV preload. Any limiting factor to right ventricular performance, e.g. dysrhythmias, would lead to reduced HP output.

Arterial Vascular Resistance

This term is probably more accurate than the term afterload to characterize another limiting factor to HP flow. Afterload incorporates elements like LV wall stress that would otherwise affect unassisted cardiac output but not HP output. The easiest way to measure arterial resistance to HP flow is by measuring the difference between arterial pressure and LV pressure, or deltaP. This difference is the pressure head against which the HP moves blood across the aortic valve. As LV pressure varies with the cardiac cycle, so does the pressure head, and consequently, HP flow rate.

In animal preparations, HP flow increases with LV ejection, as the pressure between the left ventricle and the aorta approaches zero. With isovolumic relaxation, HP flow rate decreases. As the left ventricle fills with the opening of the mitral valve, its pressure increases, thus decreasing deltaP. This leads to a gradual increase in HP flow, which persists with isovolumic contraction until ventricular ejection is reached again. Note here that with ventricular ejection, the heart ejects blood through the HP cannula itself, which leads to an increase in HP flow greater than that expected from the diminution of deltaP alone. Consequently, the deltaP-HP flow relationship that has been characterized in animal experiments displays hysteresis.[26,27]

The HP console does not provide a way to measure blood flow through the HP cannula. In clinical use, the reliance would be on methods of systemic flow measurement and on indicators of LV unloading (e.g. pulmonary capillary wedge pressure) in order to assess the function of the HP.

Another aspect of circulatory resistance relates to the rheologic characteristics of blood. Higher hematocrit values contribute to the hindrance of blood flow through the Hemopump. At maximal pump speed and at the same arterial pressure, a ten-point increase in hematocrit decreases flow by almost 100 mL/min. At a hematocrit of 30% to 40 % and at maximal pump speed, blood flow varied between 2200 mL/min and 1520 mL/min when afterload (i.e., mean arterial pressure) was raised from 60 mm Hg to 110 mm Hg.[28]

Pump Speed

With a higher pump speed the flow rate becomes greater. Since the HP cannula interrupts the integrity of the aortic valve, it induces aortic insufficiency if the pump is off. Depending on the aortic pressure (i.e., the resistance against pump flow), low pump speeds can also cause net regurgitant flow, since the action of the HP leads to an increase in aortic pressure. Aortic regurgitation is an added obstacle in the way of recovery of a failing ventricle.

At higher pump speed, the decompression of the left ventricle can reach a point where the size of the ventricular cavity is reduced to a point that hinders aspiration of blood by the HP cannula. Furthermore, with such a reduced ventricular cavity, the HP cannula is in direct contact with walls of the left ventricle, thus potentially inducing ventricular ectopy. Excessive ectopy adversely affects right ventricular function, and hence LV preload. The above factors set a plateau to the rate of flow increase with increasing pump speed after a certain level. Nonetheless, the degree to which the HP sustains circulation remains substantial even with decreased right ventricular function. In animal experiments, the HP has been shown to support the circulation completely for up to 45 minutes with the heart in ventricular fibrillation.[29] It is also important to mention that the three factors detailed above are interrelated to an extent. If one of them changes and the resulting HP flow contradicts the operator's prediction, it is useful to consider an unfavorable consequence on any of the other two determinants (Figures 3 and 4).

Clinical Experience with the Hemopump

The primary indication for the HP is cardiogenic shock. In contrast to the IABP, the HP is capable of offering greater support to the failing ventricle. In one report, cardiac index increased by about 0.5 L/min/m^2, mean aortic pressure by about 5 mm Hg, and pulmonary wedge pressure decreased about 10 mm Hg.[29] Hemopump support has been described in

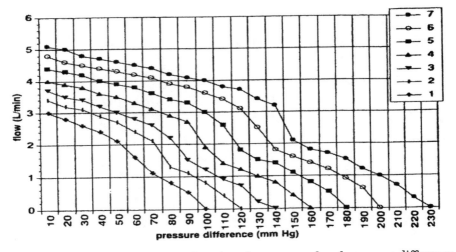

Figure 3. Hemopump flow as a function of pump speed and pressure difference between left ventricle and central aorta. (Reproduced with permission.[26])

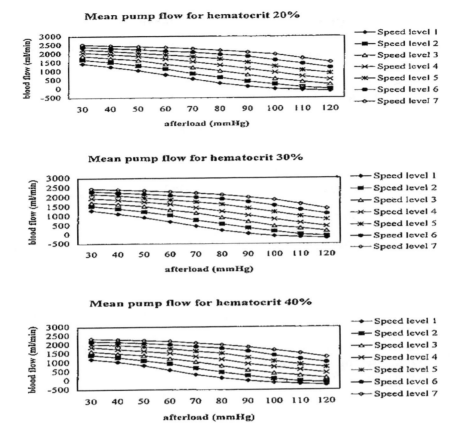

Figure 4. Hemopump flow as a function of hematocrit, pressure difference and pump speed. (Reproduced with permission.[28])

the setting of MI complicated by shock.[30] In animal experiments, the HP was noted to reduce infarct size. These experiments have also shown that, under HP support, perfusion of ischemic territory as compared to nonischemic territory increased by two-fold.[31] Postcardiotomy shock patients have also been shown to benefit from HP support.[29,32] Up to 65% of these patients were able to wean off mechanical assistance. The HP proved a reliable enough assist device to bridge these patients to transplantation, with a low incidence of device-related complications.[33,34]

The HP has been successfully used to support blood circulation during coronary angioplasty in high-risk patients, and during coronary bypass graft operations. Hemopump support blunts both the rise in pulmonary wedge pressure and the drop in cardiac output.[35] Early human trials and animal experiments have described the feasibility of coronary bypass grafting on a beating heart using the HP for hemodynamic support.[36,37] Later, a randomized trial on 32 patients compared coronary surgery using the HP with traditional surgery using cardiopulmonary bypass. The results show that the HP can be safely utilized to perform coronary bypass.[38]

Complications

As might be expected with any such intravascular device, vascular complications do occur with the HP. Patients who have pre-existing peripheral vascular disease are at higher risk. Injury to the aortic valve has been described in animals in the form of hemorrhage within the leaflets, and contusion and abrasion of leaflet margins.[24] Trauma to red blood cells occurs inevitably with the HP, but the resultant intravascular hemolysis usually does not lead to clinically significant anemia. The decreased red blood cell count is most notable in the first 24 hours of HP function with stabilization afterwards. Platelets have also been noted to drop but the ensuing thrombocytopenia is usually mild and unlikely to impair hemostasis.

A cautionary note pertains to the use of the HP in those patients who have an existing or a potential communication between the left and right cardiac chambers (i.e., atrial or ventricular septal defect or patent foramen ovule). The action of the HP is potent enough to cause shunting of blood from the right side to the left, with resultant life threatening hypoxia.[39]

Long-Term Mechanical Assist Devices

Long-term assist devices are intended for support of a failing heart for a prolonged time. The aim is not temporary support while the heart is given a chance to recover. At this point, myocardial recovery is not expected and survival of the organism without circulatory assistance is extremely improbable.

Effects of LVAD Therapy

Profound cardiogenic shock that is refractory to medical therapy is a potentially lethal condition unless cardiac transplantation is urgently performed. If transplantation is not feasible, the only option is to use a mechanical assist device. Survival until transplantation is dramatically improved by the use of an assist device versus medical therapy alone (71% vs. 36%). LVADs allow for patient rehabilitation as demonstrated by improved renal, hepatic, and physical capacity assessment.[40]

LVADs provide complete pressure and volume unloading of the left ventricle. The aortic valve usually remains in the closed position with blood moving from the assist device into the proximal aorta. The pulmonary capillary wedge pressure falls typically to values ranging from 6 to 12 mm Hg. Reports of echocardiographic examinations of the previously dilated left ventricle describe a major decrease in cavity dimensions to the point of collapse.[41]

After prolonged mechanical unloading, LV systolic function can improve, with increased ejection fraction from 11% $\pm$ 5% to 22% $\pm$ 17%, and decreased diastolic dimension (with the assist system off) in one study.[40] The pressure-volume curve, a measure of the compliance of the

LV chamber, shifts toward that of normal myocardium.[42] In some patients, LV function improves to a point that the LVAD is removed and the native heart reassumes its role. These patients are usually in New York Heart Association class I.[43] For them, the assist device is a "bridge to recovery."

Reverse ventricular remodeling describes the modification in LV dimensions and function, together with the underlying changes at the cellular level. These cellular changes are apparent from the histological examination of cardiac tissue after prolonged unloading. There is a reduction in acute myocyte damage, as evidenced by a reduction in contraction band necrosis and in the number of wavy fibers. On the other hand, fibrosis increases, probably reflecting myocardial healing, without evidence of ongoing myocyte atrophy.[44] Isolated myocardial fibers demonstrate a normalization of force-frequency relationship and a positive inotropic response to beta-receptor agonists.[45] Myocytes of a failing ventricle usually display a decremental response to repetitive stimulation and a blunted response to isoproterenol administration.[46] The intracellular handling of calcium flux normalizes. This is accomplished with the return of sarcoplasmic reticulum calcium ATPase, calcium release channels, and cell membrane sodium-calcium exchanger, membrane proteins whose genes are down-regulated in failing myocardium, to normal levels.[47,48]

Despite all the favorable myocardial changes, the vast majority of LVAD patients never recover their ventricular function. The definitive form of therapy of terminal failure at this point is still cardiac transplantation. The Food and Drug Administration granted approval to all existing devices to "bridge" patients to the final form of therapy. In the next few paragraphs, focus will be made on the guiding principles that govern the clinical use of assist devices.

Pulsatile versus Nonpulsatile Flow

Pulsatile flow is a complex, polymorphic phenomenon rather than a uniform entity. Therefore, different experiments utilizing "pulsatile flow" may actually involve totally different patterns of blood circulation. The physical nature of pulsatile flow is dependent both on the characteristics of the mechanical pump and on those of the vascular tree.[49] For instance, the pulsatile cardiopulmonary bypass pump produces nonpulsatile, continuous flow when the systemic vascular resistance is low. Conversely, the nonpulsatile roller pump produces pulsatile flow when systemic vascular resistance is elevated.[50]

It is difficult to make a firm deduction concerning the superiority of one type of artificial flow over the other. Overall, it appears that nonpulsatile flow contributes to a higher peripheral and pulmonary vascular resistance than pulsatile flow, probably because this latter has a better ability to maintain a patent microcirculation and an adequate lymphatic flow.[51] An alternative explanation is that pulsatile flow leads to greater carotid and aortic baroreceptor activity than nonpulsatile flow does, at the same mean pressure.[52] A potential role for hormones is also possible since higher levels of plasma renin and vasopressin activity have been recorded with nonpulsatile flow.[53]

As far as kidney function is concerned, it is suggested that pulsatile flow maintains renal cortical perfusion, leading to higher urine output, and prevents ischemic changes.[54] These findings, nonetheless, were not consistent. A note on coronary circulation: with both pulsatile and nonpulsatile flow devices, coronary perfusion in the beating heart is pulsatile. This is the result of changes in myocardial pressure with each systole and diastole. Only when the heart is in fibrillation is coronary flow continuous with the use of a nonpulsatile flow device.[55]

Compared to the seeming superiority of pulsatile flow, investigators were able to show that nonpulsatile flow is physiologically equivalent to 80% of the same flow if generated in pulsatile fashion.[56] Support beyond 6 weeks abolishes the need for a higher cardiac output. Interestingly, "nonpulsatile" perfusion beyond the 6 weeks generates a pulse of about 40 beats/min and a pulse pressure that increases with time. After 3 months, the pulse pressure is in the range of 15 mm Hg.[57]

Right Ventricular Function with LVAD

As the LVAD unloads the left ventricle, the pressure in the pulmonary circulation falls, thus decreasing right ventricular afterload. In addition, with the decreasing LV volume, right ventricular compliance increases, as verified in experimental preparations both with and without an intact pericardium. Finally, right ventricular contractility decreases after LVAD implantation because of ventricular interdependence.

This interdependence is the natural consequence of the fact that both ventricles have common muscle fibers, share one septum, and dwell within the same pericardial space. In diastole, as the pressure and the volume of one ventricle increase, the pressure-volume curve of the contralateral ventricle becomes steeper, indicating decreased compliance.[58] The reverse is also true, as is the case with LVAD application. This relation is observed even with an open pericardium, although it is more marked with the pericardium intact.[59] In systole, an increase in the pressure or volume in one ventricle causes an increase in both the systolic and the diastolic pressure in the other ventricle.[60] The contribution of the LV systole to the rise in right ventricular pressure during systole is much greater than the contribution of the right ventricle to the left sided pressure rise. In fact, pulmonary artery flow relies more on LV systole than on right ventricular contraction, with the left ventricle responsible for as much as two-thirds of the total right ventricular output.[61] The consequences of this interaction are of great importance when the left ventricle is assisted, since both ventricular systolic and diastolic pressure, in addition to LV volume, are sharply decreased.

Thus, the effect of the LVAD on the right ventricle is the net result of two opposing tendencies: one toward increasing output by decreasing preload and increasing compliance, the other toward decreasing output by decreasing contractility. Experimental studies have shown that, in a normal heart, right ventricular output does not change with LV bypass.[62] On the other hand, if LV assist is applied after induction of heart failure, the net effect is actually toward a decrease in cardiac output resulting from right heart failure.[63] The same is observed in situations where severe septal or right ventricular free wall ischemia is provoked.[64]

A good right ventricular function is vital for LVAD patients since the right ventricle is responsible for LVAD filling. With poor filling, LVAD output is decreased and right ventricular function is impaired even further. The result of such a situation is hemodynamic collapse. Clinically, decompensation of the right ventricle occurs in about 25% of patients receiving LVAD support,[65] with some reports quoting an incidence up to 52%.[66] The development of right ventricular failure is a major determinant of survival after LVAD placement. Clinical parameters that are found useful in predicting right ventricular failure are right atrial pressure and transpulmonary pressure gradient (the difference between mean pulmonary artery pressure and pulmonary capillary wedge pressure) prior to LVAD implantation. The change in mean pulmonary artery pressure directly after LVAD implantation is also of importance in predicting the post operative course. The presence of at least two of the following parameters: right atrial pressure $\geq$ 20 mm Hg, transpulmonary gradient $\geq$ 16 mm Hg, or decrease in mean pulmonary artery pressure $\leq$ 10 mm Hg can predict right ventricular dysfunction with a sensitivity of 82% and a specificity of 88%.[67]

In addition to the hemodynamic factors discussed above, multiple other factors are potential contributors to right-sided circulatory failure after LVAD implantation. Cardiopulmonary bypass itself is associated with a concomitant increase in pulmonary vascular resistance mediated by complement activation. Blood product infusion and vasopressors can also play a role in raising pulmonary resistance. Despite mechanical intervention in the form of mechanical right ventricular assistance, mortality in this group of patients remains quite elevated. In fact, survival to transplant among patients who require right ventricular mechanical assistance is about 27%, as compared to 83% among those who do not.[68]

Infectious Complications of LVAD Use

Infection is a common problem that affects LVAD patients. Many factors contribute to the increased incidence and the added severity of infectious complications in these patients. Firstly, patients who require LVAD support have multiple end organ damage, whether reversible or not. Their natural defenses are breached by support measures they usually require, including central access lines, intravascular monitoring catheters, and endotracheal tubes. In addition, their illness is usually advanced to the point at which their cellular and humoral immune systems cannot offer them adequate protection.

LVADs, just like any other foreign body, allow bacterial adhesion. Adhesion-mediated infections can be extremely resistant to antibiotics and host defenses. They also have the added risk of potential septic embolization. The desire for improved biocompatibility of artificial organs led to the development of biomaterial that facilitates cellular adhesion and increases their susceptibility to bacterial adhesion.[69]

Several centers have published their experience with infectious complications of prolonged LVAD use. In one such report, up to 50% of patients successfully bridged to transplantation had positive blood cultures. Organisms involved with the septicemia included, in order of prevalence, *Staphylococcus* species (9 of 12 patients), *Candida* (3 of 12 patients), *Pseudomonas*, and *Enterococcus* (2 of 12 patients each). Two of the twenty patients actually required device removal or replacement.[70] Another institution compared infection rate of patients who died during LVAD support to that of those who were successfully bridged to transplantation and found no trend for a higher number of infections in nonsurvivors.[71]

Immunobiology of LVAD

The material used in the manufacture of assist devices and their connections, though termed biologically inert, does interact with the immune system. Protein adsorption on the material surface, changes in the material induced by the host, together with the systemic effects of the material trigger multiple reactions including inflammation, coagulation, and activation of the immune system.[72]

Cellular mechanisms begin when monocyte/macrophage cells form a lining on the LVAD surface[73,74] and are functionally activated. T lymphocytes interact with these monocytic cells and express cell surface markers, including CD95 proteins.[72] When these T lymphocytes interact with antigen-presenting cells, which include activated monocytes, a sequence of events takes place and leads to apoptosis, or cell suicide, of these CD95 producing T-cells. This phenomenon is termed activation-induced cell death (AICD).[75]

T-cells that are noted to undergo AICD are predominantly those that produce Th-1-type cytokines (i.e., IL-1 and interferon gamma). T-cells that produce IL-10 and transforming growth factor beta, i.e., Th-2-type cytokine producing cells, are relatively spared. The preponderance of these Th-2-type cytokines leads to B-cell activation and resultant production of auto-antibodies directed against major histocompatibility complex (MHC) antigens of both class II and I.[73]

These antibodies increase the risk of allograft failure. HLA class I antigens are expressed on the cell surface of donor endothelium. Recipient antibodies directed against these antigens can predispose to complement-mediated humoral rejection, which occurs within the first 24 to 48 hours after transplantation. The presence of these antibodies, particularly if they are of the IgG isotype, is considered a contraindication to transplantation. Transplant candidates with anti-MHC class I antibodies have a high *panel reactive antibodies*, or PRA, level. They require donor-specific cross matching before transplantation. An important risk factor for the development of these antibodies has been identified as platelet transfusion during or around LVAD surgery.[76,77]

Anti-MHC class II antibodies, on the other hand, predispose potential graft recipients to high-grade cellular rejection post transplant. This type of rejection occurs at a median time of 70 days in those patients with IgG type antibodies. Their cumulative annual frequency of cellular rejection episodes is 85%, compared to 17% in those who do not express these antibodies. The exact mechanism that involves these IgG antibodies in high-grade cellular rejection remains poorly understood at present.[77]

The most effective regimen against anti-HLA class I antibody production is a combination of intravenous pooled human immunoglobulin (IVIg) and intravenous cyclophosphamide. Patients with anti-HLA class II antibodies respond well to intravenous cyclophosphamide, given monthly peritransplant for 2 to 6 doses, together with standard immunosuppression post transplantation.[78,79]

Anticoagulation

Thromboembolic phenomena are a serious complication of LVAD implantation. As many as 30% of patients experienced clinically apparent embolic incidents with the earlier devices.[80] The advent of textured-surface blood contacting surfaces dropped the incidence of systemic embolism to less than 4%.[81]

The need for anticoagulation per se varies with the different devices. When anticoagulation is needed, heparinization is started when chest-tube drainage falls below 150 mL/24 hours and oral anticoagulation is initiated later.

Patient Selection

In the context of cardiogenic shock, it is important to distinguish patients who necessitate mechanical assistance for survival from those who can recover from the state of shock with pharmacologic support alone. We also need to identify those patients who do not qualify for mechanical assistance either because they are not suitable candidates for heart transplantation, or because the end-organ damage that resulted from shock has progressed to an extent that makes mechanical assistance futile.

Patients who are being considered for mechanical assistance usually present with an aortic systolic pressure around 85 mm Hg, a pulmonary capillary wedge pressure > 20 mm Hg, and a cardiac index < 2 L/min/m^2, despite inotropic support. These patients also show signs of end-organ damage either because of insufficient perfusion or because of elevated cardiac filling pressure. Anuria and uremia, respiratory failure necessitating mechanical ventilation, and liver damage as evidenced by bilirubin and liver enzyme elevation are commonly present.

Early reports indicated that end-organ dysfunction by itself is not a contraindication for LVAD implantation. This was mainly based on the observation that improvement in organ function accompanied hemodynamic improvement.[82] These studies, however, were unable to distinguish indicators of irreversible organ damage that lead to poor patient survival. More recent studies indicate that preoperative uremia is indicative of poor outcome. Patients with blood urea nitrogen levels greater than 40 mg/dL have a 46% chance of survival until transplant, as compared to 76% of those whose levels are less than 20 mg/dL.[83] Furthermore, LVAD patients who require renal replacement therapy while waiting for heart transplantation have a mortality rate of 93% at 6 months.[84] Such prognoses may preclude insertion of an assist device in patients on renal replacement therapy.[85] Another predictor of poor outcome in the postoperative course of bridge to transplant patients is abnormal liver function. Direct bilirubin levels greater than three times the upper limit of normal are associated with a survival rate of 33%.[86] This degree of bilirubin elevation, or alternatively the need for renal replacement therapy, probably indicates irreversible organ damage that is unlikely to improve despite the correction of hemodynamic parameters.

Although these studies help somewhat in decision making, further questions remain to be answered. It can always be argued that liver or kidney failure is a result of delay in the application of mechanical assistance. As experience with mechanical assistance grows, this important issue will hopefully be clarified.

Operative and Perioperative Considerations

LVAD implantation is major vascular surgery that carries a high risk for bleeding. Impaired liver function and massive transfusions predispose LVAD candidates to bleeding problems. Hypothermia that can result from high volume fluid administration at room temperature contributes to a disseminated intravascular coagulation (DIC)-like picture. Cardiopulmonary bypass, which is utilized in LVAD implantation, can induce DIC as a consequence of the total body inflammatory response to the synthetic elements of the bypass circuit. Platelet dysfunction in uremic patients increases predisposition to bleeding.

Renal failure and oliguria can complicate the management of fluid balance. Volume overload and electrolyte imbalances are common problems. Aggressive pharmacologic intervention, in addition to membrane dialysis and/or fluid ultrafiltration, may be needed. As we have discussed above, peri-operative renal failure portends a poor survival.

Intraoperatively, transesophageal echocardiography can determine the adequacy of chamber de-airing and can also detect interatrial or interventricular septal defects which warrant reparative surgery because LV unloading with LVAD activation can lead to right-to-left blood shunting.[87]

The aortic valve does not open with a normally functioning LVAD, leading to stasis of blood across the valve. LVAD candidates who have had aortic valve replacement surgery are thus in danger of thrombosis of the metallic prosthesis with subsequent embolization. Re-replacement of the metallic valve with a bioprosthetic valve is one solution. Some operators suggest sewing a prosthetic patch above the mechanical valve and below the coronary ostia in order to exclude the valve. This procedure is simple and rapid; however, blood clots can still form on top of the patch itself.[88] The replacement of the aortic root with a homograft is yet another option. Significant aortic regurgitation is another problem. It permits blood re-entry into the LV cavity and the LVAD inflow, thus "short-circuiting" LVAD connection and leading to deceptively elevated LVAD flow that does not reflect systemic output. Another important valvular lesion is severe tricuspid regurgitation. This may worsen right ventricular function and precipitate failure.[88]

After successful implantation of the LVAD, attention is turned to the right ventricle. Right ventricular function is crucial for successful separation from the cardiopulmonary bypass. Dobutamine or milrinone are used for inotropic support. Dysrrhythmias can affect right ventricular output and require appropriate management. Lowering pulmonary vascular resistance improves right ventricular function. Inhaled nitric oxide is a potent vasodilator without prominent systemic effects due to avid binding to hemoglobin.[89] Patients who respond to nitric oxide administration demonstrate an increase in LVAD flow and a decrease in central venous pressure, with unchanged pulmonary pressures in view of the increased blood flow that counteracts the decrease in vascular resistance. With prolonged therapy, however, nitric oxide synthase may be suppressed, producing dependency on inhaled nitric oxide.[90]

Further care in the intensive care unit is an extension of the immediate postoperative management. LVAD patients usually progress to hemodynamic stability and improved functional status. LVAD recipients are also at risk of complications of any cardiac surgery, namely acute respiratory distress syndrome, localized or systemic infection, and acute tubular necrosis.

A comprehensive discussion of all long-term assist devices is well beyond the scope of this chapter. A few representative devices that have gained recognition through extensive clinical experience will be illustrated.

Thoratec Assist Device

History and Description

The Thoratec (thtec [Thoratec Corporation, Woburn, MA]) assist device (Figure 5) is a modified form of a device developed at the Hershey Medical Center of Pennsylvania State University and first used clinically by Dr Pierce during the late 1970s.[91] Full FDA commercial approval was granted in 1995. The thtec device comprises a rigid case encapsulating a thromboresistant polyurethane pumping chamber. This prosthetic ventricle is connected to an inflow and outflow cannula by a pair of Bjork-Shiley form of monostrut heart valves that insures unidirectional blood flow. It can be used for left or right ventricular support. A pair of thtec devices

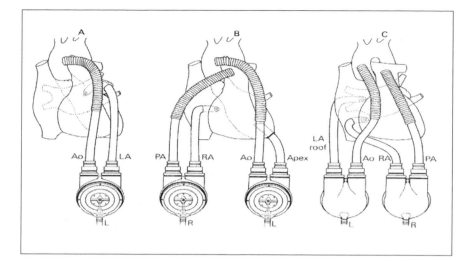

Figure 5. Diagram showing the Thoratec device used as a univentricular or biventricular assist device. The left inflow cannula can be connected to the left atrial appendage (**A**), the ventricular apex (**B**), or the left atrial "roof" via the interatrial groove. Outflow cannula connects to the ascending aorta. Right sided connections are the right atrium for the inflow and the pulmonary artery for the outflow. (Reproduced with permission from Farrar et al. *N Engl J Med* 1988;318:333-340)

can be used for biventricular support or as a total artificial heart. The inflow cannula can be connected to the atrium or to the ventricular apex in case of LV assistance or to the right atrium in case of right ventricular support. The outflow cannula returns blood from the paracorporeal prosthetic ventricle to the ascending aorta or to the pulmonary trunk.

The prosthetic ventricle incorporates a fill switch to detect when the ventricle is full and trigger prosthetic ventricle systole. Thus, the device operates on a 'fill-to-empty' mode that prevents stasis and provides a fixed stroke volume, variable rate type flow. The stroke volume of the prosthetic ventricle is 65 mL. Power to the prosthetic ventricle is derived from a vacuum pump during filling and from a compressor that applies pressure during emptying. Two independent units of vacuum pumps, compressors, drive modules and battery backup systems are incorporated in a dual drive console or in a portable driver that allows patients to ambulate. Normally, each drive unit actuates one prosthetic thtec ventricle although an emergency selector valve allows the actuation of two thtec devices by one unit. This emergency measure is helpful in case one unit fails in a patient dependent on biventricular support. Note here that despite the thromboresistant polyurethane that makes up the prosthetic ventricle and the effort to prevent blood stasis, patients should be systemically anticoagulated. Typically, intravenous heparin is started once chest tube drainage has become minimal post thtec implantation. Warfarin sodium is then utilized, with a target INR between 2.5 and 3.5.[92]

Clinical Experience with thtec

The main advantages of the thtec device are simplicity of design and suitability to a wide range of patients. In fact, there is no lower body weight limit for implantation. Pediatric patients as little as 17 kilograms in weight have been successfully assisted with the thtec device.[92] The inflow cannula can be connected either to the left atrium or to the ventricular apex. Each alternative has its advantages and its inconveniences. Atrial cannulation can be performed without need for cardiopulmonary bypass, is relatively easier, and involves a lesser degree of myocardial damage. It also allows for the insertion of the thtec device in those patients with small LV dimensions or those with an extensive area of infarction that makes implantation in the ventricular apex impossible. On the other hand, LV cannulation provides higher blood flow, presents a lower risk of thromboembolism, and imparts a greater degree of left ventricular unloading.[93]

Similarly, there are several different modes of operation: ECG synchronous, asynchronous, and "fill-to-empty" mode. The first mode is intended to create counterpulsation in a way resembling that of the IABP. The asynchronous mode operates at a fixed rate, with a stroke volume that consequently varies with the filling status of the prosthetic ventricle. The last mode, as the name implies, uses an automatic sensor that activates the device as soon as it detects a "full" prosthetic ventricle.[94] The asynchronous mode is usually selected at the initiation of pumping and during weaning of the patient from the device. The "fill-to-empty" mode provides the highest attainable flow at the prevailing hemodynamic circumstances. The ECG synchronous mode was theoretically thought to have advantages over the asynchronous and automatic modes as far as decreasing myocardial oxygen consumption through a superior degree of LV unloading. Clinically, no significant differences were noted and recent experimental studies did not reveal any meaningful advantages on the hemodynamic level.[95]

The first human implantation was performed in September 1984.[96] As of February 1999, 1048 patients had been implanted with 1590 thtec devices for single or for biventricular assistance, alone or in combination with other types of assist devices. Overall survival of those patients who received the thtec as a bridge to transplantation is around 60%, after support duration lasting up to 515 days with a mean of 38 days.[97] A recent report published the data on the 10-year survival rate of 111 patients who received thtec device from a single institution. Those who were supported by the device for an anticipated recovery of their ventricle had a 16% survival rate, compared with 22% of those who originally received the thtec as a bridge to transplant. Ten years after their operation, 33% of transplanted patients were still living.[98]

Complications of thtec support are mainly bleeding, infection, and systemic embolization. In one report, symptomatic central nervous system embolization occurred in 6 of 72 patients, a rate of about 8%. The major cause of death on the device has been mostly related to multiple organ failure.[99] It seems that this last complication is related not so much to the device itself, as it is to the condition of the patient at implantation. This is a recurring theme with almost all circulatory assist systems. The identification of the patient with end-stage myocardial failure but reversible end-organ impairment appears to be more difficult than either the choice of the assist device or its operation.

The thtec VAD has enjoyed far-reaching clinical success that bears witness to its efficacy and reliability. Currently, a titanium model is being developed to permit intracorporeal implantation. The application of this device, intended for long-term ambulatory assistance, derives from the long experience collected from its extracorporeal predecessor. Whether it will enjoy as wide a range of clinical use in the presence of newer devices remains to be seen.

Abiomed BVS 5000

The Abiomed BVS 5000 (ABIOMED Inc., Danvers, MA) was first introduced into the clinical arena in 1987. It is another pulsatile assist device capable of left, right, or biventricular support. It consists of a tubular, single use blood pump. Each incorporates an atrial and a ventricular pumping chamber, separated by a trileaflet polyurethane valve. A similar valve is positioned at the outflow of the pumping chamber to ensure unidirectional blood flow. As is the case with the thtec device, the BVS 5000 is paracorporeal and pneumatically actuated. Unlike the thtec, however, filling of the atrial chamber throughout pump systole and diastole is passive and dependent on gravity rather than vacuum. Custom-designed cannulae connect to the right or left atrium, with an outflow cannula in the pulmonary artery or aorta, respectively.

A bedside console is responsible for the pneumatic actuation, as well as for the constant optimization of pump performance. This optimization allows a near constant stroke volume of 80 mL in the face of changing afterload. Pump output is thus directly related to the frequency of ejection. Data from driveline air flow is acquired and communicated to the control algorithm. This provides important information about pump performance (i.e., stroke volume) and filling status (i.e., pump preload). Control of pump function is then accomplished automatically based on that information, without the need for timing and pump flow adjustment by the clinician. Pump ejection occurs asynchronously to the patient's own ventricular systole (Figure 6).

Pump filling is gravity-dependent. Therefore, adjusting the height of the pumping chamber regulates pump preload. The pump is typically positioned between 0 and 25 cm below the level of the patient's atria for ideal filling depending mainly on the patient's volume status, among other variables.

The pump console also provides a weaning mode that allows gradual decrease in pump flow in decrements of 0.1 L/min down to a minimum flow of 0.5 L/min. If the patient shows signs of poor tolerability to the weaning procedure, the weaning mode can be turned off and the BVS 5000 returns to full-flow.[100]

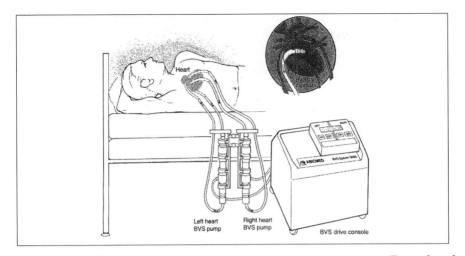

Figure 6. The Abiomed BVS 5000 as a biventricular support system. (Reproduced with permission from Shook, BJ. *Cardiac Surgery State of the Art Reviews* 1993;7:309.)

In many reviews reporting the experience of busy heart surgery programs, the Abiomed BVS 5000 has proven to be an effective and relatively inexpensive means of circulatory support. Its major advantage is comparative simplicity of design and function, without the need for a large number of specialized personnel. Its major inconvenience is limitation of patient mobility, which limits its use to a rather short period.[101]

Pusher Plate Devices

The conception and development of these pulsatile long-term mechanical assist devices began in the mid 1970s. The original idea was to create a permanent "replacement" for the failing heart. Nonetheless, the course of development together with progressive insight into the treatment of heart failure and heart transplantation led to their transformation into "bridging" devices. They convey patients over the troubled waters of terminal heart failure, onto the shore of the ultimate treatment: transplantation. In doing so, they not only improve mortality, but also provide patients with a quality of life otherwise unattainable. Successful implantation projects these patients into NYHA Class I category and allows them to be discharged home and to resume their jobs.

These two long-term assist devices are implanted in the abdominal cavity or in an extraperitoneal pocket created below the rectus muscle or behind the posterior rectus fascia. The intra-abdominal position offers better protection against infections because of the presence of the omentum. The disadvantage is a host of potential complications that may occur; namely, the risk of inadvertent visceral perforation during implantation, compression or erosion of the abdominal viscera by the LVAD, and the formation of adhesions. These latter can cause bowel obstruction and make LVAD explantation particularly difficult. The periperitoneal pocket lacks the resistance to infections that is provided by the omentum. Moreover, the surgical creation of this pocket is frequently complicated by the development of a hematoma or a seroma that acts as a culture medium for microorganisms. In the majority of cases, the LVAD is implanted periperitoneally in fear of the serious complications of abdominal insertion.[102]

Novacor Left Ventricular Assist System (Novacor LVAS)

Description

The first human implantation of the Novacor assist device (Baxter Healthcare Corp., Deerfield, IL) occurred in 1984.[103] It consists of a seamless polyurethane sac bonded to symmetrically opposed pusher plates, all of which are housed in lightweight fiberglass. Inflow and outflow Dacron grafts, measuring 25 mm in diameter, connect the blood-containing sac to the apex of the left ventricle and the ascending aorta, respectively. A pair of porcine pericardial valves (bovine valves before 1993) ensures unidirectional flow of blood. A pulsed-solenoid energy converter is coupled to the pusher plates and transforms electrical energy to mechanical energy. Power is transmitted via percutaneous electric connections to a console based or, after 1993, a wearable controller. When the patient is ambulatory, power is provided by reserve battery packs, otherwise, standard household electrical power is used. Together with the electric connection, a vent tube connects the pusher plate space surrounding the polyurethane sac with the atmosphere. It serves to equalize the pressure in the space with the atmospheric pressure, hence preventing the development of negative pressure that would otherwise impede the function of the pusher plates. The polyurethane sac fills passively. When full, a sensor activates the pusher plates and blood is thus pressurized into the ascending aorta (Figure 7).[104]

After implantation, the Novacor LVAS requires systemic anticoagulation to prevent thromboembolization. Heparin is initiated early after implantation with warfarin substitution as soon as the patient is able to ingest orally, and INR is kept between 2.5 and 3.5. Antiplatelet therapy, in the form of aspirin or dipyridamole, is added after removal of the chest drains.

Clinical Experience

By the end of 1997, 820 patients had received the Novacor system worldwide.[105] Data accumulated on 768 of these patients shows that the average support period was 85 days, with a maximum recorded at 962 days. Transplantation was performed on 58% of these patients while 41%

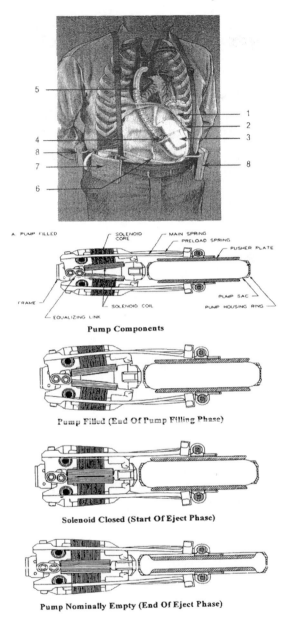

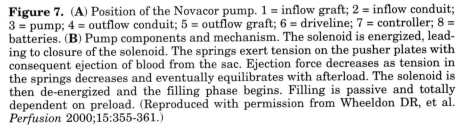

Figure 7. (**A**) Position of the Novacor pump. 1 = inflow graft; 2 = inflow conduit; 3 = pump; 4 = outflow conduit; 5 = outflow graft; 6 = driveline; 7 = controller; 8 = batteries. (**B**) Pump components and mechanism. The solenoid is energized, leading to closure of the solenoid. The springs exert tension on the pusher plates with consequent ejection of blood from the sac. Ejection force decreases as tension in the springs decreases and eventually equilibrates with afterload. The solenoid is then de-energized and the filling phase begins. Filling is passive and totally dependent on preload. (Reproduced with permission from Wheeldon DR, et al. *Perfusion* 2000;15:355-361.)

of patients died on support. About 3% of patients demonstrated sufficient LV function recovery to allow device explantation. Importantly, up to 89% of these patients could be discharged home at one point, a witness to the dramatic improvement in their quality of life resulting from Novacor support.[106]

In view of these numbers, one cannot but praise the success of long-term support achieved with Novacor. Nevertheless, the undoubted success of this form of therapy is not without adverse events. Complications consist mainly of bleeding, infection, and embolic phenomena. During the process of the clinical use of Novacor LVAS, however, modifications and improvements were continually introduced to curtail the occurrence of these complications.

In one recent report on experience with Novacor LVAS, 61 patients were supported for an average of 148 days. Perioperative bleeding occurred in 45% of cases. Infections were subdivided as to location. Driveline infections were witnessed in 26% of patients, pocket infection in 11%, and sepsis in 24%. Conduit endocarditis was recorded in two patients, or 4%. Importantly, symptomatic cerebral embolization occurred in 24 out of 61 patients, a rate of 39%. It is also notable that not a single incident of mechanical failure was noted with any of these 61 patients on Novacor, a testimony to the reliability of the design.[107]

HeartMate Left Ventricular Assist System

Description

Work on the HeartMate LVAS (Thoratec Corp.) started in 1975. The design made provision for two variants: the implantable pneumatic (IP) using pneumatic energy and the vented electric (VE) using electrical energy. In both devices, the pumping chamber and the blood contacting elements are identical. The major difference lies in portability. The Heart-Mate IP is powered and controlled by a fairly large external pneumatic drive console. The HeartMate VE contains an electric motor and connects via a percutaneous cable to a portable control system and an energy source. The electric variant has a vent tube to equalize the chamber pressure with the atmospheric pressure. This vent tube can be used to actuate the pump pneumatically in an emergency, e.g., failure of the motor or the electrical connection.

The device consists of a titanium chamber that houses the blood chamber and the air (IP) or motor chamber (VE). The two chambers are separated by a polyurethane diaphragm. The blood pump is textured to enable adherence of circulating cells and the consequent formation of a pseudo-intima. This cellular layer constitutes the blood-device interface. It reduces thrombus formation to such an extent that systemic anticoagulation is not required. Inflow and outflow conduits connect the device to the apex of the left ventricle and the ascending aorta while porcine valves ensure unidirectional blood flow.

As in the case of the Novacor LVAS, device filling is passive. Heart-Mate LVAS has two modes of operation: fixed rate and automatic. In the fixed rate mode, the device ejects blood at the rate specific time intervals, regardless of the filling status. This usually gives a constant flow. The automatic mode provides the maximal possible flow, depending on the filling status. In the automatic mode, a sensor detects when the blood chamber is completely filled and actuates the motor (VE), or the air pump (IP). The diaphragm moves toward the fixed "wall" and the blood chamber becomes pressurized. The outflow valve opens and blood is ejected into the ascending aorta. The maximal stroke volume of the HeartMate LVAS is 83 mL and the maximal rate is around 140 "beats" per minute, giving a maximal flow rate of 11.6 L/min. The control console displays pump parameters as well as visual and audible alerts for low flow and low battery. The HeartMate VE has portable controller and batteries, which allow for untethered patient ambulation. When the patient is resting, the device can be connected to a desktop power supply while batteries are recharged (Figure 8).[108]

Clinical Experience

Clinical trials with the pneumatic system started in 1985, after 10 years of development. As of July 1998, 1387 patients had undergone HeartMate implantation worldwide. Data collected on all 993 patients who had received the HeartMate by 1997 is available from 122 centers worldwide. The average flow was around 5.2 L/min with maximal flow around 10.0 L/min. The majority of patients, 753 in total, have had the IP LVAS. Their average implant duration was 82 days with a maximum of 727 days of support. The percentage of patients who survived until transplant or explantation was 68%, which implies a mortality rate of 32% on the device. As for the VE LVAS, 240 patients were supported for an average of 102 days, with a maximum of 606 days. Sixty-two percent of these survived until transplant or explantation while 38% presumably expired.[109]

Infections, bleeding and mechanical failures complicate HeartMate therapy. In a report on 100 patients, 59% had positive blood cultures at some point, while drive line infection and pocket infection occurred in 28% and 11%. Mechanical failures were noted in up to 12% of patients, 50% of whom did not survive.[110] It is important to note here that Heart-Mate patients who were discharged home did not suffer from a higher complication rate when compared to hospitalized patients.[111]

Novacor versus HeartMate

These two VADs have achieved far and wide clinical recognition for their contribution to the survival of terminal heart failure patients. Both show a mortality rate approaching 40%. At first glance, this mortality rate may seem rather elevated; however, we need to keep in mind that,

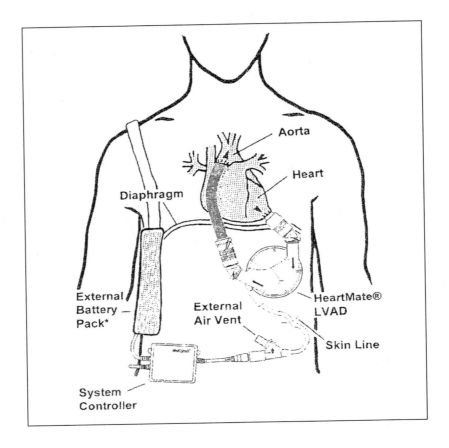

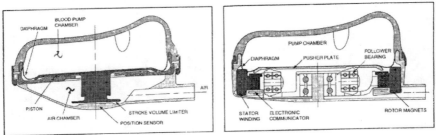

Figure 8. (**A**) The HeartMate LVAD position. (**B**) Drawing that illustrates the components of pneumatic and electric HeartMate LVAS. In the pneumatic version, the position sensor, upon contact with the stroke volume limiter, initiates air chamber pressurization and blood ejection. In its electric version, the pusher plate is lifted by conversion of the rotational motion of the rotor into linear motion. (Reproduced with permission from Wheeldon DR, et al. *Perfusion* 2000;15:355-361.)

if these devices were unavailable, the mortality rate of these unfortunate patients would approach 100% at 1 year.

Their hemodynamic performance is somewhat equivalent. The generated flow is mostly preload dependent and relatively insensitive to changes in afterload. Preload is but right ventricular output. Hence, VAD output varies directly with that of the right ventricle. This allows a rather physiologic control of total output similar to that in a normal circulation. VAD output accommodates systemic oxygen demand by following changes in right ventricular output. The extent of LV unloading is also similar, with the aortic valve remaining in the closed position with either device.

A prospective study comparing the two systems was conducted on a relatively limited number of patients (40). The results echo the conclusions of the clinical experience of each device outlined above. Hemodynamically, mean cardiac index with either of the two VADs is around 3.0 L/min/m^2, mean pulmonary pressure is about 30 mm Hg and systemic vascular resistance is normalized around 800 dynes·min·cm^{-5}. The major difference lies in the type of complications encountered.

HeartMate patients are primarily plagued by mechanical failures related to blood leakage through the diaphragm into the motor chamber, drive line failure, or controller malfunction requiring replacement (16 occurrences vs. 5 with Novacor). They also suffer more frequently from device related infections than their counterparts on Novacor support (55% vs. 20%).

On the other hand, Novacor patients tend to have a higher incidence of bleeding, not a surprising observation in view of the need for systemic anticoagulation. They also have a much higher incidence of symptomatic thromboembolic phenomena (20% vs. 0% on HeartMate), with the overwhelming majority of these emboli targeting the central nervous system.[112] It is important to note here that these devices are in constant reevaluation and revision. Newer versions of the same device are continuously being produced and evaluated with the aim of improving on the potential complication profile.

Despite the many advantages of these two devices and the substantial knowledge gained from their use, they still fall short of their original aim as a permanent replacement for the left ventricle. Nonetheless, they have helped hundreds of patients lead a dignified quality of life and survive until transplantation. Hope lies now in the next generation of assist devices to offer an alternative permanent solution to the failing ventricle.

Axial Flow Devices

Advancement in the field of mechanical assistance and the ever increasing body of knowledge that has been gathered with the years of experience have allowed the development of VADs based on the principle of axial pumps. The latest long-term assist devices, namely the MicroMed-DeBakey (MicroMed Technology, Inc., Houston, TX) and the Jarvik 2000 (Jarvik Heart Inc., New York, NY), herald the next generation of mechanical assist devices.

The basic operative and physiologic principles here are very similar to those discussed above in the section on the Hemopump, another axial pump design. The blood flow is essentially nonpulsatile and pump output is dependent mainly on afterload. As a permanent assist device, an axial pump design offers multiple advantages over pusher plate type pulsatile devices.

First, their size is substantially smaller than that of pulsatile devices, since a reservoir chamber is not needed. The pulsatile VAD chamber alone has a volume of about 80 cm^3, while the device itself may require 310 cm^3, compared to as little as 15 cm^3 of space needed for the axial pump. The smaller size makes surgical implantation technically easier, especially since access to the abdominal cavity or the creation of a preperitoneal space is not always needed. Furthermore, their smaller size allows their implantation in any patient, regardless of body habitus. Their design does not involve heart valves, which minimizes trauma to the formed elements of the blood. The control mechanism is simpler and does not require an on/off mode otherwise needed for pulsatile flow generation. In fact, contrary to what was believed in the past, monitoring the afterload dependent operation of the pump through parameters like pump output proved to be unnecessary. Control of pump speed is simply left to the patient, according to the anticipated level of activity. Finally, energy requirements of axial pumps are modest and their operation is silent to the extent of being imperceptible even to the patient.[113]

The Jarvik 2000 Heart

Description

The Jarvik heart is an axial flow impeller pump. The pump itself is inserted into the LV apex and a Dacron outflow graft is anastomosed end-to-side to the thoracic descending aorta. Circulation to the coronaries, the brachiocephalic, the left carotid and the subclavian arteries is thus provided by retrograde flow. The device measures 5.5 cm in length and has a diameter of 2.5 cm. It weighs 85 g and displaces a volume of 25 mL. The pump revolves at speeds of 8000 to 12,000 rpm. Power is delivered percutaneously from external batteries. Electrical connections extend cephalad from the device via the left pleural cavity and the neck to the base of the skull, where a percutaneous titanium pedestal transmits fine electrical wires through the scalp (Figure 9).[114]

Hemodynamic principles

In animal experiments, performed on sheep with normal hearts, the pump performing at the speed of 12,000 rpm leads to a total output greater than preimplantation cardiac output by about 33%. At 15,000 rpm, the left atrium becomes concave or even collapsed, depending on intravascular volume status (preload).

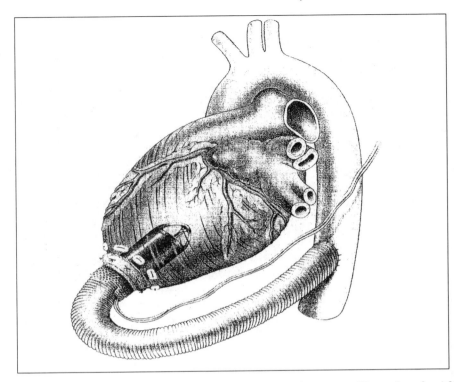

Figure 9. The Jarvik 2000 pump in the ventricular apex. (Reproduced with permission.[114])

The left ventricle is completely unloaded at 10,000 rpm, as signaled by persistent closure of the aortic valve during systole. The mean arterial pressure is noted to vary directly with pump speed. Aortic pulse pressure varies inversely with pump output. In hemodynamic systems operating with an axial pump, pulse pressure is generated by concomitant contribution of the heart itself. When the axial pump assumes total responsibility, pulsatility is somewhat maintained since pump output proper increases during systole due to the higher pump preload rendered by ventricular contraction. At 10,000 rpm, with a persistently closed aortic valve, pulse pressure is a mere 11 ± 4 mm Hg.

In the off mode, the pump allows functional aortic regurgitation via reverse flow through the pump from the descending aorta into the left ventricle during diastole. This reverse flow can amount to up to 21% of total cardiac output and leads to a significant increase in pulmonary capillary wedge pressure (from 14.0 ± 3.8 to 25.0 ± 6.9 mm Hg).[114]

Human Application

The first implantation of the Jarvik 2000 heart in a heart failure patient was performed in June 2000. The device was inserted into the ventricular apex following a left thoracotomy, under cardiopulmonary bypass via femoral arterial and venous cannulation. Immediately after discontinuation of bypass, the VAD was able to provide an output of 5-6 L/min with a mean arterial pressure of 50 to 70 mm Hg. The elevated systemic vascular resistance seen in nonpulsatile flow was treated by hydralazine and then by angiotensin converting enzyme inhibitors. Beta-receptor blockers were used to decrease heart rate, thus improving ventricular filling and, consequently, stroke volume. The higher stroke volume lead to an increase in flow pulsatility, which helped lower vascular resistance. Retrograde flow via the ascending aorta to the cardiac and cerebral circulation did not show any adverse effects. With the pump in the off mode, functional regurgitation was noted as expected. Regurgitant volume was observed to amount as much as 10% of total cardiac output. Systemic anticoagulation with warfarin was used, the international normalized ratio being kept around 2.0. Pump speed is regulated by the patient via a controller.[115]

The advantages of the Jarvik 2000 heart are multiple. Implantation is performed without median sternotomy, which, as discussed earlier, makes the eventual transplantation operation easier. There is no inflow cannula, which rids the patient of the thrombotic and hemolytic problems encountered with inflow cannulae. There is no need for an external pocket in the mediastinum or the peri-peritoneum, which decreases risk of infection. The power transmission takes place via a skull-mounted pedestal built after a cochlear stimulation model. For almost 20 years now, this latter has functioned without report of infection, according to otology reports.[116] Further experience with this VAD is of course needed to fully explore its undoubtedly tremendous impact on the future management of the end-stage heart failure patient.

The MicroMed-DeBakey VAD (MM-D VAD)

Description

The MM-D VAD and the Jarvik 2000 heart, both axial flow pumps, bear certain similarities in design and function. The MM-D device consists of a titanium inflow cannula that is inserted into the LV apex and that leads to the pump proper, which, in turn, connects to the ascending aorta via a Vascutek Gelweave (Sulzer Vascutek, Austin, TX) vascular graft. A monitoring flow probe wraps around the outflow conduit and its wiring exits the skin above the right iliac crest, together with the pump motor cable. The pump is implanted through a median sternotomy in a small extracardiac pocket. The inflow cannula is inserted into the ventricular apex and the outflow graft is sutured to the ascending aorta. Cardiopulmonary bypass is utilized during the operation. Six hours after surgery, intravenous heparin is started while antiplatelet therapy, namely aspirin and dipyridamole, is initiated after successful removal of all chest drains. Oral warfarin therapy is then substituted for intravenous heparin, with target INR levels between 2.5 and 3.5 (Figure 10).[117]

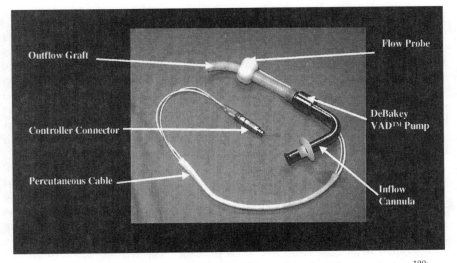

Figure 10. The MicroMed Debakey VAD. (Reproduced with permission.[122])

The pump design allows an output of 5 L/min against an aortic pressure of 100 mm Hg at a rotor speed of 10,000 rpm. The initial period after implantation is characterized by nonpulsatile flow. With time, low amplitude pulsations become detectable. These latter can be abolished at any time by increasing pump speed.[117] During both instances, the aortic valve does not open, suggesting that pulsatility is probably the result of varying pump inflow, and consequently output, with the partial recovery of LV function.

Human Application

The MM-D is the first axial-flow VAD to be used clinically. Clinical trials began as early as November 1988 in Europe. As of November 1999, 18 patients had received the device. Of these, two patients had to undergo VAD replacement with another pump and two other patients died.[118] The clinical application of the MM-D assist device is still in its initial phase. Further experience will undoubtedly add to our understanding of this important assist device.

Axial-flow VADs are the next generation of long-term assist devices. With their numerous advantages they may change the whole philosophy of mechanical ventricular assistance, perhaps to where transplantation would no longer be the only available ultimate therapy.

The Centrifugal Pump

Description

The development of a centrifugal pump goes back to 1969, when Drs. Blackshear and Bernstein designed the first commercially available pump: The Medtronic-BioMedicus pump (Medtronic, Inc.).[119] The principle is to rotate blood in a vortex, hereby imparting a centrifugal force that translates into pressure. Alternatively, one can envision the process as transformation of the mechanical energy of the impeller into kinetic energy conferred to blood. The pump consists of a plastic cone containing an impeller. This latter is set into motion by a magnet motor. Initial designs had a shaft transmit the rotational motion. However, the risk of blood seeping through the seal led to the use of magnetic coupling to put the impeller into motion. Blood is introduced via an inlet at the apex of the cone and exists via a side outlet.

Major advantages of the centrifugal pump are simplicity of design, versatility, and relatively low costs of manufacture and operation. Initial concerns regarding trauma to formed blood elements and the inadequacy of nonpulsatile flow proved not to be of clinical significance and the first application of the centrifugal pump was introduced in 1977 when the Medtronic pump was substituted for the roller pump in cardiopulmonary bypass.[120] Later, the centrifugal pump was applied for LV assistance mainly in postcardiotomy failure. It can be used as femoral-femoral bypass or as left (right) ventricular to aortic (pulmonic artery) bypass (Figure 11).

Hemodynamic Principles

The working characteristics of the centrifugal pump are reminiscent of those of the axial pump already described (Hemopump). The flow rate is dependent on preload, pump speed and, most importantly, the pressure difference (pressure head) between inlet and outlet. If applied to a circulatory system not in ventricular fibrillation, it provides "pulsatile" flow. As the ventricle contracts in systole, the pressure difference across the pump decreases and its pump flow increases. In diastole, the reverse occurs. It is also possible to witness reverse flow during diastole if the pump is operating at low speed (Figure 12).

The slope of the flow-pressure head curve is characteristic of each pump. The shallower (that is, the less negative) the slope is, the more pulsatile the flow. This is easily understandable when one looks at the plot: a shallow curve implies a more important increase in flow with a certain drop in pressure difference when compared to a pump with a steeper slope.[121] Factors that can affect the slope of the flow-pressure difference curve, for instance, are pump inlet and outlet dimensions, among others.

Clinical Experience

The centrifugal pump is widely used for circulatory support especially for post-cardiotomy shock. After failure to wean from bypass is recognized, it is perhaps easiest to apply a pump to the existing bypass cannulation in place. Cannulation can be done through the femoral vessels. The more common cannulation, however, is through the left atrium for the inflow

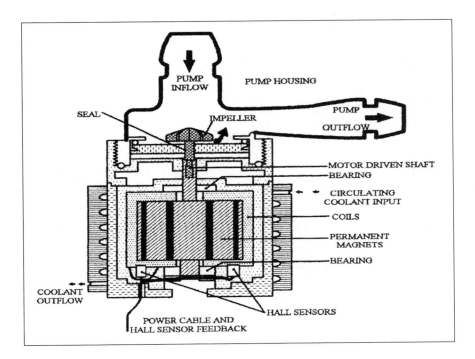

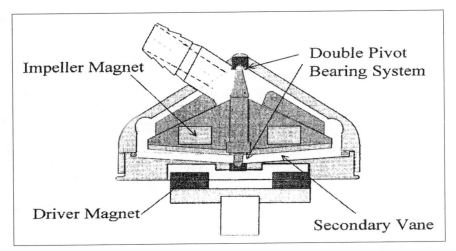

Figure 11. (**A**) The original Medtronic centrifugal pump. Note that rotational motion is transmitted to the impeller via a shaft connected to the motor. (**B**) The Gyro C1E3. Rotational motion is transmitted to the impeller using magnetic energy. Compared to earlier models, this insures better "'seal'" and a decreased thrombogenicity as the area of blood stasis around the shaft is significantly reduced. (Part **A** reproduced with permission from Nose Y, et al. *Artif Organs* 2000;24(6):412-420; Part **B** reproduced with permission from Orime Y, et al. *ASAIO J* 2000;46:128-133.)

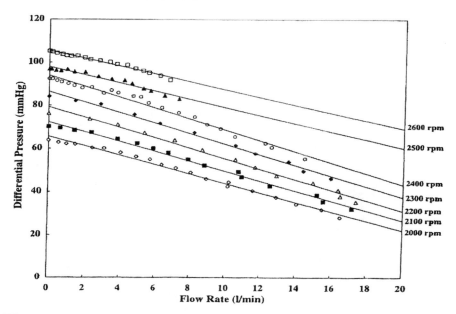

Figure 12. Example of centrifugal pump flow in relation to impeller speed and inflow-outflow pressure deferential. (Reproduced with permission.[121])

and the ascending aorta for the return. The patient requires systemic anticoagulation, usually in the form of intravenous heparin. Some centers use specialized circuits (Carmeda-coated, Medtronic, Inc.) in order to avoid the complications of systemic anticoagulation. This has been proven safe from the thromboembolic standpoint as long as pump flow is maintained above 2.0 L/min. Total duration of support with a centrifugal pump is usually limited to no more than 2 to 3 weeks.[122] After this period is elapsed and the patient still unable to wean from circulatory support, consideration is given for cardiac transplantation or for implantation of a permanent VAD.

Several reports have been published on the clinical experience with centrifugal pumps. In one such report by Joyce and co-workers, the average duration of support was 3.6 days. The proportion of patients who could be weaned or transplanted and then discharged from the hospital was 42%, while the global mortality rate was an alarming 67%.[123] These results are even better than those in the report of the International Registry for Mechanical Assist Pumps, where only 25% of patients were discharged from the hospital.[124]

A comparison of survival rates among different groups of patients is helpful to understand the underlying cause of this high mortality rate. Interestingly, it is not the performance of the centrifugal pump but the patients' underlying condition and the status of the myocardium that dictate their chances for survival. The highest mortality rate, nearing 89%, is reported in those patients who underwent cardiopulmonary resuscitation prior to implantation of the device. Patients who suffered an MI leading to cardiogenic shock fare better, with survival rates approaching

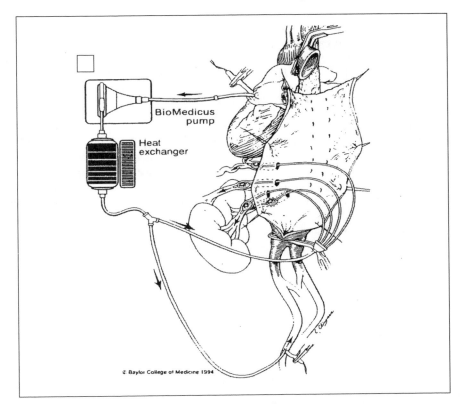

Figure 13. The centrifugal pump in Aortic surgery, refer to text for details. (Reproduced with permission.[128])

27%. The best odds for survival were for those patients who received centrifugal pump support for post-cardiotomy failure. Almost 47% were alive and well after discharge. The most common cause of death in all these patient groups is multiple organ failure.[125]

Complications do arise during the course of support with a centrifugal pump. These are no different than those already mentioned for other types of circulatory assist, namely bleeding, vascular complications, multiple organ failure, and red cell hemolysis.

As we have mentioned earlier, there exists no long-term, implantable cardiac assist device in the form of a centrifugal pump. Nevertheless, such a device has been contemplated by scientists and clinical investigators ever since the early days of centrifugal pump development. The original designers of the centrifugal pump have outlined this concept, taking advantage of the possibility of magnetic coupling in order to create a completely implantable pump with transcutaneous energy transmission.[126] Lately, animal experiments have shown the feasibility of hemodynamic support using a centrifugal pump for a period exceeding 9 months.[127]

As we have discussed above, this important support system has been successfully used in different forms of cardiogenic shock. Another application that illustrates its versatility and usefulness is in thoracoabdominal aortic aneurysm repair surgery. When used to ensure distal aortic and abdominal organ perfusion, the centrifugal pump has been found to reduce markedly the dreaded neurologic complications of this demanding surgery.[128] The long experience of cardiovascular surgeons with the centrifugal pump, together with its simple and effective mode of operation, probably led to its selection for this purpose (Figure 13.)

Mechanical circulatory assist devices have made a significant difference in the lives of many patients who otherwise would have succumbed to their state of shock. As technical advancements happen, we will hopefully reach a point where an assist device will replace the function of the failing heart without need for transplantation. As heart disease continues to top the list of potentially fatal human illness, the hope is that, when we reach that point, the advanced technology involved would be accessible to the many patients who need it.

References

1. Laks H, Ott RA, Standeven JW, et al. The effect of left atrial-to-aortic assistance on infarct size. *Circulation* 1977; 56:II38-43.
2. Laschinger JC, Grossi EA, Cunningham JN, Jr., et al. Adjunctive left ventricular unloading during myocardial reperfusion plays a major role in minimizing myocardial infarct size. *J Thorac Cardiovasc Surg* 1985; 90:80-85.
3. Van Winkle DM, Matsuki T, Gad NM, et al. Left ventricular unloading during reperfusion does not limit myocardial infarct size. *Circulation* 1990; 81:1374-1379.
4. Kantrowitz A, Tjonneland S, Freed PS, et al. Initial clinical experience with intraaortic balloon pumping in cardiogenic shock. *JAMA* 1968; 203:113-118.
5. Bregman D, Casarella WJ. Percutaneous intraaortic balloon pumping: Initial clinical experience. *Ann Thorac Surg* 1980; 29:153-155.
6. Tepe NA, Edmunds LH, Jr. Operation for acute postinfarction mitral insufficiency and cardiogenic shock. *J Thorac Cardiovasc Surg* 1985; 89:525-530.
7. Naunheim KS, Swartz MT, Pennington DG, et al. Intraaortic balloon pumping in patients requiring cardiac operations. Risk analysis and long-term follow-up. *J Thorac Cardiovasc Surg* 1992; 104:1654-1660; discussion 1660-1651.
8. Christenson JT, Badel P, Simonet F, et al. Preoperative intraaortic balloon pump enhances cardiac performance and improves the outcome of redo CABG. *Ann Thorac Surg* 1997; 64:1237-1244.
9. Peric M, Frazier O, Macris M, et al. Intra-aortic balloon pump as a bridge to tranplantation (abstract). *J Heart Transplant* 1986; 5:380.
10. Normal JC, Cooley DA, Igo SR, et al. Prognostic indices for survival during postcardiotomy intra-aortic balloon pumping. Methods of scoring and classification, with implications for left ventricular assist device utilization. *J Thorac Cardiovasc Surg* 1977; 74:709-720.
11. Gibbon J. Artificial maintenance of life during experimental occlusion of the pulmonary artery. *Arch Surg* 1937; 34:1105-1131.
12. Gibbon J. The maintenance of life during experimental occlusion of the pulmonary artery followed by survival. *Surg Gynecol Obstet* 1939; 69:602-614.

13. Shawl F, Ballentine B, Slonine D, et al. Percutaneous institution of cardiopulmonary (bypass) support: Technique and complications (abstract). *J Am Coll Cardiol* 1989; 13:159A.

14. Tommaso C. Use of percutaneously inserted cardiopulmonary bypass in the cardiac catheterization laboratory. *Cathet Cardivasc Diag* 1990; 20:32-38.

15. Kirklin JK, Westaby S, Blackstone EH, et al. Complement and the damaging effects of cardiopulmonary bypass. *J Thorac Cardiovasc Surg* 1983; 86:845-857.

16. Hashimoto K, Miyamoto H, Suzuki K, et al. Evidence of organ damage after cardiopulmonary bypass. The role of elastase and vasoactive mediators. *J Thorac Cardiovasc Surg* 1992; 104:666-673.

17. Salisbury P, Bor N, Lewin R, et al. Effects of partial and of total lung bypass on the heart. *J Appl Physiol* 1959; 14.

18. Lefemine AA, Flessas A, Moon HS. Left ventricular bypass for ventricular failure. Technical and hemodynamic considerations. *J Thorac Cardiovasc Surg* 1973; 65:758-767.

19. Axelrod HI, Galloway AC, Murphy MS, et al. Percutaneous cardiopulmonary bypass with a synchronous pulsatile pump combines effective unloading with ease of application. *J Thorac Cardiovasc Surg* 1987; 93:358-365.

20. Scholz KH, Figulla HR, Schroder T, et al. Pulmonary and left ventricular decompression by artificial pulmonary valve incompetence during percutaneous cardiopulmonary bypass support in cardiac arrest. *Circulation* 1995; 91:2664-2668.

21. von Segesser LK. Cardiopulmonary support and extracorporeal membrane oxygenation for cardiac assist. *Ann Thorac Surg* 1999; 68:672-677.

22. The use of extracorporeal circulation for circulatory support during PTCA. *J Thorac Cardiovasc Surg* 1990; 99:385-386.

23. Hill JG, Bruhn PS, Cohen SE, et al. Emergent applications of cardiopulmonary support: A multiinstitutional experience. *Ann Thorac Surg* 1992; 54:699-704.

24. Wampler RK, Moise JC, Frazier OH, et al. In vivo evaluation of a peripheral vascular access axial flow blood pump. *ASAIO Trans* 1988; 34:450-454.

25. Frazier OH, Wampler RK, Duncan JM, et al. First human use of the Hemopump, a catheter-mounted ventricular assist device. *Ann Thorac Surg* 1990; 49:299-304.

26. Meyns B, Siess T, Laycock S, et al. The heart-Hemopump interaction: A study of Hemopump flow as a function of cardiac activity. *Artif Organs* 1996; 20:641-649.

27. Wulff J, Lonn U, Keck KY, et al. Flow characteristics of the Hemopump: An experimental in vitro study. *Ann Thorac Surg* 1997; 63:162-166.

28. Lachat M, Jaggy C, Leskosek B, et al. Hemodynamic properties of the hemopump HP14. *Int J Artif Organs* 1999; 22:155-159.

29. Wampler RK, Frazier OH, Lansing AM, et al. Treatment of cardiogenic shock with the Hemopump left ventricular assist device. *Ann Thorac Surg* 1991; 52:506-513.

30. Smalling RW, Sweeney M, Lachterman B, et al. Transvalvular left ventricular assistance in cardiogenic shock secondary to acute myocardial infarction. Evidence for recovery from near fatal myocardial stunning. *J Am Coll Cardiol* 1994; 23:637-644.

31. Merhige ME, Smalling RW, Cassidy D, et al. Effect of the hemopump left ventricular assist device on regional myocardial perfusion and function.

Reduction of ischemia during coronary occlusion. *Circulation* 1989; 80:III158-166.

32. Meyns B, Sergeant P, Wouters P, et al. Mechanical support with microaxial blood pumps for postcardiotomy left ventricular failure: can outcome be predicted? *J Thorac Cardiovasc Surg* 2000; 120:393-400.

33. Meyns BP, Sergeant PT, Daenen WJ, Flameng WJ. Left ventricular assistance with the transthoracic 24F Hemopump for recovery of the failing heart. *Ann Thorac Surg* 1995; 60:392-397.

34. Wiebalck AC, Wouters PF, Waldenberger FR, et al. Left ventricular assist with an axial flow pump (Hemopump): Clinical application. *Ann Thorac Surg* 1993; 55:1141-1146.

35. Scholz KH, Dubois-Rande JL, Urban P, et al. Clinical experience with the percutaneous hemopump during high-risk coronary angioplasty. *Am J Cardiol* 1998; 82:1107-1110, A1106.

36. Sweeney M, Frazier O. Device supported myocardial revascularization. *Ann Thorac Surg* 1992; 54:1065-1070[Abstract].

37. Lonn U, Peterzen B, Granfeldt H, et al. Coronary artery operation supported by the Hemopump: An experimental study on pig. *Ann Thorac Surg* 1994; 58:516-518.

38. Lonn U, Peterzen B, Carnstam B, et al. Beating heart coronary surgery supported by an axial blood flow pump. *Ann Thorac Surg* 1999; 67:99-104.

39. Meyns B, Vanermen H, Vanhaecke J, et al. Hemopump fails as bridge to transplantation in postinfarction ventricular septal defect. *J Heart Lung Transplant* 1994; 13:1133-1137.

40. Frazier OH, Benedict CR, Radovancevic B, et al. Improved left ventricular function after chronic left ventricular unloading. *Ann Thorac Surg* 1996; 62:675-681; discussion 681-672.

41. Levin HR, Oz MC, Chen JM, et al. Reversal of chronic ventricular dilation in patients with end-stage cardiomyopathy by prolonged mechanical unloading. *Circulation* 1995; 91:2717-2720.

42. Moazami N, Argenziano M, Kohomoto T, et al. Inflow valve regurgitation during left ventricular assist device support may interfere with reverse ventricular remodeling. *Ann Thorac Surg* 1998; 65:628-631.

43. Muller J, Wallukat G, Weng YG, et al. Weaning from mechanical cardiac support in patients with idiopathic dilated cardiomyopathy. *Circulation* 1997; 96:542-549.

44. Nakatani S, McCarthy PM, Kottke-Marchant K, et al. Left ventricular echocardiographic and histologic changes: Impact of chronic unloading by an implantable ventricular assist device. *J Am Coll Cardiol* 1996; 27:894-901.

45. Burkhoff D, Holmes JW, Madigan J, et al. Left ventricular assist device-induced reverse ventricular remodeling. *Prog Cardiovasc Dis* 2000; 43:19-26.

46. Pieske B, Sutterlin M, Schmidt-Schweda S, et al. Diminished post-rest potentiation of contractile force in human dilated cardiomyopathy. Functional evidence for alterations in intracellular Ca2+ handling. *J Clin Invest* 1996; 98:764-776.

47. Arai M, Alpert NR, MacLennan DH, et al. Alterations in sarcoplasmic reticulum gene expression in human heart failure. A possible mechanism for alterations in systolic and diastolic properties of the failing myocardium. *Circ Res* 1993; 72:463-469.

48. Go LO, Moschella MC, Watras J, et al. Differential regulation of two types of intracellular calcium release channels during end-stage heart failure. *J Clin Invest* 1995; 95:888-894.

49. McDonald D. Blood Flow in Arteries. In: Nichols WW, O'Rourke MF (eds): Baltimore: Williams & Wilkins, 1974.

50. Hickey PR, Buckley MJ, Philbin DM. Pulsatile and nonpulsatile cardiopulmonary bypass: Review of a counterproductive controversy. *Ann Thorac Surg* 1983; 36:720-737.

51. Mavroudis C. To pulse or not to pulse. *Ann Thorac Surg* 1978; 25:259-271.

52. Angell James JE, Daly M. Effects of graded pulsatile pressure on the reflex vasomotor responses elicited by changes of mean pressure in the perfused carotid sinus- aortic arch regions of the dog. *J Physiol* 1971; 214:51-64.

53. Philbin DM, Coggins CH, Wilson N, et al. Antidiuretic hormone levels during cardiopulmonary bypass. *J Thorac Cardiovasc Surg* 1977; 73:145-148.

54. Goodman TA, Gerard DF, Bernstein EF, et al. The effects of pulseless perfusion on the distribution of renal cortical blood flow and on renin release. *Surgery* 1976; 80:31-39.

55. Moores WY, Hannon JP, Crum J, et al. Coronary flow distribution and dynamics during continuous and pulsatile extracorporeal circulation in the pig. *Ann Thorac Surg* 1977; 24:582-590.

56. Yada I, Golding LR, Harasaki H, et al. Physiopathological studies of nonpulsatile blood flow in chronic models. *Trans Am Soc Artif Intern Organs* 1983; 29:520-525.

57. Tsutsui T, Sutton C, Harasaki H, et al. Idioperipheral pulsation during nonpulsatile biventricular bypass experiments. *ASAIO Trans* 1986; 32:263-268.

58. Santamore WP, Lynch PR, Meier G, et al. Myocardial interaction between the ventricles. *J Appl Physiol* 1976; 41:362-368.

59. Maruyama Y, Ashikawa K, Isoyama S, et al. Mechanical interactions between four heart chambers with and without the pericardium in canine hearts. *Circ Res* 1982; 50:86-100.

60. Maughan WL, Sunagawa K, Sagawa K. Ventricular systolic interdependence: Volume elastance model in isolated canine hearts. *Am J Physiol* 1987; 253:H1381-1390.

61. Damiano RJ, Jr., La Follette P, Jr., Cox JL, et al. Significant left ventricular contribution to right ventricular systolic function. *Am J Physiol* 1991; 261:H1514-1524.

62. Farrar DJ, Compton PG, Dajee H, et al. Right heart function during left heart assist and the effects of volume loading in a canine preparation. *Circulation* 1984; 70:708-716.

63. Chow E, Farrar DJ. Right heart function during prosthetic left ventricular assistance in a porcine model of congestive heart failure. *J Thorac Cardiovasc Surg* 1992; 104:569-578.

64. Daly RC, Chandrasekaran K, Cavarocchi NC, et al. Ischemia of the interventricular septum. A mechanism of right ventricular failure during mechanical left ventricular assist. *J Thorac Cardiovasc Surg* 1992; 103:1186-1191.

65. Farrar DJ, Compton PG, Hershon JJ, et al. Right heart interaction with the mechanically assisted left heart. *World J Surg* 1985; 9:89-102.

66. Nakatani S, Thomas JD, Savage RM, et al. Prediction of right ventricular dysfunction after left ventricular assist device implantation. *Circulation* 1996; 94:II216-221.

67. Fukamachi K, McCarthy PM, Smedira NG, et al. Preoperative risk factors for right ventricular failure after implantable left ventricular assist device insertion. *Ann Thorac Surg* 1999; 68:2181-2184.

68. Chen JM, Levin HR, Rose EA, et al. Experience with right ventricular assist devices for perioperative right-sided circulatory failure. *Ann Thorac Surg* 1996; 61:305-310; discussion 311-303.

69. Gristina AG, Giridhar G, Gabriel BL, et al. Cell biology and molecular mechanisms in artificial device infections. *Int J Artif Organs* 1993; 16:755-763.

70. McCarthy PM, Schmitt SK, Vargo RL, et al. Implantable LVAD infections: Implications for permanent use of the device. *Ann Thorac Surg* 1996; 61:359-365; discussion 372-353.

71. Holman WL, Murrah CP, Ferguson ER, et al. Infections during extended circulatory support: University of Alabama at Birmingham experience 1989 to 1994. *Ann Thorac Surg* 1996; 61:366-371; discussion 372-363.

72. Itescu S, Ankersmit JH, Kocher AA, et al. Immunobiology of left ventricular assist devices. *Prog Cardiovasc Dis* 2000; 43:67-80.

73. Spanier T, Oz M, Rose E, et al. Activation of NFKb is central to the proinflammatory/procoagulant response in textured surface left ventricular assist device recipients and may be influenced by anit-inflammatory intervention with aspirin. *J Heart Lung Transplant* 1997; 17:80.

74. Spanier T, Rose E, Schmidt A, et al. Interactions between dendritic cells and T cells on the surface of left ventricular assist devices leads to a Th2 pattern of cytokine production and B cell hypreactivity in vivo. *Circulation* 1996; 94:1704.

75. Ankersmit HJ, Tugulea S, Spanier T, et al. Activation-induced T-cell death and immune dysfunction after implantation of left-ventricular assist device. *Lancet* 1999; 354:550-555.

76. Moazami N, Itescu S, Williams MR, et al. Platelet transfusions are associated with the development of anti-major histocompatibility complex class I antibodies in patients with left ventricular assist support. *J Heart Lung Transplant* 1998; 17:876-880.

77. Itescu S, Tung TC, Burke EM, et al. Preformed IgG antibodies against major histocompatibility complex class II antigens are major risk factors for high-grade cellular rejection in recipients of heart transplantation. *Circulation* 1998; 98:786-793.

78. Glotz D, Haymann JP, Sansonetti N, et al. Suppression of HLA-specific alloantibodies by high-dose intravenous immunoglobulins (IVIg). A potential tool for transplantation of immunized patients. *Transplantation* 1993; 56:335-337.

79. Brunner T, Yoo NJ, LaFace D, et al. Activation-induced cell death in murine T cell hybridomas. Differential regulation of Fas (CD95) versus Fas ligand expression by cyclosporin A and FK506. *Int Immunol* 1996; 8:1017-1026.

80. Didisheim P. Current concepts of thrombosis and infection in artificial organs. *Asaio J* 1994; 40:230-237.

81. Rose EA, Levin HR, Oz MC, et al. Artificial circulatory support with textured interior surfaces. A counterintuitive approach to minimizing thromboembolism. *Circulation* 1994; 90:II87-91.

82. Friedel N, Viazis P, Schiessler A, et al. Patient selection for mechanical circulatory support as a bridge to cardiac transplantation. *Int J Artif Organs* 1991; 14:276-279.

83. Farrar DJ. Preoperative predictors of survival in patients with Thoratec ventricular assist devices as a bridge to heart transplantation. Thoratec Ventricular Assist Device Principal Investigators. *J Heart Lung Transplant* 1994; 13:93-100; discussion 100- 101.

84. Kaltenmaier B, Pommer W, Kaufmann F, et al. Outcome of patients with ventricular assist devices and acute renal failure requiring renal replacement therapy. *Asaio J* 2000; 46:330-333.

85. Miller LW. Mechanical assist devices in intensive cardiac care. *Am Heart J* 1991; 121:1887-1892.

86. Reinhartz O, Farrar DJ, Hershon JH, et al. Importance of preoperative liver function as a predictor of survival in patients supported with Thoratec ventricular assist devices as a bridge to transplantation. *J Thorac Cardiovasc Surg* 1998; 116:633-640.

87. Savage R, McCarthy P, Stewart W, et al. Intraoperative transesophageal echocardiographic evaluation of the implantable left ventricular assist device. *Vid J Echocardiography* 1992; 2:125-136.

88. McCarthy P, Smedira N. Implantable LVAD insertion in patients with previous heart surgery. *J Heart Lung Transplant* 2000; 19:S95-S100.

89. Semigran MJ, Cockrill BA, Kacmarek R, et al. Hemodynamic effects of inhaled nitric oxide in heart failure. *J Am Coll Cardiol* 1994; 24:982-988.

90. Heath MJ, Dickstein ML. Perioperative management of the left ventricular assist device recipient. *Prog Cardiovasc Dis* 2000; 43:47-54.

91. Olsen EK, Pierce WS, Donachy JH, et al. A two and one half year clinical experience with a mechanical left ventricular assist pump in the treatment of profound postoperative heart failure. *Int J Artif Organs* 1979; 2:197-206.

92. Whittaker S, Glanville C. The Thoratec ventricular assist device system. *Perfusion* 2000; 15:363-368.

93. Holman WL, Bourge RC, Murrah CP, et al. Left atrial or ventricular cannulation beyond 30 days for a Thoratec ventricular assist device. *Asaio J* 1995; 41:M517-522.

94. Farrar D, Compton P, Lawson J, et al. Control modes of a clinical ventricular assist device. *IEEE Engr Med Biol* 1986; 5:19-25.

95. Mihaylov D, Verkerke GJ, Blanksma PK, et al. Evaluation of the optimal driving mode during left ventricular assist with pulsatile catheter pump in calves. *Artif Organs* 1999; 23:1117-1122.

96. Hill JD, Farrar DJ, Hershon JJ, et al. Use of a prosthetic ventricle as a bridge to cardiac transplantation for postinfarction cardiogenic shock. *N Engl J Med* 1986; 314:626-628.

97. Corp. TL. Thoratec voluntary registry data. St. Ives: Cambs: Thoratec Laboratories Corp., Woburn, Massachusetts.

98. McBride LR, Naunheim KS, Fiore AC, et al. Clinical experience with 111 thoratec ventricular assist devices. *Ann Thorac Surg* 1999; 67:1233-1238; discussion 1238-1239.

99. Farrar DJ, Lawson JH, Litwak P, et al. Thoratec VAD system as a bridge to heart transplantation. *J Heart Transplant* 1990; 9:415-422; discussion 422-413.

100. Wassenberg PA. The Abiomed BVS 5000 biventricular support system. *Perfusion* 2000; 15:369-371.

101. Couper GS, Dekkers RJ, Adams DH. The logistics and cost-effectiveness of circulatory support: Advantages of the ABIOMED BVS 5000. *Ann Thorac Surg* 1999; 68:646-649.

102. McCarthy PM, Hoercher K. Clinically available intracorporeal left ventricular assist devices. *Prog Cardiovasc Dis* 2000; 43:37-46.

103. Portner P, Oyer P, McGregor C, et al. First human use of an electrically powered implantable ventricular assist system (abstract). *Artif Organs* 1985; 9:36.

104. Robbins RC, Oyer PE. Bridge to transplant with the Novacor left ventricular assist system. *Ann Thorac Surg* 1999; 68:695-697.

105. de Vivo F, De Santo LS, Maiello C, et al. Novacor left ventricular assist device: Present experience. *Int J Artif Organs* 1999; 22:11-13.

106. Murali S. Mechanical circulatory support with the Novacor LVAS: Worldwide clinical results. *Thorac Cardiovasc Surg* 1999; 47 Suppl 2:321-325.

107. Minami K, El-Banayosy A, Sezai A, et al. Morbidity and outcome after mechanical ventricular support using Thoratec, Novacor, and HeartMate for bridging to heart transplantation. *Artif Organs* 2000; 24:421-426.

108. Frazier OH, Myers TJ, Radovancevic B. The HeartMate left ventricular assist system. Overview and 12-year experience. *Tex Heart Inst J* 1998; 25:265-271.

109. Poirier VL. Worldwide experience with the TCI HeartMate system: Issues and future perspective. *Thorac Cardiovasc Surg* 1999; 47 Suppl 2:316-320.

110. McCarthy PM, Smedira NO, Vargo RL, et al. One hundred patients with the HeartMate left ventricular assist device: Evolving concepts and technology. *J Thorac Cardiovasc Surg* 1998; 115:904-912.

111. DeRose JJ, Jr., Umana JP, Argenziano M, et al. Implantable left ventricular assist devices provide an excellent outpatient bridge to transplantation and recovery. *J Am Coll Cardiol* 1997; 30:1773-1777.

112. El-Banayosy A, Arusoglu L, Kizner L, et al. Novacor left ventricular assist system versus Heartmate vented electric left ventricular assist system as a long-term mechanical circulatory support device in bridging patients: A prospective study. *J Thorac Cardiovasc Surg* 2000; 119:581-587.

113. Nose Y, Kawahito K, Nakazawa T. Can we develop a nonpulsatile permanent rotary blood pump? Yes, we can. *Artif Organs* 1996; 20:467-474.

114. Westaby S, Katsumata T, Houel R, et al. Jarvik 2000 heart: Potential for bridge to myocyte recovery. *Circulation* 1998; 98:1568-1574.

115. Westaby S, Banning AP, Jarvik R, et al. First permanent implant of the Jarvik 2000 Heart. *Lancet* 2000; 356:900-903.

116. Parkin JL. Percutaneous pedestal in cochlear implantation. *Ann Otol Rhinol Laryngol* 1990; 99:796-800.

117. Wieselthaler GM, Schima H, Hiesmayr M, et al. First clinical experience with the DeBakey VAD continuous-axial-flow pump for bridge to transplantation. *Circulation* 2000; 101:356-359.

118. Noon GP, Morley D, Irwin S, et al. Development and clinical application of the MicroMed DeBakey VAD. *Curr Opin Cardiol* 2000; 15:166-171.

119. Dorman F, Bernstein EF, Blackshear PL, et al. Progress in the design of a centrifugal cardiac assist pump with trans- cutaneous energy transmission by magnetic coupling. *Trans Am Soc Artif Intern Organs* 1969; 15:441-448.

120. Lynch MF, Peterson D, Baker V. Centrifugal blood pumping for open heart surgery. *Minn Med* 1978; 61:536-538.

121. Tagusari O, Yamazaki K, Litwak P, et al. Effect of pressure-flow relationship of centrifugal pump on in vivo hemodynamics: A consideration for design. *Artif Organs* 1998; 22:399-404.

122. Noon GP, Lafuente JA, Irwin S. Acute and temporary ventricular support with BioMedicus centrifugal pump. *Ann Thorac Surg* 1999; 68:650-654.

123. Joyce LD, Kiser JC, Eales F, et al. Experience with generally accepted centrifugal pumps: Personal and collective experience. *Ann Thorac Surg* 1996; 61:287-290; discussion 311-283.

124. Pae WE, Jr. Ventricular assist devices and total artificial hearts: A combined registry experience. *Ann Thorac Surg* 1993; 55:295-298.

125. El-Banayosy A, Posival H, Minami K, et al. Seven years of experience with the centrifugal pump in patients with cardiogenic shock. *Thorac Cardiovasc Surg* 1995; 43:347-351.

126. Bernstein EF, Dorman FD, Blackshear PL Jr., et al. An efficient, compact blood pump for assisted circulation. *Surgery* 1970; 68:105-115.

127. Ohtsuka G, Nakata K, Yoshikawa M, et al. Long-term in vivo left ventricular assist device study for 284 days with Gyro PI pump. *Artif Organs* 1999; 23:504-507.

128. Safi HJ. Role of the BioMedicus pump and distal aortic perfusion in thoracoabdominal aortic aneurysm repair. *Artif Organs* 1996; 20:694-699.

Chapter 14

Myocardial Metabolic Support in Cardiogenic Shock

Carl S. Apstein, MD and Kurt W. Saupe, PhD

Introduction

Much evidence has accumulated that therapeutic manipulation of myocardial metabolism, also known as "metabolic support," can improve outcome in clinical situations in which myocardial ischemia is present. However, there are as of yet no clinical trials that investigate the safety and efficacy of metabolic support in patients with ischemic cardiogenic shock. To evaluate the possibility that metabolic support may be a useful therapy in patients with ischemic cardiogenic shock, this chapter reviews (1) evidence that metabolic support (in the form of <u>high levels of glucose and insulin</u>) is beneficial during clinical situations similar to cardiogenic shock, and (2) studies of metabolic support (again, in the form of a high level of glucose and insulin) in animal models of shock and shock-related situations. Clinical trials of glucose and insulin during both "pathological" and "surgical" ischemia and reperfusion will be reviewed as will the experimental studies which provide insight into the basic mechanisms by which glucose and insulin are beneficial during ischemia.

Myocardial Metabolism and Metabolic Support

In the healthy, well-oxygenated heart, adenosine triphosphate (ATP) is synthesized primarily by oxidation of long-chain free fatty acids (FFA), with lesser amounts of ATP synthesized from oxidation of short and medium-chain FFA, glucose, lactate, ketones, as well as by anaerobic glycolysis. The relative contribution of each substrate to total myocardial ATP

From: Hollenberg SM, Bates ER. *Cardiogenic Shock*. Armonk, NY: Futura Publishing Co., Inc.; ©2002.

production is influenced by factors including age, disease state, and the concentrations of the substrates in the arterial blood. This latter factor is exploited in the studies discussed in this chapter, in which circulating concentrations of glucose and insulin are raised to increase myocardial glucose utilization. Because the heart can generate ATP from many different substrates, and rapidly switch from one substrate to another, it has been called an "omnivore." The omnivorous behavior of the heart allows for experimental and clinical manipulation of cardiac metabolism, which has been termed "metabolic support."

When the myocardium becomes ischemic, the relative contribution of FFA oxidation to total ATP synthesis decreases, while the contribution of ATP from metabolism of glucose increases. Therapeutically, most forms of metabolic support attempt to exaggerate this switch in myocardial metabolism by inhibiting oxidation of FFA, by increasing myocardial metabolism of glucose, or some combination of both. Currently, there are two general methods for manipulating myocardial metabolism. The first involves pharmacological stimulation or inhibition of metabolic enzyme(s). Several pharmacological agents appear to directly increase glucose oxidation, reduce FFA oxidation, and confer a degree of myocardial anti-ischemic protection; these include trimetazidine, ranolazine, etomoxir, and dichloroacetate. Lopaschuk[1] has recently reviewed the anti-ischemic effects and mechanisms by which these agents influence energy metabolism.

The focus of this review will be a second, more "low-tech" approach to manipulating myocardial metabolism, by altering the concentrations of substrates in the arterial blood. Specifically, we will discuss studies where supplemental glucose and insulin (and potassium in the clinical and whole animal studies) were administered.

Concerns Regarding Use of Metabolic Support During Ischemia

The value of raising the arterial concentration of glucose as a form of metabolic support for ischemic myocardium has been hotly debated during the last 30 years. During this time several concerns have been raised. Neely warned against the damaging effects of myocardial accumulation of glycolytic products, and argued that a *reduction* of glycolysis and maintenance of a low tissue lactate level may be just as important in protecting the heart as maintenance of ATP levels via increased anaerobic glycolysis.[2] In 1970, Opie argued that increasing blood glucose levels would be good for the survival of ischemic myocardium by *increasing* the rate of anaerobic glycolysis, by reversing ion losses, by a direct membrane effect, by altering the extracellular volume, and by decreasing circulating free fatty acid levels.[3]

The key to resolving this concern regarding the advisability of increasing the rate of anaerobic glycolysis in the ischemic heart relates to a second issue, namely that for metabolic support to be efficacious, there must be adequate myocardial blood flow to both (1) deliver the substrates to the myocytes, and (2) wash out any harmful metabolites. Although there are no clinical data reporting myocardial perfusion levels specifically from cardiogenic shock patients, recent elegant measurements of myocardial perfusion during the initial hospital presentation of patients with acute myocardial infarction (MI) have demonstrated that the acute infarct region is one of moderate low-flow, not severe or zero-flow ischemia.[4-7] Thus, the level of tissue perfusion in a significant fraction of the acutely infarcting region appears to be more than adequate for successful metabolic manipulation. The transmural distribution of the residual ischemic flow is heterogeneous. This condition of heterogeneous low-flow ischemia creates a "mixed" metabolic milieu where both anaerobic glycolysis and oxidative phosphorylation actively coexist, creating a situation where provision of alternate substrates can influence glycolytic or oxidative pathways. It is likely that myocardial perfusion is also heterogeneous in the setting of cardiogenic shock. The ventricle in shock usually initially consists of a large area of acute severe ischemia, or a mixture of chronic infarction and recent ischemia, and a relatively nonischemic region that becomes progressively underperfused as systemic arterial pressure decreases.

Clinical Studies of Glucose-Insulin-Potassium

There are no clinical studies of post-MI cardiogenic shock that use any type of myocardial metabolic support. Until such studies are performed, only tentative conclusions can be made by extrapolation from studies of metabolic support in closely related clinical settings. There is now substantial clinical evidence (see Table 1) favoring the use of myocardial metabolic support with glucose-insulin-potassium (GIK) in the management of (1) acute MI without distinction as to the presence of shock, (2) the ischemia and reperfusion which accompany cardiac surgery, and (3) left ventricular (LV) pump failure as a complication of coronary artery bypass graft (CABG) surgery, which represents a specific form of cardiogenic shock.

Table 1.

Major Clinical Trials where GIK Has Decreased Mortality Risk

Study	Clinical Condition	Sample size	Mortality Decrease
GIK meta-analysis:[8]	Acute MI; No Reperfusion	1932	28% (p = 0.004)
DIGAMI;[9]	Acute MI ± Reperfusion	620	29% (p = 0.027)
ECLA[10,11]	Acute MI + Reperfusion	252	66% (p = 0.004)
Post-op cardiogenic shock[12]		322	34% (p < 0.02)

DIGAMI = Diabetes Insulin-Glucose in Acute Myocardial Infarction
ECLA = Estudios Cardiologicos LatinoAmerica
GIK = Glucose-Insulin-Potassium

GIK in Acute Myocardial Infarction: Trials from the Pre-Thrombolytic Era

In 1962, Sodi-Pallares et al.[13] reported in a small nonrandomized trial that GIK improved some of the ECG abnormalities associated with acute MI, reduced ventricular arrhythmias, and improved early survival. Subsequent clinical trials yielded conflicting and inconclusive results, but many of these trials were of poor study design, often due to inadequate knowledge of the pathophysiology of acute MI. For example, several trials initiated therapy as late as 48 hours after the onset of chest pain, too late to influence MI size. Others used inadequate glucose and did not achieve the glucose and insulin plasma levels required to maximally decrease plasma FFA levels. It is not surprising that such studies showed no benefit.[8] Moreover, none of these pre-thrombolytic trials had a large sample size, and therefore lacked the statistical power to rigorously assess GIK.

Nonetheless, one of the best early randomized trials, done by Rackley and colleagues,[14] reported that GIK improved cardiac function, decreased ventricular arrhythmias, and was associated with a trend toward a decreased mortality risk. The Rackley GIK regimen consisted of a solution of 30% glucose (300 gm/L), 50 units of regular insulin per liter, and 80 mEq of KCl/L, given intravenously at 1.5 mL/kg/hour, or approximately 2.5 L per day for a 70 kg patient. This protocol was developed from dose-response studies of glucose and insulin whose goal was to maximize myocardial glucose uptake and decrease arterial FFA levels and myocardial FFA uptake.[5] The successful effects of this regimen on myocardial energy metabolism are summarized in Table 2. During the first 24-48 hours of treatment of patients with acute MI, despite a significant infusion of volume, pulmonary capillary pressure decreased and cardiac output and ejection fraction increased. This clinical functional improvement could have resulted from either improved systolic or diastolic function, consistent with experimental studies (see below) which have shown that glucose and insulin treatment can improve both systolic and diastolic dysfunction during ischemia and reperfusion.

To overcome the historical deficits of small sample size and poor study designs, a retrospective meta-analysis overview was done for all

---

Table 2.

Effects of the Rackley GIK Regimen on Myocardial Metabolism

- Blood glucose levels increased to 200-250 mg/100mL
- Myocardial glucose uptake increased by 250%
- Blood free fatty acid (FFA) levels decreased by 70%, from 950 to 300 μM.
- Myocardial FFA uptake decreased by 90%
- Myocardial oxygen consumption: no change
- Myocardial respiratory quotient ($CO_2:O_2$) increased from 0.70 to 0.93, indicating a shift from fat to carbohydrate oxidation
- Blood K^+ increased from 4 to 5 mEq/L

---

randomized placebo-controlled trials of GIK for acute MI done in the pre-fibrinolytic era.[8] This analysis concluded that GIK was highly likely to reduce mortality risk in acute MI. Trials were included for the meta-analysis only if GIK (or placebo) was started within 48 hours of chest pain. In nine such trials, involving 1932 patients, in-hospital mortality was reduced by 28% relative to the placebo group by the GIK therapy (p = 0.004).

GIK in Acute Myocardial Infarction: Trials With Reperfusion

Urgent reperfusion by thrombolytic therapy or primary angioplasty is now standard care for acute MI, and several studies have reported significant mortality reductions when GIK was used in such a clinical setting. In a small nonrandomized study,[15] 44 patients with acute MI treated with fibrinolysis also received GIK, carnitine and magnesium by peripheral intravenous infusion. Those patients receiving this combined "metabolic support" had a significantly lower incidence of death or heart failure development than historical control patients treated with throm-bolysis but without concomitant metabolic support. This study also dem-onstrated that a central venous line is not required for GIK delivery.

Similarly, in the Swedish Diabetes Insulin-Glucose in Acute Myocar-dial Infarction (DIGAMI) trial[9] half of the patients received fibrinolytic therapy for acute MI and were randomized to receive either glucose plus insulin (G+I) followed by multi-dose insulin therapy or standard care. In the G+I group, there was a trend towards a decrease in mortality at 3 months post-MI, and this became significant at 1 year post-MI (29% relative mortality reduction, p = 0.027). Although the DIGAMI trial specif-ically enrolled diabetics, its results may be applicable to nondiabetics as well, because the most dramatic benefit of the G+I therapy was seen in the patients with only "borderline" or mild diabetes, i.e., patients who did not require insulin prior to their hospitalization for acute MI. In this subgroup of patients, the in-hospital mortality was reduced by 58% by G+I (p < 0.05) and the 1-year mortality was reduced by 52% (p < 0.02)

The strongest evidence for the benefits of GIK in the treatment of acute MI in the era of emergent reperfusion therapy comes from the recent ECLA (Estudios Cardiologicos LatinoAmerica) study.[10,11] This was the largest prospective, randomized trial of GIK for the treatment of acute MI ever carried out , and the only such trial done in the era of thrombolytic therapy. There was a remarkable 66% reduction (2p = 0.008) in the relative in-hospital mortality risk when GIK was added to reperfusion (95% of those reperfused had thrombolysis, 5% had primary percutaneous translu-minal coronary angioplasty [PTCA]) relative to reperfusion alone; the absolute mortality risk decreased from 15.2% to 5.2%.

The ECLA study also compared high dose GIK (the Rackley regimen) to a lower dose. During the 1-year follow-up period the high dose GIK group had a statistically significant survival advantage relative to the control group, but the low dose GIK group did not, suggesting a greater degree of myocardial salvage by the high dose GIK. There was no difference in the in-hospital mortality risk between the high and low dose GIK groups, but this result is not conclusive because the small group sizes, with 8-10 deaths per group, provided little statistical power for ruling out a dose-related difference. The superiority of the high dose GIK in the ECLA study is consistent with the recent meta-analysis of GIK usage in acute MI. In the nine trials that used a variety of GIK regimens, the acute MI mortality risk was reduced by 28% by GIK relative to controls, but in the four trials that used high dose GIK, (i.e., the Rackley regimen) the relative acute MI mortality reduction was 48%.[8] Furthermore, a recent Polish study of low-dose GIK for acute MI showed no beneficial effect; this study's regimen delivered only approximately 15% of the glucose of the Rackley regimen.[16] Thus, the Rackley GIK regimen appears to be the current best choice.

Glucose and Insulin During "Surgical" Ischemia and Reperfusion

During most cardiac surgery procedures, the myocardium is subjected to ischemia and reperfusion. GIK has been studied both pre- and postoperatively and has generally been associated with beneficial effects.

Preoperative GIK

In a prospective, randomized trial, GIK was beneficial in unstable angina patients when the GIK was given as adjunctive therapy prior to and for 12 hours after CABG surgery. During the 18-hour immediate postoperative period, the GIK group had a 40% greater cardiac index than the controls (p < 0.001), despite receiving significantly less inotropic pharmacologic support than the controls. Atrial fibrillation, a relatively common postoperative arrhythmia, occurred in 53% of the control patients, but in only 13% of the GIK patients (p = 0.02).[17] The mechanism for GIK's reduction of postop atrial fibrillation was not studied specifically; possibilites include an atrial anti-arrhythmic action of GIK, or by prevention of an acute increase in atrial afterload by reducing a post-ischemic increase in LV stiffness[18] associated with CABG surgery.[19] Similarly, in a double-blind placebo controlled study, preoperative GIK was associated with a 24% greater postoperative cardiac index in a mixed group of CABG and valve surgery patients; GIK caused the greatest relative increase in cardiac index in those patients with depressed LV function.[20]

Postoperative Cardiogenic Shock

Severe LV dysfunction immediately after cardiac surgery represents a particular form of cardiogenic shock[12,21,22] with profound post-ischemic and anesthetic 'stunning,' and/or extensive ischemic injury. Marked systemic metabolic abnormalities are often present, including high concentrations of FFAs, lactic acidosis, hypoxemia, and high levels of catecholamines from both endogenous and exogenous sources. Treatment usually consists of mechanical cardiovascular support (e.g., intra-aortic balloon counterpulsation or LV assist device), and/or maximal pharmacologic inotropic therapy, but despite such therapy, the acute mortality rate in this syndrome is approximately 30%.[12]

Taegtmeyer and colleagues[12,21,22] have been pioneers in demonstrating the beneficial effects of GIK in this syndrome. In an initial trial in 22 consecutive patients, GIK markedly decreased plasma FFA levels, and increased cardiac index by nearly 40% in the first 12 hours (p < 0.005) with no significant increase in inotrope dosage; in the control "standard care" group, over the same time period, there was no significant increase in cardiac index despite a doubling of inotrope dosage. Similarly, in a small series of post-operative CABG patients, GIK enhanced the inotropic effect of dopamine while concomitantly decreasing circulating FFA levels, myocardial FFA uptake, and increasing metabolic-mechanical efficiency.[23] And in a small, nonrandomized series, 16 postoperative cardiac surgery patients with severe heart failure were treated with GIK and glutamate and had a rapid improvement in hemodynamic function relative to historical controls.[24] Based on these promising results, a larger trial comparing a control (standard care) regimen to GIK and to GIK plus an amino acid supplement (Calamine) was undertaken in 322 consecutive patients with postoperative refractory heart failure. The addition of GIK to the standard regimen (inotropic support with catecholamines and/or phosphodiesterase inhibitors plus intra-aortic balloon counterpulsaton) reduced in-hospital mortality by 34% (from 26.6 to 17.6%, p < 0.02) and also reduced the lengths of stay in the intensive care unit and in the hospital.[12]

Myocardial Metabolic Support During Experimental Cardiogenic Shock

Metabolic support has been studied in experimental preparations ranging from intact animals to isolated myocytes. Each preparation provides a tradeoff between clinical applicability and ability to identify basic molecular mechanisms. In this section we focus on studies that used increased glucose and insulin in (1) intact animal models of cardiogenic shock, and (2) isolated blood perfused hearts.

Metabolic Support During Cardiogenic Shock: Intact Animals

Only a very limited number of studies have examined metabolic support in intact animal models of cardiogenic shock. This is likely due, at least in part, to the difficulty of studying a preparation with the inherently unstable hemodynamics associated with a large acute MI. Two studies have managed to overcome that difficulty and determine the effects of metabolic support on survival.[25,26] The first, by Beyersdorf et al.,[26] followed mongrel dogs for 6 hours after ligation of the LAD in combination with a 50% occlusion of the circumflex. These restrictions to coronary flow resulted in a progressive decrease in arterial blood pressure, cardiac index and stroke work index. Mortality at 6 hours post-occlusion in the untreated dogs was 36% with the remaining 64% demonstrating steady declines in cardiac output, blood pressure and stroke work index. In 12 dogs, infusion of a "metabolic cocktail" containing glucose, insulin, potassium, glutamate, aspartate, MPG and CoQ_{10} was initiated 2 hours post surgery. This treatment group had a 6-hour mortality of only 17% (2 of 12). More impressively, the 10 survivors demonstrated not only stable, but also improving systemic hemodynamics and "hypercontractility" in the remote (noninfarcting) myocardium. Part of this was likely due to the increase in blood flow to the remote myocardium that was measured in dogs that received the treatment. Additionally, the concentrations of high-energy phosphates (ATP and phosphocreatine [PCr]) in the remote myocardium were increased by the treatment.

While combining several different metabolic interventions simultaneously may (or may not) be the most efficacious type of metabolic support, determining which components of a metabolic cocktail exert which effects can be daunting. The effects of GIK without other metabolic interventions were examined during ischemic cardiogenic shock in rabbits by Coven et al.[25] Their experimental model consisted of ligating coronary arteries until a 50% decrease in cardiac output from baseline occurred. If the animal was hemodynamically stable for the next 5 minutes, either metabolic support (GIK), inotropic support, saline, or combined inotropic and metabolic support were administered. These authors found that GIK increased survival time from 1 hour in the placebo group to 4 hours in the GIK group, and to 5 hours if dobutamine was given together with the GIK. Hemodynamic function was also improved by the GIK, and the combination of GIK+dobutamine increased cardiac output in the shock state more than either agent alone.[25]

Metabolic Support in Severely Ischemic Myocardium: Isolated Hearts

In whole animal models of cardiogenic shock, complex temporal changes in the neuroendocrine system, coronary vascular tone, and cardiac mechanics make it difficult to examine mechanisms of action of increased G+I in a detailed manner. For this, we and others have turned to isolated, (Langendorff) perfused heart preparations where factors such as preload, the composition of the coronary perfusate, and the coronary flow rate can be controlled. This experimental model allows one to answer questions such as:

1) Are the beneficial effects of metabolic support due to effects on the severely ischemic (infarcting) region, on the hypoperfused (noninfarcting) region, or both?

2) Are these beneficial effects of metabolic support manifest in improved systolic function, diastolic function, or both?

3) What are the molecular events that underlie the beneficial effects of metabolic support?

4) Is metabolic support complementary with standard pharmacological therapy for cardiogenic shock such as inotropic support?

5) Are the beneficial effects of G+I solely due to its ability to decrease coronary vascular resistance and thus improve myocardial blood flow?

Eberli et al. studied increased G+I (19.5 mM glucose, 250μU/mL insulin) as a form of metabolic support in isolated hearts undergoing severe ischemia (coronary perfusion pressure [CPP] of 8 mm Hg).[18] They found that G+I had three main effects: (1) decreased coronary vascular resistance allowing more coronary flow at a given CPP; (2) increased LV developed pressure; and (3) prevented any stiffening of the LV (increase in end-diastolic pressure in the isovolumic heart). Interestingly, these effects were observed not only during the ischemic period, but also during the period of post-ischemia reperfusion. Because all of these beneficial effects might have been the result of the increased coronary flow, the studies were repeated at a constant level of coronary flow (approximately 10% of baseline). With coronary flow held at this constant level, improved systolic and diastolic function were still observed when increased G+I were present. In summary, this study by Eberli et al. demonstrates that even in severe ischemia (as indicated both by the level of perfusion and amount of creatine kinase released upon reperfusion) metabolic support is able to reach the ischemic tissue, increase perfusion by lowering coronary vascular resistance, provide an inotropic benefit, prevent contracture, improve LV function upon reperfusion, and that the beneficial effects of increased G+I are not all due to its ability to increase coronary blood flow.

One interesting aspect of using G+I as a form of metabolic support is that only a small portion of myocardial ATP is derived from glucose. Thus it has been speculated that the increase in glucose utilization with G+I is not acting to improve myocardial energetics. To evaluate whether G+I does improve myocardial energetics during ischemia, and investigate the molecular mechanism(s) underlying the beneficial effects of G+I, Cave et al.[27] used ^{31}P NMR to measure myocardial energetics (ATP, PCr, P_i, pH, ADP, free energy released from ATP hydrolysis) in the presence and absence of increased G+I during constant flow, severe ischemia. Consistent with the findings of Eberli et al.,[18] they found that in ischemic hearts, G+I lowered coronary vascular resistance while improving LV systolic and diastolic function. These effects were also seen during post-ischemia reperfusion. Additionally, the study found that G+I preserved high-energy phosphates (both ATP and PCr) while lessening the accumulation of inorganic phosphate. Interestingly, increased G+I increased glucose uptake and lactate production as expected, but <u>did not</u> worsen the degree of acidosis that developed during the ischemia, likely because even the small amount of residual flow is able to "wash out" protons.

Metabolic Support in Hypoperfused Myocardium: A Useful Adjunct to Inotropic Support?

The standard treatment for cardiogenic shock includes inotropic support of the myocardium in an attempt to increase cardiac output, arterial blood pressure and perfusion of the periphery. This "whipping the heart to save the body" tradeoff has long troubled physicians attempting to treat cardiogenic shock. To determine whether metabolic support might be a useful adjunct to inotropic support, Saupe et al.[28] studied isolated, blood perfused rat hearts using ^{31}P NMR spectroscopy to measure myocardial energetics. They chose a level of hypoperfusion (CPP of 30-35 mm Hg) that modeled the <u>non-MI</u> region of the heart during cardiogenic shock. This level of hypoperfusion caused significant systolic dysfunction (a decrease in LV developed pressure of approximately 50%) that could be almost completely reversed with inotropic support (dobutamine) (Figures 1 and 2). However, the negative consequences of restoring systolic function with dobutamine were a rapid stiffening of the LV, depletion of ATP and PCr, and accumulation of P_i.

Providing the hearts with increased G+I as an adjunct to the dobutamine completely prevented the stiffening of the LV. Additionally, increased G+I prevented the rapid depletion of ATP and PCr and accumulation of

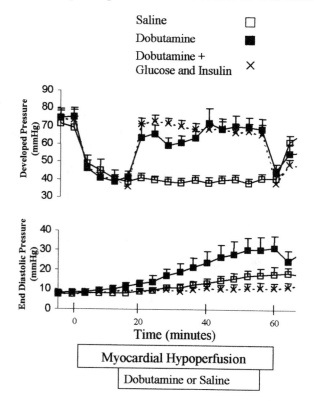

Figure 1. See text for discussion.

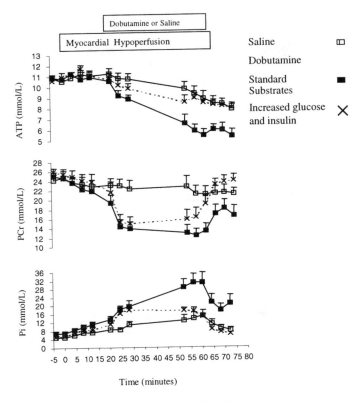

Figure 2. See text for discussion.

P_i that inotropic support had caused. Similar to what was reported in the study by Cave et al.[27] discussed above, myocardial pH was not affected by the increased G+I, again demonstrating that increasing the rate of anaerobic glycolysis in a setting of significant residual myocardial flow does not worsen myocardial acidosis. However, in the setting where dobutamine had already restored LV developed pressure to 95% of baseline, addition of G+I did not increase LV developed pressure further. This lack of benefit of G+I on LV systolic function was apparent not only during the hypoperfusion, but also during reperfusion. In summary, the study of Saupe et al.[28] demonstrates that the "cost" of inotropically stimulating the hypoperfused heart is accelerated LV stiffening and energetic depletion, and that these costs can be reduced by using G+I (metabolic support) as an adjunct to inotropic support.

Possible Molecular Mechanisms for Beneficial Effects of Increased Glucose and Insulin

The observed benefits of increased glycolytic substrate provision and utilization have been attributed to a number of mechanisms that are summarized in Table 3.

Table 3.

Possible Molecular Mechanisms for Beneficial Effects of Increased Glycolytic Substrate During Low-Flow Ischemia and Reperfusion

1. The yield of moles of ATP per mole of oxygen consumed is 12% higher for glucose than for FFA oxidation[29]
2. Anti-FFA effects:[30-33]
   a. Decrease of circulating FFA levels and myocardial FFA uptake
   b. Increased esterification of intracellular FFA by increasing the supply of alpha-glycerophosphate
3. Increased rate of ATP synthesis via anaerobic glycolysis with consequent beneficial effects:[18,27,28,34,35]
   a. Increased concentrations of phosphocreatine and ATP
   b. Blunting of an increase in inorganic phosphate concentrations
   c. Increased free energy yield from ATP hydrolysis
4. Increased myocardial glycogen[36-38]
5. Improved sodium and calcium homeostasis[39-42]
6. Increased tolerance to increases of intracellular calcium[43]
7. Replenishment of citric acid cycle intermediates by anaplerosis[12]
8. Increase of glucose and decrease of FFA oxidation during reperfusion[44,45]

The number of moles of ATP produced per mole of carbon oxidized is approximately 29% higher for FFA relative to glucose, but the number of moles of ATP produced per mole of oxygen consumed is 12% higher for glucose than for FFA oxidation.[29] Thus, when oxygen is abundant during normal perfusion conditions, it is more efficient for the aerobic myocardium to utilize and oxidize FFA, but during ischemia glucose appears to be a better myocardial substrate than FFA.

Anti-FFA actions may be the most important effects of GIK administration.[30] During clinical ischemia syndromes FFA levels are often increased secondary to the lipolytic action of endogenous or therapeutically administered catecholamines and/or heparin. High levels of FFA depress myocardial contractility, inhibit glycolytic flux, increase cyclic AMP levels, accumulate as toxic fatty acid derivatives, cause membrane damage and arrhythmias, and increase myocardial oxygen consumption without a concomitant increase in myocardial work (oxygen wasting effect of FFA).[30-33] During ischemia, the reduced beta-oxidation of FFA results in intracellular accumulation of acylcarnitine and acyl CoA. Acylcarnitine inhibits the sarcoplasmic reticular Ca^{2+} pump and the sarcolemmal Na^+/Ca^{2+} exchanger and Na^+ pump and can also activate Ca^{2+} channels, and increase cyclic AMP levels. These actions can lead to cell calcium overload, oxygen wasting, and arrhythmia generation. However, in the presence of a high glucose and insulin substrate, the inhibition of glycolysis by FFA is minimal, and high circulating levels of glucose and insulin both depress plasma levels of FFA and decrease myocardial FFA uptake at any given plasma FFA level.[30,31]

Increasing glycolytic substrate during low-flow ischemia results in increased glycolytic ATP synthesis, but to a relatively small degree,[18] and its significance has been questioned. However, this effect was sufficient to attenuate the ischemia-induced decrease in ATP and phosphocreatine, to blunt the ischemic increase in inorganic phosphate (P_i), and maintain slightly lower ADP levels.[18,27,28] The combination of a higher [ATP] and lower [P_i] and [ADP] resulted in a significantly higher calculated free energy yield from ATP hydrolysis in the presence of the G+I substrate. This increase in free energy is available to all cellular ATPase reactions. Thus, the increase in ischemic glycolytic ATP synthesis, even if relatively small, has the consequence of acting as a "trap" for inorganic phosphate and ADP with a resulting amplification of free energy yield beyond that contributed by the increase in glycolytic ATP synthesis *per se*.

Glycolytic ATP protects membranes,[39] drives the transport of Ca^{2+} into the sarcoplasmic reticulum,[38,40] improves sodium homeostasis of ischemic myocardium[41] and regulates ATP-sensitive K+ channels.[42] Recent work from our lab has also shown that a high glucose substrate increases myocyte resistance to the toxic effects of the increase in cell calcium concentration that occurs during hypoxia.[43]

GIK may be beneficial by increasing myocardial glycogen. Pre-operative GIK increased myocardial glycogen, and reduced postoperative hypotension and arrhythmias in patients who had mitral valve replacement.[36] Myocardial glycogen was also increased by a preoperative fat loading diet and overnight glucose loading and the increased glycogen levels were associated with fewer post-op infarctions, arrhythmias, and need for inotropic support.[46] A positive correlation among enhanced glucose uptake, glycogen levels, and contractile function has been shown in patients undergoing surgery for coronary artery disease.[37]

Insulin is probably a critical component of the GIK combination. The combination of glucose and insulin is more effective than either alone in stimulating glycolysis under ischemic conditions.[18] Insulin may also stimulate pyruvate dehydrogenase and increase pyruvate entry into the citric acid cycle,[47] increase glycogen synthesis[10] and have direct ionic and inotropic effects.[48-51] In recent studies of low-flow ischemia insulin improved contractile function and myocardial metabolic efficiency without alteration of ATP, PCr, or P_i levels.[52,53] In clinical practice, however, administration of insulin without glucose in nondiabetics can cause hypoglycemia. Therefore combined glucose and insulin administration is the practical clinical regimen.

In clinical ischemic settings, where a level of oxidative metabolism persists, and/or during post-ischemic reperfusion, an increased glycolytic flux can potentially deliver more substrate (pyruvate) to the citric acid cycle, thereby providing additional oxidative substrate and also replenishing citric acid cycle intermediates by a process of "anaplerosis."[12] Furthermore, during reperfusion, increasing glucose oxidation and decreasing FFA oxidation results in improved cardiac function and efficiency of the reperfused, post-ischemic heart.[44,45]

Summary

The studies reviewed here demonstrate that metabolic support, in the form of increased glucose and insulin, is efficacious in protecting the myocardium in many clinical and experimental settings where myocardial ischemia is present. In so doing, metabolic support may be a promising treatment for ischemic cardiogenic shock. However, until appropriate clinical trials are conducted, the efficacy of metabolic support in treating clinical ischemic cardiogenic shock will remain unknown.

While metabolic support may be promising as a treatment of cardiogenic shock, many questions remain unanswered. For example, what is the optimal form of metabolic support, i.e., is there some "metabolic cocktail" that provides more benefits than any single component? Does the optimal form of metabolic support depend on the etiology of the heart disease? Is metabolic support efficacious in chronic (as well as in acute) heart failure? It is our hope that studies in the near future will address these important questions.

References

1. Lopaschuk G. Fatty acid and glucose metabolism: A target for intervention. In: Hearse DJ, ed. Metabolic Approaches to Ischemic Heart Disease and Its Management. London: Science Press, 1998:44-57.

2. Neely JR, Grotyohann LW. Role of glycolytic products in damage to ischemic myocardium. Dissociation of adenosine triphosphate levels and recovery of function of reperfused ischemic hearts. *Circ Res* 1984; 55:816-824.

3. Opie L. The glucose hypothesis. Its relation to acute myocardial ischemia. *J Mol Cell Cardiol* 1970; 1:107-115.

4. Milavetz JJ, Giebel DW, Christian TF, et al. Time to therapy and salvage in myocardial infarction. *J Am Coll Cardiol* 1998; 31:1246-1251.

5. Christian TF, O'Connor MK, Schwartz RS, et al. Technetium-99m MIBI to assess coronary collateral flow during acute myocardial infarction in two closed-chest animal models. *J Nucl Med* 1997; 38:1840-1846.

6. Sabia PJ, Powers ER, Ragosta M, et al. An association between collateral blood flow and myocardial viability in patients with recent myocardial infarction. *N Engl J Med* 1992; 327:1825-1831.

7. Chareonthaitawee P, Christian TF, O'Connor MK, et al. Noninvasive prediction of residual blood flow within the risk area during acute myocardial infarction: A multicenter validation study of patients undergoing direct coronary angioplasty. *Am Heart J* 1997; 134:639-646.

8. Fath-Ordoubadi F, Beatt KJ. Glucose-insulin-potassium therapy for treatment of acute myocardial infarction: An overview of randomized placebo-controlled trials. *Circulation* 1997; 96:1152-1156.

9. Malmberg K, Ryden L, Hamsten A, et al. Effects of insulin treatment on cause-specific one-year mortality and morbidity in diabetic patients with acute myocardial infarction. DIGAMI Study Group. Diabetes Insulin-Glucose in Acute Myocardial Infarction. *Eur Heart J* 1996; 17:1337-1344.

10. Diaz R, Paolasso EA, Piegas LS, et al. Metabolic modulation of acute myocardial infarction. The ECLA (Estudios Cardiologicos Latinoamerica) Collaborative Group. *Circulation* 1998; 98:2227-2234.

11. Apstein CS. Glucose-insulin-potassium for acute myocardial infarction: Remarkable results from a new prospective, randomized trial. *Circulation* 1998; 98:2223-2226.

12. Taegtmeyer H, Goodwin GW, Doenst T, et al. Substrate metabolism as a determinant for postischemic functional recovery of the heart. *Am J Cardiol* 1997; 80:3A-10A.

13. Sodi-Pallares D, Testelli M, Fishleder F. Effects of an intravenous infusion of a potassium-insulin-glucose solution on the electrocardiographic signs of myocardial infarction. *Am J Cardiol* 1962; 9:166-181.

14. Rackley C, Russell R, Rogers W, et al. Clinical experience with glucose-insulin-potassium therapy in acute myocardial infarction. *Am Heart J* 1981; 102:1038-1049.

15. Arsenian MA, New PS, Cafasso CM. Safety, tolerability, and efficacy of a glucose-insulin-potassium- magnesium-carnitine solution in acute myocardial infarction. *Am J Cardiol* 1996; 78:477-479.

16. Ceremuzynski L, Budaj A, Czepiel A, et al. Low-dose glucose-insulin-potassium is ineffective in acute myocardial infarction: Results of a randomized multicenter Pol-GIK trial. *Cardiovasc Drugs Ther* 1999; 13:191-200.

17. Lazar HL, Philippides G, Fitzgerald C, et al. Glucose-insulin-potassium solutions enhance recovery after urgent coronary artery bypass grafting. *J Thorac Cardiovasc Surg* 1997; 113:354-360; discussion 360-352.

18. Eberli FR, Weinberg EO, Grice WN, et al. Protective effect of increased glycolytic substrate against systolic and diastolic dysfunction and increased coronary resistance from prolonged global underperfusion and reperfusion in isolated rabbit hearts perfused with erythrocyte suspensions. *Circ Res* 1991; 68:466-481.

19. McKenney PA, Apstein CS, Mendes LA, et al. Increased left ventricular diastolic chamber stiffness immediately after coronary artery bypass surgery. *J Am Coll Cardiol* 1994; 24:1189-1194.

20. Girard C, Quentin P, Bouvier H, et al. Glucose and insulin supply before cardiopulmonary bypass in cardiac surgery: A double-blind study. *Ann Thorac Surg* 1992; 54:259-263.

21. Coleman GM, Gradinac S, Taegtmeyer H, et al. Efficacy of metabolic support with glucose-insulin-potassium for left ventricular pump failure after aortocoronary bypass surgery. *Circulation* 1989; 80:I91-96.

22. Gradinac S, Coleman GM, Taegtmeyer H, et al. Improved cardiac function with glucose-insulin-potassium after aortocoronary bypass grafting. *Ann Thorac Surg* 1989; 48:484-489.

23. Svedjeholm R, Hallhagen S, Ekroth R, et al. Dopamine and high-dose insulin infusion (glucose-insulin-potassium) after a cardiac operation: Effects on myocardial metabolism. *Ann Thorac Surg* 1991; 51:262-270.

24. Svedjeholm R, Huljebrant I, Hakanson E, et al. Glutamate and high-dose glucose-insulin-potassium (GIK) in the treatment of severe cardiac failure after cardiac operations. *Ann Thorac Surg* 1995; 59:S23-30.

25. Coven D, Suter T, Eberli F, et al. Dobutamine and glucose-insulin-potassium (GIK) improve cardiac function and survival in a randomized trial of experimental cardiogenic shock (abstract). *Circulation* 1994; 90:I-480.

26. Beyersdorf F, Acar C, Buckberg GD, et al. Studies on prolonged acute regional ischemia. V. Metabolic support of remote myocardium during left ventricular power failure. *J Thorac Cardiovasc Surg* 1989; 98:567-579.

27. Cave AC, Ingwall JS, Friedrich J, et al. ATP synthesis during low-flow ischemia: Influence of increased glycolytic substrate. *Circulation* 2000; 101:2090-2096.

28. Saupe KW, Eberli FR, Ingwall JS, et al. Metabolic support as an adjunct to inotropic support in the hypoperfused heart. *J Mol Cell Cardiol* 2001; 33:261-269.

29. Opie LH. The Heart. NY: Raven Press, 1991:p. 211.

30. Oliver MF, Opie LH. Effects of glucose and fatty acids on myocardial ischaemia and arrhythmias. *Lancet* 1994; 343:155-158.

31. Opie LH. Metabolism of free fatty acids, glucose and catecholamines in acute myocardial infarction. Relation to myocardial ischemia and infarct size. *Am J Cardiol* 1975; 36:938-953.

32. Neely J, Morgan H. Relationship between carbohydrate and lipid metabolism and the energy balance of heart muscle. *Ann Rev Physiol* 1974; 36:413-459.

33. Liedtke AJ. Lipid burden in ischemic myocardium. *J Mol Cell Cardiol* 1988; 20 Suppl 2:65-74.

34. Apstein CS, Gravino FN, Haudenschild CC. Determinants of a protective effect of glucose and insulin on the ischemic myocardium. Effects on contractile function, diastolic compliance, metabolism, and ultrastructure during ischemia and reperfusion. *Circ Res* 1983; 52:515-526.

35. King LM, Boucher F, Opie LH. Coronary flow and glucose delivery as determinants of contracture in the ischemic myocardium. *J Mol Cell Cardiol* 1995; 27:701-720.

36. Oldfield GS, Commerford PJ, Opie LH. Effects of preoperative glucose-insulin-potassium on myocardial glycogen levels and on complications of mitral valve replacement. *J Thorac Cardiovasc Surg* 1986; 91:874-878.

37. Depre C, Vanoverschelde JL, Melin JA, et al. Structural and metabolic correlates of the reversibility of chronic left ventricular ischemic dysfunction in humans. *Am J Physiol* 1995; 268:H1265-1275.

38. Xu KY, Zweier JL, Becker LC. Functional coupling between glycolysis and sarcoplasmic reticulum Ca2+ transport. *Circ Res* 1995; 77:88-97.

39. Weiss JN, Lamp ST. Glycolysis preferentially inhibits ATP-sensitive K+ channels in isolated guinea pig cardiac myocytes. *Science* 1987; 238:67-69.

40. Jeremy RW, Koretsune Y, Marban E, et al. Relation between glycolysis and calcium homeostasis in postischemic myocardium. *Circ Res* 1992; 70:1180-1190.

41. Cross HR, Radda GK, Clarke K. The role of Na+/K+ ATPase activity during low flow ischemia in preventing myocardial injury: A 31P, 23Na and 87Rb NMR spectroscopic study. *Magn Reson Med* 1995; 34:673-685.

42. Weiss JN, Lamp ST. Cardiac ATP-sensitive K+ channels. Evidence for preferential regulation by glycolysis. *J Gen Physiol* 1989; 94:911-935.

43. Kondo RP, Apstein CS, Eberli FR, et al. Increased calcium loading and inotropy without greater cell death in hypoxic rat cardiomyocytes. *Am J Physiol* 1998; 275:H2272-2282.

44. Lopaschuk GD, Wambolt RB, Barr RL. An imbalance between glycolysis and glucose oxidation is a possible explanation for the detrimental effects of high levels of fatty acids during aerobic reperfusion of ischemic hearts. *J Pharmacol Exp Ther* 1993; 264:135-144.

45. Lopaschuk GD. Alterations in fatty acid oxidation during reperfusion of the heart after myocardial ischemia. *Am J Cardiol* 1997; 80:11A-16A.

46. Lolley DM, Ray JF, 3rd, Myers WO, et al. Importance of preoperative myocardial glycogen levels in human cardiac preservation. Preliminary report. *J Thorac Cardiovasc Surg* 1979; 78:678-687.

47. Kobayashi K, Neely JR. Effects of ischemia and reperfusion on pyruvate dehydrogenase activity in isolated rat hearts. *J Mol Cell Cardiol* 1983; 15:359-367.

48. Moore RD. Effects of insulin upon ion transport. *Biochim Biophys Acta* 1983; 737:1-49.

49. Gupta MP, Makino N, Khatter K, et al. Stimulation of Na+-Ca2+ exchange in heart sarcolemma by insulin. *Life Sci* 1986; 39:1077-1083.

50. Kato M, Kako KJ. Na+/Ca2+ exchange of isolated sarcolemmal membrane: Effects of insulin, oxidants and insulin deficiency. *Mol Cell Biochem* 1988; 83:15-25.

51. Farah AE, Alousi AA. The actions of insulin on cardiac contractility. *Life Sci* 1981; 29:975-1000.

52. Tune JD, Mallet RT, Downey HF. Insulin improves cardiac contractile function and oxygen utilization efficiency during moderate ischemia without compromising myocardial energetics. *J Mol Cell Cardiol* 1998; 30:2025-2035.

53. Tune JD, Mallet RT, Downey HF. Insulin improves contractile function during moderate ischemia in canine left ventricle. *Am J Physiol* 1998; 274:H1574-1581.

Chapter 15

Epilogue: New Directions in the Future

This is a time of great promise in the field of cardiogenic shock. Recent developments have produced tremendous progress in averting shock in the course of myocardial infarction and in treating cardiogenic shock once it develops. Progress has resulted from the interplay of increased understanding of pathogenesis, more rapid and aggressive application of supportive measures, and, most importantly, institution of a strategy of early revascularization therapy.

Improved understanding of the pathophysiology of cardiogenic shock has led to the realization that some myocardium which appears akinetic on initial evaluation may still be viable, because of either stunning, hibernating, or a combination of the two. Understanding these concepts has worked to counteract the fatalistic attitude that once a certain degree of myocardial dysfunction was present, any therapeutic modality was futile since recovery was impossible.

Application of newly elucidated concepts regarding the pathophysiology of cardiogenic shock has led to renewed emphasis on the importance of expeditious initiation of supportive measures to maintain blood pressure and cardiac output. This entails pharmacotherapy based on hemodynamic parameters, and most often also includes mechanical support with intra-aortic balloon counterpulsation. In appropriate settings, more intensive support with mechanical assist devices may also be implemented.

Most importantly, we now have good evidence to support early coronary revascularization for patients with cardiogenic shock secondary to acute myocardial infarction. An extensive body of observational and registry studies showed consistent benefits from revascularization, but could not be regarded as definitive due to their retrospective design. We now have available the results of two randomized controlled trials of revascularization for patients with myocardial infarction. Although statistical significance was not achieved for the primary endpoint in either the

From: Hollenberg SM, Bates ER. *Cardiogenic Shock*. Armonk, NY: Futura Publishing Co., Inc.; ©2002.

SHOCK or SMASH trials, the results of the two studies were consistent and strongly support a strategy of expeditious revascularization. Both trials showed an absolute mortality reduction of 9% with an early invasive strategy, implying that 11 patients needed to be treated to save one life. In the SHOCK trial, a larger difference in mortality beyond 30 days was seen, with a statistically significant 13% absolute reduction in mortality at 6 months and 1 year. It is important to realize that this absolute benefit (7.6 patients treated to save one life) is more than twice the number of lives saved by the administration of thrombolytic therapy within 1 hour after the onset of infarction, and is in fact comparable in magnitude to the benefit of coronary artery bypass surgery for left main coronary artery disease.

Thus, early revascularization for cardiogenic shock in the setting of acute myocardial infarction represents one of the most significant new advances in the treatment of coronary artery disease. What further advances can we look forward to in the near future? Coronary artery stenting is becoming routine, both in elective cases and as a component of primary angioplasty for acute myocardial infarction. Adjunctive glycoprotein IIb/IIIa inhibition is also becoming more routine in high-risk patients undergoing percutaneous coronary intervention. Recent data indicate that abciximab added to stenting improves outcomes in patients with myocardial infarction undergoing coronary stenting. Although this approach has not been tested formally in patients with cardiogenic shock, early results of consecutive cases are very promising, and it seems likely that this strategy will improve outcomes. Techniques of surgical revascularization are improving as well, particularly with respect to strategies to minimize post-bypass myocardial dysfunction, and this will likely translate into improved outcomes for patients with cardiogenic shock taken emergently to the operating room. Finally, adjunctive therapies such as metabolic interventions are being reexamined, and have the potential to further improve outcomes after revascularization.

We have come a long way in the therapy of cardiogenic shock. We still have a long way to go, but what was once regarded as a uniformly fatal condition is now proving treatable. We can only hope that progress in the next few years is as rapid as the last few, and that this will lead to even more significant reductions in morbidity and mortality from cardiogenic shock.

Index